Praise for *Llewellyn's Complete Formulary of Magical Oils*

"This book is a testament to Celeste Heldstab's passion for all things aromatic as well as her generosity of spirit. Her passion is infectious and absolutely pervades these pages. Celeste skillfully demystifies the process of using and blending oils by providing lucid, detailed, and easy-to-read instructions while simultaneously emphasizing the magical power inherent in plants. Celeste will inspire you to concoct your very own magical oils and potions."

—Judika Illes, author of *The Encyclopedia of 5,000 Spells*

"Kudos to Celeste Heldstab! Jam-packed with a wealth of information and easy-to-follow recipes, *Llewellyn's Complete Formulary of Magical Oils* provides everything the magical practitioner needs to know about oils—and then some. No magical library is complete without it!"

—Dorothy Morrison, author of *Utterly Wicked*

"Celeste has delivered a fabulous compendium brimming with insightful how-to's. This book is a must-have for anyone interested in creating homemade blends and remedies for everyday use. Having purchased many of Celeste's oils, I can attest to her talent for creating redolent masterpieces. Now she is generously sharing her knowledge and years of experience with the rest of us!"

—Lisa Hunt, creator of *Animals Divine Tarot* and *The Fairy Tale Tarot*

— LLEWELLYN'S —

· COMPLETE ·

FORMULARY

— OF —

MAGICAL

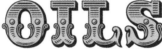

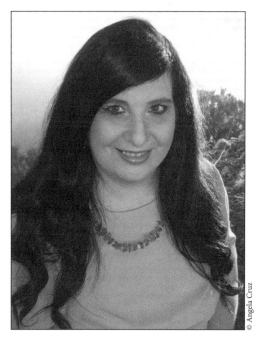

© Angela Cruz

About the Author

Celeste Rayne Heldstab (Monroe, LA) has over twenty-five years of experience creating oils and incense for companies and individuals. Since 2000, she has taught many workshops on how to utilize essential oils in magical applications, along with tarot reading and incense making. She follows an eclectic spiritual path that incorporates Native American beliefs and voodoo, and manages an online store that sells incense, oils, and other products.

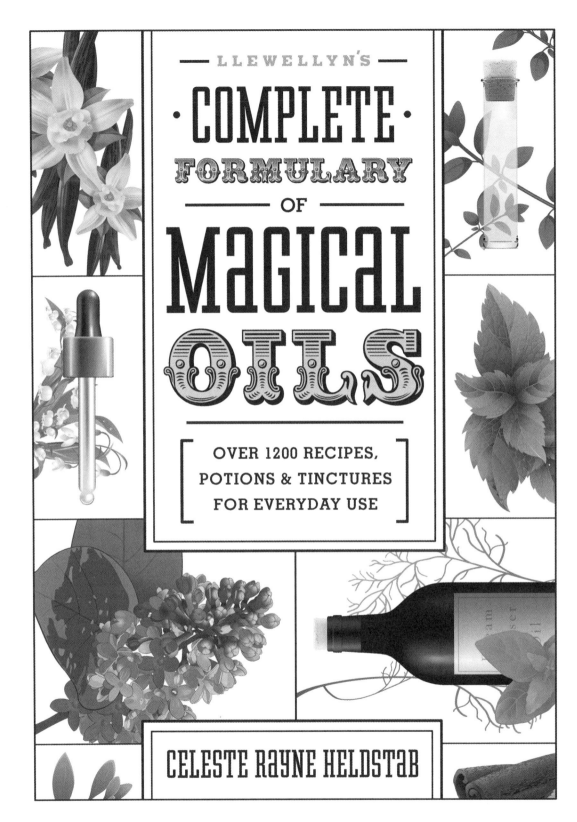

LLEWELLYN'S
·COMPLETE·
FORMULARY
OF
MAGICAL
OILS

OVER 1200 RECIPES,
POTIONS & TINCTURES
FOR EVERYDAY USE

CELESTE RAYNE HELDSTAB

Llewellyn Publications
Woodbury, Minnesota

FIRST EDITION
Thirteenth Printing, 2022

Book design by Donna Burch
Cover art: Cinnamon with vanilla and mint, Vanilla Flower, Mint Herb © iStockphoto.com/elapela,
Lilac © iStockphoto.com/Tatyana Andreevna Kurilina, Serum Dropper © iStockphoto.com/
Peggy Koh, Spring Flowers © iStockphoto.com/Addan, Basil Herb © iStockphoto.com/Joan
Loitz, Wine Bottle © iStockphoto.com/Martin Spurny, Herbs © iStockphoto.com/stdemi,
Flask © iStockphoto.com/Sergii Kostenko
Cover design by Kevin R. Brown

Llewellyn Publications is a registered trademark of Llewellyn Worldwide Ltd.

Library of Congress Cataloging-in-Publication Data
Heldstab, Celeste Rayne.
  Llewellyn's complete formulary of magical oils : over 1200 recipes,
potions & tinctures for everyday use / Celeste Rayne Heldstab. — 1st ed.
     p.   cm.
  Includes bibliographical references (p.   ).
  ISBN 978-0-7387-2751-6
1. Essences and essential oils—Miscellanea. 2. Magic—Miscellanea.
I. Title. II. Title: Complete formulary of magical oils.
  BF1442.E77H45 2011
  133.4'4—dc23
                    2011045557

Llewellyn Worldwide Ltd. does not participate in, endorse, or have any authority or responsibility concerning private business transactions between our authors and the public.
  All mail addressed to the author is forwarded, but the publisher cannot, unless specifically instructed by the author, give out an address or phone number.
  Any Internet references contained in this work are current at publication time, but the publisher cannot guarantee that a specific location will continue to be maintained. Please refer to the publisher's website for links to authors' websites and other sources.

Llewellyn Publications
A Division of Llewellyn Worldwide Ltd.
2143 Wooddale Drive
Woodbury, MN 55125-2989
www.llewellyn.com

Printed in the United States of America

To my Father, who gave me courage to conquer mountains, and to my Mother, who gave me strength to do anything I desire. To Josh, Hannah, and Matt…I miss you, my children, and we will meet again one day. There is a place in my Soul for your hearts, and know that everything I do, everything I say, every place I am, know I am with you in Spirit, always. May you never walk alone…

Book Blessing

Hearken as the Witch's word
Calls the Lady and the Lord
Moon above and earth below
Sky's cool blue and sun's hot glow,
In this right and ready hour,
Fill these pages with thy wisdom.
May those in need eye to see
The secrets which entrusted be.
To those who walk the hidden road
To find the hearthstone's calm abode.
Guardians from the four directions,
Hear us and lend Thy protection:
May these truths of Earth and Skies
Shielded be from darker times.
But to the witches whose map this be
May the way be plain to see;
And through all the coming ages,
May we find home in these pages.

Acknowledgments

When it comes to thanking people, I never can remember names, only faces … but this book brings about many exceptions to that rule. Judika Illes … my dear woman, you have brought light back into my eyes and my life, you are a dear friend and a Sister of the Craft. The gifts you have given me, I can never truly return in this life. But be assured, dear Lady, they will be returned. As far as music goes, life would not be the same without my headphones and Bluebeat.com. Dawn Henry—you literally saved my life. To Kim Landers from Adriel's Alchemy, without you none of this would have ever happened … you taught, apprenticed, and mentored me in the art of incense, herbs, and oils, as well as tarot, channeling, and other magics … I wish I knew where you were now, for your teachings live on, in this book. To Misty-Eve*, my mentor in the Druidic Craft of the Wise. The wisdom I have acquired has made my life richer, and I have come to realize that perfection is within our reach, if we only have the guts to go for it! My husband, Mark, for creating a website to feature my book—www.BayouWitchIncense.com. It is AMAZING … my four dogs, Luna, Misha, Bella-Donna, and Oliver … my five cats, Georgie Girl, Tobie, Dora, Maxwell, and Charlie … my dear familiars. You were always at my feet and forced me to take breaks when I REALLY needed them, gave me comfort when my mind was completely blocked, and licked my face or purred contentedly when something went well … I love you. And to the goddess Hecate. Mother, thank you.

Contents

Emotional & Physical Healing . . . 71

Morrigan Oil, Obeah Oil, Obitzu Oil, Oshun Oil, Osiris Oil, Pan and Astarte Oil, Pan Oil, Pomona Oil, Rhiannon Oil, Rites of Isis Oil, Sekmet Oil, Seven African Powers Oil, Star of the Sea Oil, Strega Oil

Saints & Angels . . . 197

All Saints' Oil, Angel Blessing Oil, Angel Brilliance Oil, Faith, Hope, and Charity Oil, Four Angels Oil, Gran Poder Oil, Guardian Angel Oil, Justice Judge Oil (Justo Juez), La Candelaria Oil, Madonna Loretto Oil, Mercedes Oil, Milagrosa Oil, Ocean Mother Oil, Our Lady of Fatima Oil, Our Lady of Lourdes Oil, Our Lady of Mount Carmel Oil, Sacred Heart Oil, Saint Alex Oil (An Alejo), Saint Anna Oil, Saint Anthony Oil, Saint Barbara Oil, Saint Christopher Oil, Saint Clara Oil, Saint Elijah Oil, Saint Expedito Oil, Saint Francis of Assisi Oil, Saint Helena Oil, Saint Joseph Oil, Saint Jude Oil, Saint Lazarus Oil, Saint Lucy Oil, Saint Martha Oil, Saint Martin Oil, Saint Michael Oil, Saint Peter Oil, Saint Teresa, Seven African Powers Oil, Nine African Powers Oil, Virgin Guadaupe

Hexing, Banishing & Uncrossing . . . 211

Agarbatti Chandan Oil, Banishing Oil, Banishing Oil II, Banishing/Exorcism Oil, Bat's Blood Oil, Bat's Eye Oil, Bend Over Oil, Black Arts Oil, Black Arts Oil II, Black Arts Oil III, Black Devil Oil, Compelling Oil, Confusion Oil, Confusion Oil II, Conquering Glory Oil, Conquering Glory Oil II, Controlling Oil, Controlling Oil II, Controlling Oil III, Crossing Oil, Curse-Breaker Oil, Do As I Say Oil, Domination Oil, Domination Oil II, Double-Cross Oil, Double XX (Hexing Oil), Dragon Protection Oil, Dragon's Blood Oil, Druid's Curse Oil, Escaping Oil, Espanta Muerta Oil, Evil Eye Oil, Excalibur Oil, Exodus Oil, Exorcism Oil, Exorcism Oil II, Fast Action Oil, Fiery Command Oil, Fiery Wall of Protection Oil, Fiery Wall of Protection Oil II, Flying Devil Oil, Go Away Evil Oil, Graveyard Oil/Goofer Oil, Gris-Gris Oil, Hell's Devil Oil, Hindu Oil (see Van Van), Hot Foot Oil, House Blessing Oil, I Can, You Can't Oil, I Tame My Straying Animal Oil, Inflammatory Confusion Oil, Jinx-Killer Oil, Jinx Oil, Jinx-Removing Oil, Jockey Club Perfume, Lost and Away Oil, Love-Breaker Oil, L Magus Oil, Mandrake Perfume, Mint Bouquet Oil, Mogra Oil (Sheik), Most Powerful Hand Oil, Pentatruck Oil, Purification Oil, Purification Oil II, Quitting Oil, Reveal Truth Oil, Reversing Oil, Reversing Oil II, Root Oil, Separation Oil, Seven-Day Uncrossing Oil, Shut Up Oil (Tapa Boca), Spell Breaker Oil, Spell Weaver Oil, Spider Oil, Squint Drops, Stray No More Oil, Tar Perfume (not to be worn), Tipareth Oil, Truth Oil, Unbinding Oil, Uncrossing Oil, Uncrossing Oil II, Uncrossing Oil III, Uncrossing Oil IV, Uncrossing Oil V, Uncrossing Oil VI, Unfaithful Oil, Witchbane Oil, X-Hex Oil, Yuza Yuza Oil

The Mother Moon . . . 233

January: Full Wolf Moon Oil, February: Full Snow or Storm Moon Oil, March: Full Worm or Chaste Moon Oil, April: Full Pink or Seed Moon Oil, May: Full Flower or Hare Moon Oil, June: Full Strawberry or Dyad Moon Oil, July: Full Buck or Mead Moon Oil, August: Full Green Corn or Wyrt Moon Oil, September: Full Harvest or Barley Moon Oil, October: Full Hunters or Blood Moon Oil, November: Full Beaver or Snow Moon Oil, December: Full Cold or Oak Moon Oil, Blue Moon (2nd Full Moon in a Month)

Sabbats & Rituals . . . 237

Abramelin Oil, All-Purpose Blessing and Anointing Altar Oil, All-Purpose Oil, Altar Oil, Altar Oil II, Ambrosia Oil, Anointing Oil, Anointing Oil II, Anointing Oil III, Anointing Oil IV, Arabian Bouquet Oil, Arch Druid Oil, Beltane Oil, Beltane Oil II,

Bible Oil, Black Moon Oil, Candlemas/Brid's Oil, Circle Oil, Conjure Oil, Consecration Oil, Consecration Oil II, Dark Moon Oil, Dressing for Candles, Enochian Oil, Esbat Oil, Esbat Oil II, Full Moon Oil, Full Moon Oil II, Full Moon Oil III, Full Moon Oil IV, Full Moon Oil V, General Anointing Oil, Gibbous Moon Oil, God Oil, God Within Oil, Goddess Oil, Goddess Oil II, Goddess Within Oil, Golden Lion Oil, High Altar Oil, High Altar Oil II, High Altar Oil III, High Priestess Oil, High Priestess Initiation Oil, Holy Oil, Holy Oil II, Hoodoo Oil, Imbolc Oil, Imbolc Oil II, Initiation Oil, Lammas Oil, Lammas Oil II, Litha Oil, Litha Oil II, Loban Oil, Lugh Oil, Lugh Oil II, Lughnasadh Oil, Lunar Oil, Lupercalia Oil, Mabon Oil, Mabon Oil II, Mabon/Autumn Equinox Oil, Macha Oil (Lughnasadh), Magic Circle Oil, Magical Power Oil, Mermaids Oil, Midsummer Oil, Midsummer Oil II, Midsummer Oil III, Midsummer Faerie Oil, Moon Priest Cologne, Moon Priestess Perfume, Mystic Rites Oil, New Moon Oil, Oil for the Dark of the Moon, Ostara Oil, Ostara Oil II, Ostara Oil III, Ostara Oil IV, Power Oil, Power of Old Oil, Priestess Oil, Purification Oil, Rosy Cross Oil, Sabbat Oil, Sabbat Oil II, Sabbat Oil III, Sacred Circle Oil, Sacred Oil, Samhain Oil, Self-Love Oil, Spirituality Oil, Spring Goddess Oil, Spring Time Oil, Stone Circle Power Oil, Summer Oil, Summer Breeze Oil, Summer Solstice Oil, Sun Goddess Perfume, Sun King Anointing Oil, Talisman Consecration Oil, Taper Perfume Oil, Temple Oil, Tetragrammaton Oil, Tool Cleansing Oil, Voodoo Oil, Wicca Oil, Winter Solstice Oil, Witch Oil, Witch Blood Anointing Oil, Yule Oil, Yule Oil II, Yule Oil III, Yule Oil IV

Oil, Peppermint Oil, Petitgrain Oil, Pine-Needle Oil, Rosemary Oil, Rosewood Oil, Savory Oil, Tea Tree Oil, Vetiver Oil, Violet Oil, White-Camphor Oil, Yarrow Oil, Ylang-Ylang Oil,

PART ONE

Introduction to Oils

Introduction

I have always been fascinated with smells. It seems they dominate my life and also my memory. Are you aware that smell is the last sense to leave our bodies as we pass into the next realm? Smells bring back times of joy, sorrow, weddings, children being born, friendships, romances, vacations, and so much more.

One day in the early 1990s, I was walking down a strip mall and saw a door propped open by a cauldron. Smoke was wafting from the cauldron, and I was hypnotized by the smell. I walked into the store and asked the woman behind the counter what it was and how could I make it … and so my life in the occult began.

Ariel was a witch from the Druidic Craft of the Wise. She taught me how and when to blend (the best time of day). Most important of all, she taught me to use my inner senses. I read book after book on herbs, potions, notions, tarot, astrology, astronomy, and correspondences. I was a sponge. I had come home.

After a few years we pulled away from each other. I went my way into the metaphysical world of Denver. Ariel fell into the horrific world of drugs and street life (due to a divorce). I tried to assist her, but she was too far gone and didn't desire my help. I still light incense for her every day and hope that she finds her way back.

When my husband and I moved to Littleton, Colorado, I went to a delightful store called Metamorphosis (it's been renamed Spirit Wise). I read cards, made oils and incenses, and helped run the store. It was by far one of the best times of my life. When I left Metamorphosis, I was a changed witch. I was well read on many different subjects, and knew I could do this on my own. And then …

We moved to the Buckle of the Bible belt in Louisiana. I had never been down here, and the culture shocked me … I wouldn't be able to make my store happen in this environment, so I decided to write, make incense, and enjoy the slower lifestyle.

Llewellyn's Complete Formulary of Magical Oils is the result of working with oils, mentors, people, and groups over the years. I have organized the information in a comprehensive manner so you can create your own potions. I placed essential oils and their medicinal information here for one reason only, which is to remind people that these oils are medicines—not just pretty smells—that need to be respected for their ability to heal, as well as to harm.

This book will assist you in rediscovering a lost art. Your oils can help make something happen today, and help you deal with what is to come tomorrow. They can help heal, hex, and banish. They can bring love or money to pay your bills. Only your intention and time hold you back!

Learning how to make oils is like learning to ride a bike. You learn by doing. You take a little time each day to practice, glance through the book, read a chapter, or look up an essential oil. Pretty soon you will have it mastered. There is no dogma or special rules; although, the information is here to assist you in making the process as ritualistic or as simple as you desire it to be. You can make oils by the hour of the day, phase or sign of the Moon, and even by the herbs involved. It's all up to you.

Discover how making magical oils can help you lead a better, more fulfilling life. Each oil is fully defined, and tested over time by people who have made them and experienced *much* success. This formulary will fit your lifestyle with style and magical grace. Best of all, you don't need to be a trained initiate or have special powers to use of the material in this book. All you need is an open mind and a desire to succeed.

You decide what you want, and then you create a spell or magical rite to go along with your oil, which will help you to get what you desire. You are in control at all times. The outcome depends upon your will and intent to get it.

There is much information regarding the best time to make your oils, and how to coordinate your magical operation to coincide with the phases of the Moon. I encourage you to explore and try to work with this incredible energy that is available to you. A simple rule of thumb is: use the New Moon to begin projects, attract money, help relationships, and aid in health problems; use the Full Moon to bring energy to projects that involve success in career, love, and partnerships; and use the Waning Moon to get rid of negative things in your life, bad situations, even losing weight.

When you experiment with oil blends, it is wise to write down what you add, how much you add, as well as time of day, and Moon phase and sign. Otherwise, you may create the most wonderful, delicious-smelling love oil that works like a charm and not be able to re-create it when you want to make more. If you keep track of what you do, you will know the exact steps to make your fabulous creations again. You will also know what smelled delicious and what smelled like crap, so you don't have to try that combination again. Keep the recipes in a notebook, or in your Book of Shadows, for later reference.

Two cautions: First, it is possible to be allergic to essential and fragrance oils as well as tinctures. If you plan to anoint yourself with them, test your skin in a small patch before using them to be sure you won't have a reaction. Don't use the essential oils straight, as most will cause skin irritation if used at full strength. You have been warned! Second, essential oils and tinctures will stain. Both will leave oily residues and greasy marks on any surface. The alcohol in the tinctures can bleach the color out of some fabrics and all papers, and it will damage the finish on wood furniture. Keep this in mind when anointing to be sure you don't ruin anything precious or delicate.

Some herbs will not be available as a true essential oil. There are several possible reasons for this. Some herbs or flowers are so difficult to extract oils from that it is not done commercially. Many herbs or flowers produce toxic essential oils, or oils that cause reactions severe enough to warrant that they not be sold. Some oils should *not* be used during pregnancy. Some oils cause what is known as phototoxicity upon exposure to ultraviolet light, which can cause anything from mild brown blotches to a severe burning of the skin. Many essential oils are irritating to the skin if not properly diluted.

Fortunately, there are numerous synthetic oils available that are created through chemical means and smell like the flower or herb they represent. This is especially true of the different musk, civet, and ambergris oils that were originally derived from animals. There are also many flowers and fruits that are only available in synthetic oils and that truly smell like the herb, flower, or fruit they represent. It has been my discovery over the years that they will work for magical endeavors, and in some cases, the synthetic oils are quite a bit cheaper.

I prefer to use a combination of both essential and fragrance oils, and because I charge each oil as I make it, I feel this is appropriate. A fragrance oil may have synthetics in it, but they don't come from outer space. They are made here, on Earth, and as such are derivatives of the Mother. Intent, as with any magic, is what counts. And if it smells good, it will affect your magic in a much more powerful way than something that doesn't smell so nice. Another thing to consider is that the shelf life of synthetic oils is quite a bit longer, too.

Before attempting any of the healing techniques represented in the Essential Oils section, be sure to consult your doctor or health care practitioner. Remember that even though it may come from a plant, it may not be safe.

Last, but not least, try not to get disillusioned if your magic and oils don't turn out perfect the first time. Some oils, just like some spells, take longer to work and master than others do. You must have faith, otherwise you will block the flow of energy needed to succeed. Remember that thoughts manifest themselves in each and every moment in the etheric world, which is the world of angels, the gods and goddesses, and other forms of energy that communicate with us. So if you believe in what you are doing, and it smells like what *you* think it should, then it will happen. B-E-L-I-E-V-E.

Measuring Mojo

Over the years I have had recipes that have had drops, pinches, cups, liters, and parts. Dang, it's so confuzzling! This section is to help you come to a common-sense method of making potions, oils, and such by using the "part" method.

The standard bottle I use for the recipes in this book is a one-dram bottle, which is equal to ⅛ of an ounce or 1.77 grams. Most oils come in a bottle this size. They can also be found online. I recommend always using colored glass bottles. They can be amber, cobalt blue, green—any color that will not allow light in. Light affects the oils, as will heat. Refrigeration may be a good idea.

Parts are used to standardize all the recipes. You can make a dram, an ounce, a liter, a gallon, or whatever you prefer to make, so you don't have to worry about adding too much or too little of an ingredient. You can look at the bottle and tell what you are measuring and come out with something that is perfect every time.

Pick up about a dozen glass eyedroppers at a pharmacy or online to get started. The eyedroppers can be cleaned by soaking in isopropyl alcohol (do not cover the entire dropper, just the glass section) and used again and again. Let the droppers soak for about an hour, then let them air dry. Another good investment is a Pyrex measuring cup. This can be a lifesaver when you prepare larger quantities. Do not ever use plastic, because the oils will literally eat through the plastic after a period of time, and then you will have oil everywhere. Remember, you don't want "banishing" oil all over your witches' cabinet with all your tools and other precious items. That would be a very bad thing.

When I state "add a few drops," I mean a drop from an eyedropper that is intended for use with the one dram bottle. If you use a larger container to make your oils, you may use your intuition and creativity until you achieve the right smell for your oil. Remember, this oil is for you, and you only, so make it something you truly love.

And please remember to write everything down. The Moon phase, the day of the week, and time of day, along with the ingredients used. This is so you can duplicate it later and not end up with something entirely different. Believe me, when you think you can remember it—nope, nada, zilch—you can't. I have done that and lost many treasured, beautiful, and very magical recipes. I've never been able to duplicate them when asked, or when I needed something on the fly for a ritual or spell.

Adding Herbs and Gemstones to Your Oil

I encourage you to try this, as it adds a very magical "punch" to your oils. You need not fill the bottle to the brim with herbs, just a few leaves, a petal, or a teardrop of resin is all you need. As for the gemstones, one chip from a gemstone chip necklace is all you need, even for the larger bottles.

Although adding herbs and gemstones is not mandatory, it is something I have always had very good luck with. Give it a try, and see if it makes a difference in your oils!

I also suggest using fragrance oils to begin with; they are less costly and you might be surprised at the outcome. When you decide to use essentials, you will have a better understanding of how to blend and use fragrances and essentials without spending a lot of money in the beginning. I suggest going to www.SaveOnScents.com, as they have bottles, droppers, and scents, as well as a delightful selection of fragrance oils. New Directions Aromatics at www.newdirectionsaromatics.com is a good source for essential oils. Both companies ship worldwide and have an incredible customer service team to assist you, not to mention stellar prices.

If a recipe states to use essential oils only, please do so. Otherwise, your blend may not come out as the initial intentions were written.

Using Carrier Oils in Your Blends

I recommend using a carrier oil, and it is a must if you are using essential oils only. A fragrance and essential oil blend will last longer and have a better scent "throw" (the way it smells) if it has a carrier oil added. Look over the list of carrier oils in this book and choose one that you feel works well with your magical intention. In this way, you can be certain that you are crafting a well-rounded fragrance if you decide to use it as a personal scent.

I hope this will help you enjoy making your magical oils. It has simplified the process for many I have taught, and they all have had very good results time after time with this method.

Precautionary Safety Notes

- Essential oils are the extensions of living plants, and as such, they have many safety concerns, just as living plants do. Many plants are dangerous or harmful to humans and pets. Pennyroyal and deadly nightshade come to mind.

- Essential oils should NEVER be taken orally.

- Consult a licensed aromatherapist before using them with someone who has epilepsy, heart disease, or high blood pressure.

- Use sparingly with children. Essential oils are generally not recommended for use on infants, and it is best to use them only therapeutically on young children.

- Never apply an essential oil directly onto the skin; always use a carrier oil.

- People with sensitive skin, or who have allergic reactions, should always perform a skin test on the inside of the elbow for twenty-four hours before use.

- Keep essential oils away from eyes and ears.

- Photosensitivity is also a concern with some essential oils, especially the citrus oils and Angelica. They should *not* be applied before going out into direct sunshine.

- These essential oils *should not* be used under *any* circumstances (you may substitute fragrance oils):

Bitter Almond	Sassafras
Boldo Leaf	Savin
Calamus	Southernwood
Horseradish	Tansy
Jaborandi Leaf	Thuja
Mugwort	Wintergreen
Mustard	Wormseed
Pennyroyal	Wormwood
Rue	Yellow Camphor

Relating to Pregnancy and Breastfeeding

Most of the following herb oils and herbs have been known to cause uterine contractions that can lead to miscarriage. Also avoid taking these herbs as teas during pregnancy. Never use these oils to induce a miscarriage, because they may lead to serious hemorrhaging. This list is not exhaustive, so always talk to your health care practitioner before using any oils not mentioned.

Angelica	Mustard
Anise	Musk
Basil	Pennyroyal
Camphor	Peppermint
Champa	Rosemary
Citronella	Sage
Hyssop	Savory
Jasmine	Spanish Thyme
Juniper	Tarragon
Lemon Balm	Thyme
Lovage	Raspberry
Marjoram	Wintergreen
Melissa	

Fragrance oils should be looked over carefully and also talked about with your health care practitioner. It's never worth taking a chance on your health or that of your unborn child.

PART TWO

TWO

Magical Formulations

Magical Charge for Oil

Oil of wonder; Oil of power
Increase in potency by minute and hour
I conjure you now; I charge you with strength
I give you life of infinite length
And boundless magical energy
As I will, charged you be.

The Elementals

Elementals are the little creatures that animate the four elements. You cannot ordinarily see, hear, feel, taste, or touch them, but this doesn't mean they don't exist. After all, X-rays exist, even though you cannot sense them. You may, however, get to know the elementals through the use of your extraordinary senses.

The four types of elementals are Salamanders (Fire), Sylphs (Air), Undines (Water), and Gnomes (Earth).

Elementals are experts in their own realms. The Salamander knows everything there is to know about the Fire element, both physical and psychological. Sylphs are experts on the subject of Air. Undines are experts regarding Water. Gnomes specialize in Earthy subjects. Elementals are one-element creatures, and as long as they remain imprisoned, so to speak, in their own element they are incapable of learning anything about those elements to which they don't naturally belong.

Elementals aren't entirely happy with this situation. They'd like to progress and evolve, but the only way they can do so is through vicarious association with multi-element creatures, such as human beings. For this reason, elementals seek human companionship. In return for a favored human's "tutelage," they are very willing to give service. The magician who is able to attract a helpful Undine can look forward to expert assistance in matters relating to love, friendship, healing, and the psychic arts. Gnomes will help with career and financial matters, Sylphs with intellectual pursuits, and Salamanders with creative and spiritual issues.

Elemental assistance is desirable because it makes it easier to pursue a goal. Called upon for help, an elemental gladly goes to work on his companion's project. You still need to do affirmations, incantations, visualizations, and all of the other work covered to this point—you can never expect anyone or anything to do all of your work for you. Your path to the goal will be greased, however, and you'll see speedier results than if you had no elemental help. Magical practitioners who are able to attract elemental companions have a great advantage over those who are not.

4 Winds Oil

One part of each oil is needed to make this recipe:

East Wind, the wind of intelligence: Lavender

South Wind, the wind of passion and change: Musk

West Wind, the wind of love and emotions: Rose

North Wind, the wind of riches: Honeysuckle

Wear the appropriate oil when desiring a change in that area of your life. Also wear it to boost spells you may be working. South Wind is the catch-all; if your wish doesn't fall into any of the other categories, use South Wind.

Abtina Oil

¼ part Musk   ⅛ part Balm of Gilead

⅛ part Myrrh   ⅛ part Cassia

⅛ part Olibanum   ⅛ part Lotus

⅛ part Storax

A powerful ancient and sacred blend especially for working with all four elements at once. The origin of this mixture is unknown though I do know it's very old—use carefully!

Air Oil

½ part Lavender

½ part Sandalwood

Neroli, a drop or two

Wear to invoke the powers of Air and to promote clear thinking, for travel spells, and to overcome addictions.

Air Oil II

¼ part Benzoin

½ part Lavender

¼ part Lily of the Valley

Air is the sphere of the intellect, reason, new beginnings, and change.

Air Oil III

⅔ part Lavender

⅓ part Sandalwood

Rosemary, a few drops

Communication, learning, ideas, solutions.

Angelic Wings Oil

½ part Sandalwood
¼ part Magnolia
¼ part Myrrh

Powerful ancient sacred blend especially for working with all four elements at once; the origin of this mixture is unknown. I do know it's very old—use carefully!

Apparition Oil

This oil is made with herbs (buy online or in any health-food store).

3 parts Wood Aloe	1 part Anise
2 parts Coriander	1 part Cardamom
1 part Camphor	1 part Chicory
1 part Mugwort	1 part Hemp
1 part Flax	

Enough carrier oil to cover.

Let sit in a dark place for two weeks to blend; shake occasionally. Anoint black and white candles. Causes apparitions to appear if you really want this to happen.

Crystal Woodlands Oil

¼ part Fir
⅛ part Pine
¼ part Juniper

Communication with the astral or animals.

Dryad Oil

½ part Musk	⅛ part Civet
¼ part Oak Moss	⅛ part Vanilla

An excellent blend for pursuing the arts of natural magic. This preparation was especially designed for contacting the elemental spirits of the Earth.

Earth Oil

½ part Patchouli
½ part Cypress

Wear to invoke the powers of the Earth to bring money, prosperity, abundance, stability, and foundation.

Earth Oil II

Patchouli, a few drops
½ part Magnolia
½ part Honeysuckle
Pine, a few drops

To attract the qualities of the element: endurance, stability, strength. Also for grounding, for working with astrological and elemental signs of Earth.

Earth Oil III

⅛ part Sandalwood
¼ part Patchouli
¼ part Vetiver
⅛ part Honeysuckle
¼ part Myrrh

A very powerful oil to assist you in contacting the Earth elementals. A very good oil to use in stability, grounding, and also money magics.

Fire Oil

½ part Ginger
½ part Rosemary
Petitgrain, a few drops
Clove, a few drops

Wear to invoke the powers of Fire, such as energy, courage, strength, love, passion, and so on.

Fire Oil II

⅛ part Cinnamon
⅛ part Clove
¾ part Orange
¼ part Nutmeg

Fire is associated with transformation, passion, leadership, and personal success.

Gossamer Wings Oil

¼ part Violet
¼ part Lemon
½ part Lavender
Cajuput, a few drops

Useful for contacting Faeries connected with the Air element: sylphs, elves, etc.

Gnomes Oil

½ part Sandalwood
½ part Musk
Pine, 1 to 3 drops

Gnomes are Earth elementals of the watchtowers of the North. If you like playing with them and do not mind that they can cause a little chaos now and then in your home, they can be very handy to have around. They will guard your space, and in general keep things tidy. In other words, they inspire you to pick up after yourself.

Nature-Spirit Attracting Oil

½ part Carnation
½ part Gardenia

I personally feel this oil has a very high vibration to it and, therefore, can work with the Elementals and with the Angelic Realm.

Pan's Delight Oil

¼ part Musk
¼ part Pine
¼ part Lavender

To bring out the playful, frolicking Earth spirits. Sprites, elves, and pixies love to come and join in the party when Pan is called on.

Siren Song Oil

⅛ part Lemon
¼ part Lavender
⅛ part Primrose
½ part Camphor
Rose Geranium, a few drops

To work with Water elementals. Also very good to use when learning or in the creation of music; and also when meditation is used with music.

Water Oil

½ part Palmarosa
½ part Ylang-Ylang
Jasmine, a few drops

Wear to promote love, healing, psychic awareness, purification, and so on.

Water Oil (Elemental) II

½ part Sweet Pea
⅛ part Jasmine
¼ part Camellia
⅛ part Lotus

Water is the realm of hidden mysteries, psychic senses, and peace.

Water Oil III

⅓ part Bergamot
⅓ part Jasmine
⅓ part Myrrh

Dreams, psychic ability, sensuality, increasing emotions. Helps to dispel fear from psychic attacks and helps with recovery from emotional abuse.

Love, Attraction & Sex

When you feel like making love, there is nothing better to attract your lover than smooth skin with an alluring aphrodisiac scent. Making love oil is not only a treat for your skin, it offers an olfactory sensation that is sure to help spice things up.

There are many different ways to bring romance into your life. Use love oil with an aromatherapy burner to scent the room, rub into pressure points on your lover's body, or add to your potpourri. If you wish to bless your candles, as I do, there is a special technique for applying the oil for magical purposes. Place the oil on your fingertips, and then rub the oil from the top of the candle down to the middle and from the bottom up to the middle. In this way you draw energy into your life and into your ritual.

Adam and Eve Oil
⅓ part Apple Blossom
⅓ part Rose
⅓ part Lemon

To ensure fidelity between married couples, bring sweethearts closer, and attract a lover to a single person.

Adonis's Ardor Oil
½ part Jasmine
¼ part Musk
¼ part Vanilla

This mixture is designed to stimulate and prolong sexuality and stamina. It's one of my favorites. (Not to be taken internally.)

All Night Long Oil
½ part Jasmine
⅛ part Vanilla
⅛ part Musk

A combination of oils said to completely relieve sexual problems and inhibitions, to simultaneously relax and inflame. Use in potpourri to scent the bed chamber, or as personal anointing oil.

All Night Long Oil II
¼ part Jasmine
¼ part Honeysuckle
¼ part Vanilla
¼ part Cinnamon

This is great in a diffuser for those nighttime escapades. Also good in the bath or in massage oils. When using in a massage blend, add just a few drops of this blend to about ½ cup of carrier oil. *Note: Because of the cinnamon in this blend, test a little on the inside of your elbow. Then wait twenty-four hours to see if it irritates you or your partner's skin. Do NOT use this oil internally.*

Alsatian Sex Oil—Female
⅓ part Musk
⅓ part Civet
⅓ part Ambergris
Patchouli, a few drops

Created for women to sexually attract men. Wear as a personal oil.

Alsatian Sex Oil—Male
¾ part Musk
¼ part Ambergris
Muguet, a few drops

Worn by men to sexually arouse and attract women.

Ambergris Bouquet
Cypress, 6 drops
Patchouli, a few drops

This scent, used in aphrodisiac-type oils and perfumes, is the product of sperm whales. True ambergris is best avoided because of its origins. If you can't find artificial ambergris oil, try substituting the above bouquet, or compound, which is very close to true ambergris.

Amor Oil

¼ part Orange
¼ part Almond
¼ part Cinnamon
¼ part Balm of Gilead
Piece of coral in bottle

A classic New Orleans love recipe. Sure to make heads turn when you walk into a room.

Amore' Oil

½ part Apple Blossom
⅛ part Ambergris
⅛ part Cinnamon

An attraction oil to bring you love. Be careful with this one. It has a habit of making people desire to follow you around.

Aphrodite Oil

½ part Cypress
¼ part Cinnamon
¼ part Ambergris bouquet

To invoke or worship the Goddess, or for any pursuit of romance or love.

Aphrodite Oil II

⅓ part Geranium
⅓ part Lilac
⅓ part Apple Blossom

To attract a male. Can be used by either sex.

Aphrodite Oil III

¾ part Cypress
½ part Cinnamon
Small piece of Orris Root
Olive Oil as a carrier oil

Add the true essential oils and the Orris Root to an Olive Oil base (about 1 cup). Anoint your body to bring a love into your life. *Note: Please test inside of elbow first. Cinnamon and Cypress essential oils can be very irritating to skin.*

Aphrodite's Love-Drawing Oil

¼ part Carnation
¼ part Lilac
¼ part Musk
¼ part Lily of the Valley (or Magnolia)
Cinnamon, a few drops

To invoke the goddess in all her forms and encourage love to be drawn to you.

Aphrodisiac Oil

½ part Ylang-Ylang
¼ part Orange
¼ part Jasmine
Cinnamon, a few drops

To attract passion and romance of the most intense kind.

Aphrodisiac Oil II

⅓ part Patchouli
⅓ part Sandalwood
⅓ part Ylang-Ylang

Sexy, sexy, sexy! Should be used sparingly and only when the person near you is someone you wish to arouse.

Arabian Nights Oil

⅓ part Myrrh
⅓ part Rose
⅓ part Lilac

Attracts many new friends. Can be depended upon to force others to find you stimulating and extremely appealing. It is very good for potential lovers. Add to rituals and to love charms, and to anoint hands. Great for those nights when you are on the prowl for a new playmate.

Arabian Nights Oil II

¼ part Jasmine
½ part Musk
⅛ part Honeysuckle
⅛ part Hyacinth

Creates a harmonious and festive atmosphere. A beautiful oil to use in a diffuser at a small gathering.

As You Please Oil

⅓ part Orange Blossom
⅓ part Mint
⅓ part Musk

Sprinkled on the ground or placed where a loved one will come in contact with it, this will cause that person to return to you. It will cause others to wish to please you at all costs, but it can cause stalking, so be careful.

Attraction Oil

¼ part Allspice
¼ part White Musk
¼ part Lemon, Lime, or Orange
¼ part Sweet Pea

Place an Amber stone in the master bottle and a Coriander seed in the bottles you will have for sale. Attracts money, business, and success.

Attraction Oil II

¼ part Rose
¼ part Lavender
¼ part Vanilla
¼ part Sandalwood

Touch to pulse points when in the presence of the one you want to attract. Works for both males and females.

Attraction Oil III

½ part Musk
¼ part Lilac
¼ part Jasmine
Almond, a few drops

Incites passion and draws intimate love into your life. A very good oil to present to someone who has just been handfasted or married.

Aura of Venus Oil

½ part Jasmine

⅛ part Frangipani

⅛ part Lavender

⅛ part Rose

⅛ part Musk

Used as an aid in prosperity spells or love spells. When mixing these oils, focus on confidence and success. Best to make on a Friday.

Bast Cat Oil

Cinnamon (use only one or two drops of this—it's very strong!)

½ part Sandalwood

½ part Musk

Catnip in master bottle

Blend in desired quantities. Used to invoke playfulness and sexuality, and for being on the prowl.

Bast Oil

½ part Ylang-Ylang

½ part Frankincense

Catnip in master bottle

To invoke or worship the goddess, to stimulate creativity, to encourage hedonism and playfulness.

Bewitching Oil

½ part Patchouli

½ part Vetiver

Lime, a few drops

Bay, a few drops

A "gray" purpose oil, binds others to you, causes the wearer to become enticing and beguiling, creates bonds of love and affection. Another one of those oils that I truly enjoy creating and wearing. It has a very beguiling scent and has everyone asking, "What is that you're wearing?"

Binding Love Oil

½ part Jasmine
½ part Gardenia
Vetiver, a few drops

To aid in securing long-term love. A wonderful oil to use in a marriage or handfasting ceremony.

Black Cat Oil

First three items are to be placed in master bottle before adding oils.

3 black cat hairs
Steel wool—just a few threads (not an SOS pad with soap)
Iron powder (lodestone dust)
⅓ part Sage
⅓ part Myrrh
⅓ part Bay

Compels the opposite sex to strongly desire you. Also used for breaking bad spells and unhexing.

Blue Sonata Oil

⅓ part Vanilla
⅓ part Rose
⅓ part Jasmine

This oil is used to encourage romantic admirers.

Caliph's Beloved Oil

¼ part Musk
¼ part Ambergris
¼ part Coriander
¼ part Cardamom
Carnation, a few drops

A special oil that was developed to incite sexual feelings and attract lovers. A popular aphrodisiac.

Caliph's Beloved Oil II

½ part Ambergris
½ part Rose
Apricot carrier oil to fill bottle

Lovely-smelling mixture. Excites sexual passions and attracts new lovers to the wearer. Powerful aphrodisiac. Nice to burn in a diffuser.

Call Me Oil

½ part Frangipani
½ part Musk
Cinnamon, a few drops

This oil will encourage that person you want to hear from to call you. Works very well for long-distance relationships.

Candle Oil for Love

¼ part Rose
¼ part Honeysuckle
½ part Musk
Sweet Almond carrier oil
1–2 drops Benzoin Tincture

Blend all the ingredients and then use to dress candles, or as a scented oil in an oil diffuser. Keep oil in refrigerator to extend the scent.

Cernunnos Oil

⅛ part Amber
⅛ part Patchouli
⅛ part Rose geranium
¼ part Musk
¼ part Ambergris
⅛ part Pine
Clove, a few drops

A wonderful blend. Use to align with and direct the primal, fertile, active energy of nature.

Charlotte's Web Oil

½ part Musk
¼ part Rose
¼ part Wisteria

An intoxicating love blend. Try using to dress pink or red figure candles—one to represent you and one to represent a potential lover.

Position the figures so they are facing one another; allow them to burn for fifteen minutes at a time. Each time you burn them, move them closer to one another. Continue until they are touching; then let them burn completely.

Circe Oil

¼ part Lotus
¼ part Lily of the Valley
¼ part Musk
¼ part Muguet
Clove, a few drops
Eucalyptus, a few drops
Wintergreen, a few drops

A romantic enchantment. Use to cause someone to become enthralled with you.

Circle of Flame Oil

½ part Rose
½ part Violet
Musk, a few drops

Brings about a feeling of intense and erotic love. Wear when you feel you need to bring those intense passions to the bedroom.

Cleo May Oil

¼ part Jasmine
¼ part Gardenia
¼ part Yellow Rose
¼ part Egyptian Musk

Prepare this blend by pouring the oils in a 10-ounce bottle and then adding organic vegetable oil to fill. Anoint the third eye, sacrum, and solar plexus. Pour a few drops into the palm of your hands and inhale deeply. May use in the bath as well. The ultimate seduction oil.

Cleopatra Oil

⅓ part Heliotrope
⅓ part Cedarwood
⅓ part Rose
Frankincense, a few drops

An especially favored scent of Voudoun practitioners. Cleopatra Oil may be used in a love spell to anoint a pink candle, worn to strengthen and enhance the relationship between lovers, or worn to attract a secretly desired stranger.

Cleopatra Oil II

½ part Balm of Gilead
¼ part Musk
⅛ part Orange
⅛ part Frankincense

An oil only for lovers. It entices the stranger you secretly desire. Excites and arouses those you love to come forth and respond. A powerful aphrodisiac. (Use to anoint pink candles in love rituals.)

Cleopatra Oil III

¼ part Lotus
¼ part Honeysuckle
¼ part Sandalwood
¼ part Ylang-Ylang

Very seductive blend—use carefully! And most of all have fun with this oil; it can be *very* playful and flirty.

Come-and-Get-Me Oil

⅛ part Cinnamon
¼ part Patchouli
⅛ part Rose
½ part Sandalwood

This is an incredibly powerful oil mixture that many people swear by when it comes to attracting a partner. It sends a signal similar to a cat in heat, and you will be noticed from wherever you dwell.

Come-and-See-Me Oil

¾ part Patchouli

¼ part Clove

To attract the ideal mate, mix these true essential oils in an Olive Oil base, smear on a white image candle of the appropriate sex and burn with visualization.

Come-and-See-Me Oil II

¼ ounce Olive Oil
¼ part Patchouli
¼ part Rose
¼ part Sandalwood
Cinnamon, a drop or two

Same as above, but this blend adds a bit of a romantic twist with the Rose; it is not so hard core, but a much softer version if you desire to be a little more coy.

Come-to-Me Oil

¼ part Rose
¼ part Jasmine
¼ part Bergamot
¼ part Damiana

Float nine Jasmine flowers in the master bottle. Damiana oil can be hard to find, so if you desire, you may leave this ingredient out. Another option is to add a few pieces of the herb to the bottle.

Come-to-Me Oil II

⅓ part Rose
⅓ part Jasmine
⅓ part Gardenia
Lemon, a few drops

A very powerful attraction recipe used only when you desire to force a certain stranger to feel strong sexual responses toward you.

Come-to-Me Oil III

⅛ part Wisteria

⅛ part Musk
⅛ part Jasmine
¼ part Narcissus
⅛ part Rose Geranium
⅛ part Sandalwood
⅛ part Rose
Gold leaf flakes in master bottle

This is designed for use by either sex when they desire to draw a specific person for love or sex. You can find gold leaf flakes at any arts and crafts store. It's also okay to leave them out if you desire. Remember, it is the intent with which you make this oil that makes it yours.

Come-to-Me Oil IV

⅓ part Sweet Pea
⅓ part Rose
⅓ part Patchouli

Float a bit of Catnip or a few Saffron strands (for gay men) in the master bottle. This blend is lovely and has been a favorite among gay men who have been my clients for years.

Come-to-Me Oil V

¼ part Cinnamon
¼ part Ambergris
¼ part Ylang-Ylang
¼ part Vanilla

Float a piece of Queen Elizabeth Root in your bottle, if possible. Try to make this oil on a Friday evening.

Come-to-Me Oil VI

⅓ part Rose
⅓ part Jasmine
⅓ part Vanilla
10 drops Opium fragrance oil

This oil is for commanding attention. There are many formulas for Come-to-Me Oil, but this one is the best, by far. Opium fragrance oil can be found online and in some craft stores; it's worth looking for.

Commanding Love Oil

½ part Vetiver
¼ part Jasmine
¼ part Gardenia

Used to attract a stable relationship or a potential husband or wife. Also good for bringing back home stray lovers.

Courting Oil

½ part Lily of the Valley
½ part Lilac
10 drops Musk
5 drops Cinnamon

This oil will help you attract the right mate for you.

Delight Oil

½ part Apple Blossom (alternatives: Magnolia or Mimosa)
¼ part Sweet Pea
¼ part Rose
Lavender, a few drops

Removes inhibitions and increases pleasure.

Desert Nights Oil

¼ part Frankincense
½ part Honeysuckle
¼ part Gardenia

Use to aid you in love spells. When mixing this oil, focus on confidence, success, romance, and your heart feeling full.

Desire Me Oil

½ part Jasmine
¼ part Lotus
¼ part Musk

This a strong oil to used for sexual attraction to someone you know and desire. Use with caution.

Desire Me Oil II

¾ part Rose

¼ part Vanilla

5 drops Ambergris

5 drops Cinnamon

Strong attraction oil for love and sex. Powerful—and fun!

Devil's Master Oil

¾ part Vetiver

⅛ part Rose

⅛ part Musk

A Southern potion used by men to entice women. Make this oil with the intent to find the type of woman you desire. If you don't you will bring all types to you, and you may end up with your hands full of women you may not want—and they will be very difficult to be rid of.

Dionysus Oil

⅓ part Amber

⅓ part Pine

⅓ part Musk

Dionysus, the inspirer of intoxication, madness, and ecstasy. This perfume is a fusion of sensual Amber oil, invigorating Pine, and soothing Musk. This aroma inspires the anointed to follow their imaginations, unleash their creativity, and let loose. Yeah, it's one of those kind of oils … have fun!

Dionysus Oil II

⅓ part Lilac

⅓ part Carnation

⅓ part Wisteria

This oil is for parties and celebrations. Dionysus is a complex god, as so many of them are. He loves wine and joy. But the other side of him is rage from too much alcohol. If you throw a party and wear this oil, make sure there is plenty of food and bread to help absorb the drink.

Dixie Love Oil

⅓ part Rose
⅓ part Gardenia
⅓ part Neroli

The ultimate attraction oil. A true Southern tradition that is sure to work every time. Bring that soul from the Deep South into your realm to help you find or intensify love.

Dixie Love Oil Perfume

½ part Patchouli
¼ part Cinnamon
¼ part Jasmine

Powerful attraction oil that induces the opposite sex to readily give in to your every whim. It inspires romance and lovemaking. Makes all charms even more appealing. Great for anointing rose quartz and garnet.

Draw Across Oil

¾ part Patchouli
¼ part Cinnamon

Increases the wearer's sexual magnetism. You'll attract anyone who passes or walks near you. Wear it and watch what happens. As with all Cinnamon-based oils, try it on the inside of your elbow overnight and make sure it doesn't irritate your skin. If it does, try making it again using less Cinnamon.

Enchantment Oil

¼ part Ginger
¼ part Ylang-Ylang
¼ part Sweet Pea
¼ part Musk

An aphrodisiac blend. To make your lovers see you differently than you really are. Be careful with this; it has the affect of letting others see you as they wish to see you. I know some of you have woken up the next morning and went "what the hell was I thinking?" This is one of those oils.

Enchantment Oil II

½ part Neroli
½ part White Musk

To make things appear to be different than they really are. Good for magics that require a bit of a twist. Good for job interviews.

Enchantment Oil III

¼ part Sandalwood
¼ part Ambergris
¼ part Honeysuckle
¼ part Violet
Orange, a few drops (optional)

Go ahead, send out that message for love! A sensuous scent that is sure to intoxicate anyone around you; good for both men and women.

Enchantment Oil IV

⅛ part Sandalwood
⅛ part Ambergris
⅛ part Orange
⅛ part Violet
½ part Honeysuckle

If you are feeling disenchanted with life, wear this oil and you'll see the world begin to change. The world will have more spark, more wonder.

Enchantress Oil

¼ part Acacia
¾ part Wisteria

A very compelling oil. It will tempt and taunt those around you. Good for job seeking, love, and bringing things to you that you desire.

Endless Love Oil

½ part Magnolia
½ part Orchid
Ylang-Ylang, a few drops
Benzoin, a few drops

An oil for those seeking love that lasts forever. Be careful—you just may get what you wish for, and more!

Enticement Oil

½ part Patchouli

⅛ part Cinnamon

⅛ part Lemon

¼ part Rose Musk

Causes another to desire the wearer. I created this oil for a client and she swore it worked every time she wore it. Sure enough, within six months, she had met the man of her dreams.

Eros Oil

Use equal amounts of each of the following oils:

Cinnamon

Mastic

Styrax

Benzoin

Rose

Sandalwood

Deer's Tongue

Orris

Musk

Patchouli

Amber

Ambergris

Add the following herbs to the bottles:

Lavender Flower

Orange Peel

Violet Flowers

Lovage Root

Although a complicated oil to make, it is well worth the effort. To invoke the god Eros in order to enchant a lover to your side. Wait nine days for the herbs to steep before using this oil. Shake the bottle each day while keeping your intention in mind.

Erotic Exotic Oil

⅓ part Bergamot

⅓ part Lemon

⅓ part Ylang-Ylang

To heighten passions and bring lust. Fun, lusty, and very good for fertility spells.

Erotic Patchouli Oil (Melissa's Blend)

½ part Patchouli
¼ part Musk
¼ part Myrrh (can substitute Angel perfume oil)
Opium, a few drops
Add Patchouli leaves and a Vetiver root to the bottle

A blend for Patchouli lovers everywhere.

Erzulie Oil

Equal parts:
Rose
Geranium

Erzulie is the Haitian goddess of love and dreams. For letting more sensuality into your life, and to increase your bliss and tolerance. Also good for women business owners to ensure success.

Erzulie La Flambeau Oil

¾ part Rose
¼ part Lavender
Strawberry, a few drops
Cinnamon, a few drops

To revitalize your partner's love. Refresh and bring passion back to your life. Best used in a diffuser.

Erzulie Rose Fleur Oil

⅓ part Tea Rose
⅓ part Gardenia
⅓ part Carnation

Add 1 drop of real honey to the bottle and shake until well blended. To bring harmony and peace into your life and to those around you. A great scent to wear at family gatherings.

Eve Oil

½ part Apple Blossom
½ part Rose
Lemon, a few drops

Used to attract a man's attention. Love-drawing oil with a history of making men swoon.

Eve Oil II

½ part Rose
½ part Musk
Vetiver, a few drops

The ultimate temptation oil. Temptress extraordinaire! Place a few drops in a bottle of unscented lotion and experience the art of temptation.

Eyes-for-Me Oil

¼ part Musk
¼ part Civet
¼ part Gardenia
¼ part Ambergris
Myrrh, a few drops

This blend was created in response to a request to stimulate fidelity in a lover. It keeps the partner focused solely on you. Can become rather obsessive, as well. So be careful when using this oil for more than a few days of the month.

Fertility Oil

½ part Geranium
3 parts Olive Oil
1 part Pine
2 parts Sunflower carrier oil

To increase fertility and creativity in body, mind, or spirit. Use essential oils only in this blend.

Fire and Ice Oil

¾ part Cool Water fragrance oil
¼ part Ambergris fragrance oil

Passion with an edge. This oil has a very intoxicating feel to it. I personally like to wear this during a Waning Moon because it helps me feel a bit more "in tune" with my surroundings.

Fire of Love Oil

⅓ part Opium fragrance oil
⅓ part Musk
⅓ part Magnolia

This oil will make someone feel the heat of searing love for you or wake up a passionate, relentless longing.

Fire of Passion Oil

¼ part Patchouli
¼ part Civet
¼ part Musk
¼ part Pine or Ambergris

Will cause the opposite sex to desire the wearer more passionately; this potent formula overcomes resistance to your romantic advances.

Fire of Passion Oil II

¾ part Gardenia
¼ part Ambergris
10 drops Peach
Cinnamon, a few drops

For exploring more adventurous things in the bedroom.

Fire of Love Oil

¼ part Patchouli
¼ part Civet
½ part Musk

Creates a mystical love spell and draws others to you; helps to increase your sexuality.

Fire of Love Oil II

¼ part Egyptian Musk
⅛ part Civet
¼ part Frankincense
⅛ part Patchouli
⅛ part Clove
⅛ part Vetiver

To excite passionate feelings (rather than simply friendly ones!). The original potion that is true to its name.

Fire of Lust Oil

¼ part Orange oil
¼ part Citronella
¼ part Carnation
¼ part Rose Geranium

Be careful with this oil; you can manifest stalkers! Wear sparingly. Better yet, use in a diffuser in the bedroom with a partner you adore.

Flower Oil for Attraction

¼ part Honeysuckle
¼ part Jasmine
¼ part Carnation
¼ part Violet

Wear as a personal fragrance to attract love and friendship and to honor the goddesses Flora and Maia.

Follow Me Boy Oil

½ part Jasmine
½ part Rose
Vanilla, a few drops
Piece of coral
Gold glitter

The traditional version of this product also contains a piece of coral and gold glitter. It was favored by New Orleans prostitutes to ensure they would make plenty of money through the appreciation of their passions.

Follow Me Boy Oil II

½ part Jasmine
½ part Opium fragrance oil

A great oil to wear if you work for tips! When I worked as a server, I would wear this oil. It is truly a miracle worker when you need that extra cash, not to mention a new partner in your life!

Follow Me Girl Oil

¼ part Myrrh
¼ part Patchouli
⅛ part Vetiver
⅛ part Lemon
⅛ part Vanilla
⅛ part Sandalwood

Based on the traditional New Orleans formula, this oil was worn by men to attract women.

Fragrance of Venus Oil

½ part Jasmine

½ part Red Rose
Drop of Lavender (no more)
A few drops of Musk and Ylang-Ylang

This oil should only be worn by women wishing to attract men. Best prepared on a Friday evening. Then let it sit and "brew" for a week before using.

French Bracelet Oil

⅓ part Rose
⅓ part Frangipani
⅓ part Lavender
Dittany of Crete, a few drops

Wear to bring good fortune and romance.

French Bracelet Oil II

⅓ part Rose
⅓ part Frangipani
⅓ part Honeysuckle
Narcissus, a few drops

To allure prospective lovers. Also good for wearing to job interviews!

French Creole Oil

¼ part Lilac
¼ part Musk
¼ part Bay
¼ part Lime

Special oil designed to make your dreams come true. It helps to interpret dreams prophetically. Will arouse desire in others, and assist you in making the right decisions when it comes to finding a new partner.

French Love Oil

½ part Wisteria
¼ part Violet
¼ part Orris

Helps to overcome shyness and meet new people.

Freya Oil

½ part Ambergris

½ part Musk

Add a few drops of:

Benzoin

Narcissus

Patchouli

To invoke or worship the goddess Freya (Germanic version of Venus); for pursuits of love, luxury, and beauty.

Full Bloom Oil

½ part Jasmine

¼ part Musk

⅛ part Sandalwood

⅛ part Gardenia

Muguet, a few drops

Use to aid you in love spells. When mixing these oils, focus on confidence, success, romance, and your heart feeling full.

Gay Love Oil

¾ part Vanilla

¼ part Ambergris

Cinnamon, a few drops

Devised for gay couples, both male and female.

General Love Oil

½ part Rosemary

¼ part Lavender

⅛ part Cardamom

⅛ part Yarrow

Use to aid you in love spells. The corresponding color for this potion is pink, so you may prefer to use a candle or bottle of this color.

Gigolo Oil

½ part Frankincense

¼ part Heliotrope

¼ part Hyacinth

For male "players." Yes, this oil is for you—enjoy! But please, be safe!

Goddess of Love Oil

½ part Rose
½ part Musk
Mint, a few drops

Helps in romantic pursuits.

Goddess of Love Oil II

⅓ part Hyacinth
⅓ part Rose
⅓ part Narcissus
10 drops Musk
Vanilla, a few drops

To invoke your favorite love goddess to help you meet someone new.

Great Goddess Oil

⅓ part Myrrh
⅓ part Lotus
⅓ part Lily

Causes the wearer to be treated royally, for those who wish respect more than affection.

Haitian Lover Oil—Male

¼ part Cinnamon
¼ part Anise
¼ part Orris
¼ part Clove
Sassafras, a few drops

An excellent formula for men only. Very effective when used on a red female figure candle to attract the opposite sex.

Haitian Lover Oil—Female

¼ part Patchouli
¼ part Rose
¼ part Dark Musk
¼ part Opium fragrance oil
Vetiver, a few drops

The female version of the oil above. Very effective when used to dress a male figure.

Handfasting Oil

¼ part Gardenia
⅛ part Musk
½ part Jasmine
⅛ part Rose
Rose petals

This is often given to witch couples on the evening of their handfasting. They then can use it in a massage oil (do not use internally), in a bath, or in a diffuser in the honeymoon bedroom.

Handfasting Oil II

¼ part Palmarosa
¼ part Ylang-Ylang
⅛ part Ginger
¼ part Rosemary
⅛ part Cardamom

To bless or create a marriage. Wear as personal oil and anoint candles during hand-fasting rituals.

Handfasting Oil III

¼ part Gardenia
¼ part Lily of the Valley
¼ part Lavender
¼ part Magnolia

For one the most sacred times of your life: blessing a couple's love.

He's Mine Oil

⅓ part Orange Blossom
⅓ part Jasmine
⅓ part Musk

Used to produce or increase a marriage or binding love.

Heavenly Nights Oil

White Musk
Hibiscus, a few drops

To inspire sex and fidelity.

Hummingbird Oil

¼ part Cinnamon

¼ part Anise

¼ part Orris

¼ part Clove

Sassafras, a drop or two

An excellent formula for men only. Very effective when used on a red female figure or candle.

India Bouquet Oil

¼ part Ginger

¼ part Cinnamon

¼ part Coriander

⅛ part Myrrh

⅛ part Cinnamon

Cardamom, a few drops

A blend designed to draw the opposite sex. Creates an atmosphere of attraction, brings harmony to quarreling couples, and ends the problem of marital infidelity. Use in love rituals to ensure tranquility.

India Bouquet Oil II

½ part Sandalwood

½ part Lotus

Cinnamon, about 5 drops

Vanilla, about 10 drops

An old-fashioned blend for fidelity.

Irresistible Oil

½ part Myrrh

¼ part Peppermint

¼ part Carnation

Makes the wearer irresistible!

Irresistible Oil II

⅓ part Rose
⅓ part Magnolia
⅓ part Lily of the Valley
Romeo Gigli, a few drops (optional)

This is to be worn as a perfume. If you can find the fragrance oil Romeo Gigli, wear it together with this oil when going out to make you totally irresistible.

Isis Oil

¼ part Myrrh
¼ part Lemon
⅛ part Frankincense
⅛ part Muguet
⅛ part Mimosa
⅛ part Lotus

To invoke or worship the goddess; increases passion or affection, sexually stimulating; a popular blend for married couples who need to recapture romance.

Isis Oil II

¼ part Hyacinth
¼ part Rose
½ part Myrrh
Camphor, a few drops
1 Myrrh nugget

Develops mild passion in the user. A sexually stimulating perfume. Popular with married couples who have lost the magic of the feeling of love. Guaranteed to bring on unexpected prowess and sexual pleasures.

Isis Oil III

⅓ part Narcissus
⅓ part Sandalwood
⅓ part Frankincense

To invoke the worship of the Goddess; increases passion or affection, sexually stimulating: a very popular blend for handfasted or married couples who need to recapture romance.

Jade's Lust Oil
⅓ part Jasmine
⅓ part Rain
⅓ part Musk
10 drops Rose
5 drops Ambergris
5 (or more) drops Opium fragrance oil

Very potent lust-invoking blend.

Jealousy Oil
⅓ part Cinnamon
⅓ part Galangal
⅓ part Bay

Makes you more exciting to those of the opposite sex, but will make those of the same sex quite intent on playing the "game" with you. Be prepared.

Jezebel Oil
⅓ part Ylang-Ylang
⅓ part Jasmine
⅓ part Rose
Rose Petals, in bottle
Red Jasper, in bottle

"Priestess of Baal," used by a woman to control a man. Can cause people to offer you things that you need.

Jezebel Oil II
⅓ part Frankincense
⅓ part Frangipani
⅓ part Heliotrope

A secret formula used by women who wish to have their way with any man, as it can cause males to do their bidding without question.

Jezebel Oil III (Do As I Say/Man Tamer)
½ part Palma Christi
¼ part Bergamot
¼ part Ginger Blossom
Dark Musk, a few drops

Another secret formula which, when used by women, can cause any male to do their bidding.

Joy Oil

⅓ part Grapefruit
⅓ part Mandarin Orange
⅓ part Tangerine
Lemongrass, a few drops

Stimulates sexual pursuits and increases the wearer's attractiveness; restores happiness to you when you're depressed.

Khus Khus Oil

¾ part Jasmine
¼ part Oleander

Add to bathwater and it will make you irresistible to the opposite sex. Also increase sales in business.

King of the Woods Oil

Saturn Root—in bottle
¼ part Civet
¼ part Musk
¼ part Vanilla
¼ part Cypress

Used by men, it is a sexual domination formula. Homosexual men seeking to attract other males should see Satyr Oil on page 63.

King of the Woods Oil II

½ part Vetiver
¼ part Musk
¼ part Sandalwood
Allspice, a few drops

An oil to attract lusty, eager women.

King's Perfume Oil

Frankincense

To be worn by men to improve lovemaking ability. Also helps the wearer to locate a better job. Will help a man get assistance from women—expect great change when using this oil. The Viagra of oils for men. And here you thought it would be this long and drawn-out recipe. Nope. Just true Frankincense Oil.

King's Perfume Oil II

¼ part Dark Musk
¼ part Frankincense
¼ part Orange
¼ part Allspice

A blend to attract love, luck, and wealth.

The Kiss Oil

White Musk
Ambergris, a few drops
1 drop Almond

Shy and alluring, great to anoint a pink candle with to attract that special person.
—Lady Rhea

Kore Oil

⅛ part Almond
¼ part Rose
⅛ part Lavender
¼ part Bay
¼ part Lemon

To invoke or worship the goddess of spring; or in romantic pursuits.

Kyphi Oil

Equal amounts of the following:
Frankincense
Myrrh
Orange
Lemon
Cinnamon
Rose

This name was probably derived from Kypris, the Cypriot goddess of love—and analogous to the Greek goddess of love, beauty, generation and fertility, Aphrodite. Use as a perfume—particularly at the nape of the neck and on the ear lobes—when you are interested in attracting a love partner.—Anna Riva

Lady of the Green Oil

⅓ part Vanilla

⅓ part Musk
⅓ part Sandalwood
Cedar, a few drops

To invoke or worship the goddess of spring; helps with the pursuit of fertility.

Lady of the Lake Oil

¼ part Lavender
¼ part Lilac
¼ part Earth
⅛ part Rose Geranium
⅛ part Carnation
Jasmine, 2–3 drops
Rosemary, 2–3 drops

Wear this oil to attune yourself with the love and strength of the Lady of the Lake and to reconnect with the goddess within.

La Flamme Oil

⅔ part Musk
⅓ part Ambergris
Bay, a few drops
Mimosa, a few drops

Will force a loved one to think of the wearer only and often; carries an enticing odor of promise. Use on talismans or candles. This blend is reported to fix you firmly in your lover's mind; it may be used to enhance a lover's sense of excitement toward the user or to bring home a lover that has strayed.

La Flamme Oil II

¼ part Musk
¼ part Ambergris
¼ part Rose
¼ part Opium fragrance oil

A great oil for love-drawing spells. Great for capturing a man who might be just a little unwilling.

Leather and Lace Oil

½ part Musk
¼ part Lilac

⅛ part Night Queen
⅛ part Amirage (optional)

Celebrate every facet of your fantasy sex life with this sensual oil. Use it when you need give a few new things a try in the bedroom.

L'Homme Oil

½ part Opium fragrance oil
¼ part Obsession fragrance oil
⅛ part Frankincense
⅛ part Wisteria

Best when worn as a cologne, it is a masculine blend for drawing a wife to you. Although it has well-known fragrance oils, the blend is very intoxicating.

Love and Protection Oil

¼ part Myrrh
¼ part Vetiver
¼ part Opium fragrance oil
¼ part Rose

For protecting the love that two people have. A wonderful handfasting gift.

Love Me Now Oil

¼ part Jasmine
¼ part Rose
¼ part Frangipani
¼ part Vetiver
Cinnamon, a few drops

A demanding and compelling oil for when love and lust cannot wait.

Love Oil

¼ part Sandalwood
¼ part Patchouli
¼ part Rose
¼ part Vetiver

Wear to draw love. Anoint pink candles and burn while visualizing the love that you desire.

Love Oil (Women)

½ part Rose

¼ part Jasmine
¼ part Palmarosa

Increases sexual magnetism and potency; very strong, men will be around you. Be safe!

Love Oil II

¼ part Rose
¼ part Apple Blossom
¼ part Gardenia
⅛ part Jasmine
⅛ part Ylang-Ylang

General-purpose oil for romantic pursuits.

Love Oil III

⅓ part Jasmine
⅓ part Musk
⅓ part Lemon Verbena

Used to make the one you love want to be near you. Apply to your "love centers."

Love Oil IV

½ part Rose
⅛ part Jasmine
⅛ part Violet
⅛ part Musk
⅛ part Lemon Verbena

Used to attract someone already taken by another.

Love Oil V

½ part Musk
½ part Frangipani

Brings luck in all love matters. Makes you more attractive to the opposite sex.

Love and Attraction Oil (Louisiana Style)

⅓ part Lemon

⅓ part Rose
⅓ part Vanilla
Almond, a few drops
Gold glitter or two gold stars

This oil will help you to attract a spiritual partner and soulmate.

Love and Success Oil

½ part Allspice
⅛ part Orris
⅛ part Cinnamon
⅛ part Bay
⅛ part White Sandalwood

Assists in locating happiness in marriage and great success in all things attempted. Use for anointing red and pink candles.

Love Me Perfume

⅓ part Vanilla
⅓ part Cinnamon
⅓ part Jasmine
Khus Khus, a few drops

Increases sexual magnetism and potency. Use sparingly, for it is extremely strong. May be used to anoint candles in love rituals; also makes a fine aromatic bath mixture.

Love Potion

½ part Vanilla
½ part Ginger
Sap from tree, just a little, to make things stick
Soil, enough to make a paste

Add ingredients together and mix. Spread on inside of arm from elbow to wrist. Chant details of your intentions. Step into the shower and rinse.

Love Shots Oil

⅓ part Musk
⅓ part Opium fragrance oil

⅓ part Carnation

Peach, a few drops

Apple Blossom, a few drops

To invoke Cupid's presence. Wear it to attract someone special.

Love Uncrossing Oil

½ part Vanilla

¼ part Carnation

¼ part Apple Blossom

Peach, a few drops

For removing the negativity people throw at your relationship.

Love's Messenger Oil

¼ part Rose

¼ part Cinnamon

¼ part Jasmine

¼ part Sandalwood

Vanilla, about 10 drops

To deliver a message of love straight to the heart of the one you desire, no matter how far or near they are.

Love's Whisper Oil

¼ part Frangipani

¼ part Jasmine

¼ part Honeysuckle

¼ part Wisteria

Clove, 2 to 3 drops

An oil of desire and love that is best used as a massage oil.

Lover's Oil

¼ part Musk

¼ part Civet

¼ part Ambergris
¼ part Patchouli
Bergamot, a few drops

Increases the wearer's personal magnetism and charisma.

Lover Come Back Oil
½ part Patchouli
¼ part Myrrh
¼ part Clove

This oil was created to bring back a wandering lover.

Lucky Spirit Oil
⅔ part Bitter Orange
⅓ part Citronella

A hex-breaker to place in all corners of the house and on the altar. Attracts helpful forces and can be used to reverse a curse.

Lust Oil
½ part Orange
¼ part Carnation
⅛ part Citronella
⅛ part Rose Geranium

Brings about passion in those you care about. Great for bringing some fire back to your current relationship.

Lust Oil II
½ part Cinnamon
½ part Clove

Because it may irritate the skin, it is best used in a diffuser. Creates a lust that cannot be satiated.

Lust and Seduction Oil
¼ part Musk
¼ part Civet

¼ part Ambergris
¼ part Patchouli or Cassia

This oil will assist you in seducing the object of your desires. He or she will continue to lust after you for days to come, so be careful!

Lust Potion Oil

Equal amounts of all:
    Patchouli
    Sandalwood
    Rose
    Clove
    Nutmeg
    Olive Oil

Wear as a perfume whenever you'll be in the presence of the person you're trying to attract. Be careful if you find others eyeing you as well. I find it's effective for getting a man's attention. Substitute Amber for the Rose in order to attract a woman.

Lust Promotion Oil

    ⅔ part Sandalwood
    ⅓ part Patchouli
    Cardamom, a few drops

Use this mixture to promote lustful desires. The corresponding color for this potion is red, so you may prefer to use a candle or dab a little on a towel of this color and have it lying around.

Luv Luv Luv Oil

    ½ part Rose
    ¼ part Angelica
    ⅛ part Clove
    ⅛ part Cucumber

A special blend of oils used to attract those already taken by someone else. Use of this oil makes him notice you. May also be used to attract women.

Luv Luv Luv Oil II

    ⅓ part Jasmine
    ⅓ part Ylang-Ylang

⅓ part Rain

Blended to attract someone who is out there alone and waiting for you.

Magic Massage Oil
¼ part Rose
¼ part Jasmine
¼ part Bergamot
¼ part Sandalwood
2 cups sweet almond carrier oil

Begin by massaging yourself until the aroma, warmed by your body, gets to him. Then start to massage him. Let him massage you next. Soon the magic mixture will have the two of you singing love's old, sweet song. *Note: It is not recommended that you substitute fragrance oils for this blend.*

Magic Carpet Oil
¼ part Violet
¼ part Lilac
¼ part Narcissus
¼ part Vanilla

Same as Lucky Lodestone Oil. Attracts all forms of luck and love. Draws forth wealth and success in all endeavors.

Magical Lust Oils
To attract a woman
½ part Ylang-Ylang
¼ part Cinnamon
¼ part Patchouli

To attract a man
⅓ part Sandalwood
⅓ part Ylang-Ylang
⅓ part Ginger
Patchouli, a few drops

Oils to bring about passion. Allows for a passionate and joyful love affair to manifest.

Magnetic Blade Oil
¼ part Musk
¼ part Patchouli
¼ part Ambergris

¼ part Civet
Cinnamon, a few drops

This blend was especially designed for use for love and attraction by gay men.

Maiden's Ruin Oil
⅓ part Patchouli
⅓ part Rose
⅓ part Amber
Southernwood, in bottle

Intoxicating and intriguing, this oil is to be worn by men who are looking to find romance and sexual liaisons.

Male Attraction Oil
¼ part Musk
¼ part Ambergris
¼ part Amber
¼ part Sandalwood

A love oil for men to attract a permanent mate.

Marriage Mind Oil
¼ part Neroli
¼ part Carnation
¼ part Lily of the Valley
¼ part Rose
Orris, 10 drops
Chamomile, 9 drops

To bring about a proposal and the proper response.

Marriage Oil
¼ part Rose
¼ part Pine
¼ part Myrrh

¼ part Muguet

Based on a traditional blend, this scent was intended to help an unsure suitor gain confidence to propose. It can also be use to scent a home to keep a marriage peaceful and happy.

Master of the Woods Oil

¾ part Sandalwood
¼ part Dark Musk
Civet, a few drops

To help invoke the female object of your desire. This is a compelling oil designed for men.

Melusine Oil

Equal amounts of each of the following:

Lily of the Valley
Lotus
Opium
Rose
Rain
Night Queen

Melusine is a Minoan goddess and a sea witch who answers prayers for love. Use her oil to make a love call to the one you want.

Midnight Blue Oil

⅓ part Rose
⅓ part Opium fragrance oil
⅓ part Musk
Ambergris, a few drops
Carnation, a few drops
1 drop real honey

Promotes sexual arousal between men and women.

Midnight Passion Oil

½ part Ginger
¼ part Patchouli
⅛ part Cardamom
⅛ part Sandalwood

For those late-night escapades. Place in diffuser in the bedroom and let your passions run wild.

Mystere Oil

½ part Musk
¼ part Narcissus
⅛ part Jasmine
⅛ part Rose

To invoke the mysterious aspect of the Goddess Erzulie and imbue you with the secrets of love.

Mysterious Oil

¾ part Patchouli
¼ part Jasmine

Haunting, enchanting, and intoxicating. Try this oil in a diffuser.

Nefertiti Oil

¼ part Myrrh
½ part Lotus
⅛ part Gardenia
⅛ part Lemon
Muguet, a few drops

For the pursuit of sexual love.

New Orleans Desire Oil

½ part Magnolia
¼ part Carnation
⅛ part Rose
⅛ part Orange
Civet, a few drops
Vanilla, a few drops

Based on a blend originally used by ladies of the night in nineteenth-century New Orleans, this blend is designed for sexual attraction.

Night Haunt Oil

½ part Vanilla
½ part Gardenia
1 Rosebud (crushed up if it will not fit in the bottle whole)

An attraction and compelling oil for those types that haunt the night.

No. 20 Love Oil
¼ part Almond fragrance oil (not base oil)
¼ part Rose
¼ part Lavender
¼ part Bay
Lemon, a few drops

A special oil formula from New Orleans. A favorite among prostitutes.

Nymph Oil
¼ part Ambergris
¼ part Gardenia
¼ part Jasmine
¼ part Tuberose (or Rose)
Violet, a few drops

Mix and wear on yourself. For women only. To attract men.

Nymph Oil II
¾ part Lilac
¼ part Lavender
Civet, a few drops

An extremely powerful drawing oil that attracts men, and may be worn by either sex. A personal favorite of mine just to wear on an everyday basis. Be easy on using the Civet Oil, or you could end up smelling like a male cat.

Nymph and Satyr Oil
½ part Rose
⅛ part Anise
⅛ part Violet
¼ part Jasmine
⅛ part Ylang-Ylang
⅛ part Narcissus

Brings youthfulness and playfulness back into relationships.

Oscar Wilde Oil
½ part Sandalwood
¼ part Hyacinth
⅛ part Musk

⅛ part Opium

This oil is all about being free to be who you are and love as you will. Wear it when you go to Gay Pride events, or when you are out on the town and looking for a little adventure.

Pan Oil

¼ part Juniper
½ part Patchouli
¼ part Vervain
Cedar, a few drops
Pine, a few drops

Use to aid you in love spells and seduction of women.

Passion Oil

¾ part Patchouli
¼ part Ylang-Ylang

Exotic blend to arouse passion.

Passion Oil II

¼ part Gardenia
¼ part Neroli
¼ part Apple Blossom
¼ part Ambergris

To help you bring passion back to your relationship.

Pleasure Me Oil

½ part Musk
⅛ part Opium fragrance oil
$\frac{1}{16}$ part Patchouli
$\frac{1}{16}$ part Narcissus
$\frac{1}{16}$ part Lotus

Designed to promote pleasure—both the giving and receiving of it.

Polynesian Love Oil

½ part Gardenia
¼ part Jasmine
¼ part Rose
Musk, about 10 drops

Similar to Come-to-Me Oil. Used for enticement.

"Q" Perfume Oil

¾ part Myrrh

⅛ part Peppermint

⅛ part Carnation

A highly stimulating oil used to entice anyone you deeply desire. Impossible to resist.

"Q" Perfume Oil II

½ part Musk

¼ part Wisteria

¼ part Ambergris

Designed for bisexual couples, this oil is meant to entice.

Queen Oil

½ part Honeysuckle

¼ part Jasmine

⅛ part Vanilla

⅛ part Ylang-Ylang

For women only. This procurer of passion attracts both love and success. Use with care.

Queen Bee Oil

Same as Queen Oil.

Queen of Tibet Oil

⅓ part Musk

⅓ part Lotus

⅓ part Sandalwood

Jasmine, a few drops

Exotic, tantalizing, a producer of passions; this is a special and powerful blend used by those who want, need, and expect the most from everything life has to offer!

Rafael's Love Oil

3 ounces sunflower base oil

⅓ part Sweet Pea

⅓ part Lavender

⅓ part Musk "3" blend (a blend of equal parts: Green Musk, Amber Musk, Dark Musk fragrance oils)

This oil arouses passion in your lover and is useful as massage oil. If you cannot find all three musk oils, substitute Egyptian Musk.

Sappho Oil

⅓ part Jasmine
⅓ part Rose
⅓ part Opium
Hibiscus (or Angel perfume oil), a few drops

This oil is for women looking for a special same-sex love.

Satyr Oil

¼ part Musk
⅛ part Patchouli
⅛ part Civet
⅛ part Ambergris
⅛ part Cinnamon
⅛ part Allspice
⅛ part Carnation

Said to incite the passions of anyone who comes near you; use with extreme caution. Anoint candles in any love ritual; may also be used as a bath or powder. Place oil at the heart and throat, and behind the ears.

Scarlet's Seduction Oil

¼ part Musk
¼ part Opium fragrance oil
¼ part Magnolia
¼ part Vetiver

A compelling and intense love-drawing potion.

Self-Love Oil

¼ part Tuberose
¼ part White Rose
¼ part Geranium
¼ part Rose
Palmarosa, a few drops

Prepare and empower the oil before a self-love ritual. Also use to enhance self-esteem.

Sensual Oil

¼ part Jasmine

¼ part Rose

¼ part Sandalwood

¼ part Ylang-Ylang

Use to arouse passion in a lover. Nice to use in a diffuser.

Sensual Satyr Oil

¼ part Carnation

¼ part Musk

¼ part Patchouli

¼ part Vanilla

Cinnamon, 2 to 3 drops

Use to aid in love spells and lust spells.

Sexual Chakra Oil

¼ part Ylang-Ylang

¼ part Jasmine

¼ part Sandalwood

¼ part Tangerine

Add jasmine blossoms to fill bottle

An oil to increase sexual stamina and desire. Incites passions; use to dress candles or in the bath.

Sexual Energy Oil

¼ part Ginger

¼ part Patchouli

¼ part Cardamom

¼ part Sandalwood

For couples, to enhance their experience together and bring them closer.

Siren Song Oil

¼ part Lotus

¼ part China Musk

¼ part Rose

¼ part Honeysuckle

1 small sea shell crushed in the bottle, if desired

Wear to bewitch the one you desire.

Special Favors Oil
⅓ part Coconut
⅓ part Vanilla
⅓ part Almond fragrance oil (not carrier oil)

This blend will help you call in those *really* special favors—should you ever need them.

Spellbound Oil
⅓ part Lilac
⅓ part Vanilla
⅓ part Musk

This oil will captivate someone to the point of dreaming of and desiring only you.

Soul Mate Oil
¼ part Jasmine
¼ part Musk
¼ part Patchouli
¼ part Sandalwood
Ambergris, a few drops

To aid the wearer in attracting the *right* person, but not necessarily the person they had in mind.

Spicy Love-Drawing Oil
¼ part Rose Geranium
¼ part Lavender
¼ part Rosemary
⅛ part Chamomile
⅛ part Cinnamon

Wear to attract love.

Sweet Pea Bouquet
¼ part Neroli
¼ part Ylang-Ylang
¼ part Jasmine

¼ part Benzoin

Diluted with base oil, Sweet Pea Bouquet is worn to attract new friends and to draw love. (Note that generally pure Sweet Pea Oil is not available.)

Tabu Oil

¼ part Patchouli
¼ part Oak Moss
¼ part Bergamot
¼ part Ylang-Ylang
Musk, a few drops
Neroli, a few drops

For pursuits of romantic love, especially long term. This blend is created after the commercial fragrance of the same name.

Tantra Oil

⅛ part Lavender
⅛ part Rose
¼ part Sandalwood
¼ part Frankincense
¼ part Amber

A blend designed to increase sexual stamina and desire.

Taper Perfume

⅓ part Jasmine
⅓ part Cinnamon
⅓ part Patchouli
Olive Oil

Used to float wicks. Usually no more than perfumed Olive Oil, it's more for decoration than for ritual purposes, but the oils tend to attract love, healing, and positive forces.

Think of Me Oil

⅓ part Rose
⅓ part Musk
⅓ part Opium fragrance oil
10 drops Narcissus

10 drops Lotus

Makes someone think of you obsessively; it can drive them wild!

To Attract Love Oil

¾ part Palmarosa

⅛ part Rose

⅛ part Cardamom

For drawing to you what you most desire.

To Attract Love Oil II

¾ part Patchouli

¼ part Cinnamon

2 ounces carrier oil (look at the section on carrier oils to choose the best one for your intentions)

Same as above.

To Attract Love Oil III

½ part Sandalwood

¼ part Patchouli

⅛ part Rose

⅛ part Vetiver

An oil blend to attract a male life partner.

To Attract Men Oil

½ part Sandalwood

¼ part Ylang-Ylang

¼ part Ginger

2 drops Patchouli

2 ounces carrier oil (look at the section on carrier oils to find the best one for your intentions)

An oil blend to attract a male life mate.

To Attract Women Oil

⅓ part Sandalwood

⅓ part Cinnamon

⅓ part Patchouli

This blend is used to attract a female life mate.

Tramp Oil

¾ part Night Queen
⅛ part Rain
⅛ part Opium

This oil will make your partner crave nothing but you. You will be amazed at the results! Remember that intention is everything when you create your oil.

True Love Oil

½ part Lily of the Valley
¼ part Rose
¼ part Patchouli
Cinnamon, a few drops

Used as a personal oil to attract and bind lasting love.

Tryst Perfume

⅓ part Rose
⅓ part Honeysuckle
⅓ part Vanilla

The oil of lovers, use this blend when you want passion to enter the relationship; this will help. Also develops clairvoyant power in anyone who uses it. This blend also helps to conjure the love of your dreams.

Tuberose Bouquet

⅓ part Ylang-Ylang
⅓ part Rose
⅓ part Jasmine
Neroli (just a hint)

True Tuberose Oil is rarely available. This bouquet is a wonderful relaxer and so is used in peace blends. The scent also induces love.

Vini Vin Oil

⅓ part Jasmine
⅓ part Honeysuckle
⅓ part Carnation
Cinnamon, a few drops

The Latin version of Come-to-Me Oil.

Voudoun Night Perfume Oil
½ part Myrrh
¼ part Patchouli
¼ part Vetiver
Lime, a few drops
Vanilla, a few drops

This oil is designed to draw others to you and makes them unable to resist your temptations.

Voudoun Nights Oil
¼ part Jasmine
¼ part Honeysuckle
¼ part Vanilla
¼ part Wisteria

This oil is reminiscent of a night of mystery and magic. When preparing this oil, have the intent of lust in your mind … one of my favorite standbys.

Willow World Oil
⅓ part Rose
⅓ part Musk
⅓ part Lotus
Neroli, a few drops

Use this oil for a night of passionate, intense, romantic love. Be careful what you ask for!

Witch Love Oil
½ part Light Musk
¼ part Honeysuckle
⅛ part Gardenia
⅛ Wisteria

Brings out that magic moment just when you need it. Bewitch someone you desire when you need a little miracle.

Witches Obsession Oil
½ part Musk
⅛ part Cassia
⅛ part Myrrh
¼ part Sandalwood

Use to aid in love spells for women. When mixing these oils, focus on confidence, success, romance, and your heart feeling full.

Wolf Heart Oil

⅓ part Lilac
⅓ part Narcissus
⅓ part Rose
Frankincense, a few drops

If you are looking to settle down and find a more serious relationship. This oil will give you the courage to enact that choice.

Youth Dew Oil

¼ part Frankincense
¼ part Patchouli
⅛ part Vetiver
¼ part Musk
⅛ part Clove

This oil is designed after the commercial fragrance of the same name. Gives people the illusion that you are younger than you are.

Emotional & Physical Healing

Some of the oils listed here helped me through my own challenging life transitions and to bring about necessary changes. Now, I am extremely happy to be able to share with you their immense benefits and incredible powers.

There are a number of ways you can use your oils in a ritual setting. They are often rubbed on candles for use in spellwork—this blends the powerful energies of the oil with the magical symbolism of the candle's color and the energy of the flame itself.

Sometimes, oils are used to anoint the body. If you are blending an oil to use for this purpose, be sure that you're not including any ingredients that are irritating to the skin. Some essential and fragrance oils, such as frankincense and clove, will cause a reaction in sensitive skin and should only be used very sparingly. Oils applied to the body bring the wearer the energies of the oil—an Energy Oil will give you a much-needed boost; a Courage Oil will give you strength in the face of adversity. Finally, crystals, amulets, talismans, and other charms may be anointed with the magical oil of your choice. This is a great way to turn a simple mundane item into an item of magical power and energy.

For Optimum Results

Visualize daily your desired outcome while using a few drops of the oils, until your ambitions are achieved. Feel free to use your intuition regarding using more than one oil at a time. Sometimes this can even strengthen the effects of each oil. The rule of thumb would be: don't use stimulating and pacifying oils together, such as Study and Sleep, as they would cancel each other out. Trust your instincts, don't be afraid try combinations, and you'll find—you just "know."

Acceptance Oil

½ part Geranium
¼ part Blue Tansy
⅛ part Frankincense
⅛ part Sandalwood
Neroli, a few drops
Rosewood, a few drops

Used to help one through difficult times. Helps calm the mind so you can focus on a solution or get closure on a situation.

Accepting One's Identity Oil

⅓ part Sandalwood
⅓ part Frankincense
⅓ part Jasmine

This blend is effective for people who shut down their communication by isolating themselves in their own world. It will help them better express their desires and emotions.

Aesculapius Oil

¼ part Rose
¼ part Carnation
¼ part Citron
¼ part Gardenia

To invoke or worship the god of the medical arts; for healing work.

Aiding Communication Oil

⅓ part Sage
⅓ part Lavender
⅓ part Chamomile

Overcomes shyness and eases communication.

Amethyst Oil for Clear Thinking

Immerse an amethyst crystal in about 2–3 tablespoons of Olive Oil.

Set in the Sun for about 2–3 days. Remove amethyst from the oil and pour oil into a bottle with tight-fitting lid.

Whenever you need a fast spurt of clear and logical thinking, place a dot of the oil on each of your temples.

Angel Brilliance Oil

¾ part Bergamot
¼ part Neroli
Rose, a few drops
Cinnamon, a few drops

To assist you in calling upon the angelic realm to bring you vigor and strength during difficult times.

Anger Be Gone Oil

½ Chamomile
¼ Violet
¼ Sandalwood

For soothing angry tempers. If you've had a fight with someone and wish to reconcile, this blend can certainly help.

Anger Oil (Do Not Wear)

¼ part Chili Powder
¼ part Black Pepper
¼ part Sulfur
¼ part Asafetida
2 ounces carrier oil (see section of carrier oils to see which would be best for your intentions)

Sprinkle around the room to overcome feelings of irritation. Averts fights which may occur in the future and helps to cleanse the mind of evil thoughts. Keep away from furniture and material that might stain. I place in all four corners of the room.

Anti-Depressant Oil

½ part Bergamot
¼ part Petitgrain
¼ part Rose Geranium
Neroli, a drop or two

Helps with menopause, PMS, and times that may be trying and causing strife.

Asclepius Healing Oil

½ part Rose
¼ part Hyssop
1⁄16 part Juniper
1⁄16 part Anise

To bring about the healing energies of Asclepius, the mortal healer who became a god. If you can, add some of these dry herbs to the bottle: Hyssop, Juniper, and Anise.

Autumn Leaves Oil

¼ part Sandalwood
⅛ part Pine
⅛ part Nutmeg
¼ part Musk
¼ part Cinnamon
Allspice, a few drops

Use this calming and quieting oil to soothe ruffled feelings and tensions.

Balsamo Tranquilo Oil

⅓ part Sandalwood
⅓ part Violet
⅓ part Cucumber

The name means "tranquil balm" or "quieting and calming oil." This blend can settle a straying mate or quiet the ghosts of your house. It stops all beings in their tracks but calmly, like a giant tranquilizer.

Blessing Oil

½ part Jasmine
½ part Juniper
Jasmine Blossoms in master bottle

Great for keeping on your personal altar for magical workings.

Blessing Oil II

1 to 4 lavender blossoms
⅓ Sage
⅓ Basil
⅓ Patchouli
Carrier oil can be Olive Oil (used for protection) or almond, sunflower, etc.

Use a small dark vial. Place all but the oil together in the vial, then add enough oil to fill the bottle. Shake thoroughly. Use for anointing ritual candles, self, consecrating tools, etc.

Lavender is used for purification, happiness, love, and peace. Basil brings protection and love. Sage brings purification, protection, healing, wealth, longevity. Patchouli brings prosperity, wards off evil and negativity, and aids divination. All of these are desirable generic attributes, so this recipe is a good general-purpose blend.

Blessing Oil III
½ part Lily
¼ part Rose
¼ part Narcissus

If used on the body, it is believed to purify the soul. The most popular use is to anoint altars, candles, implements, incense burners, or any ritual tools.

Bliss Oil
¼ part Lavender
¼ part Geranium
¼ part Neroli
¼ part Clary Sage

Helps with hyperventilation, calms, relaxes, and is euphoric.

Buddha Oil
½ part Sandalwood
¼ part Orris
⅛ part Mastic
⅛ part Cinnamon

To invoke or worship the Buddha and stimulate latent mystical powers.

Calming Oil
¼ part Lavender
¼ part Geranium
¼ part Mandarin Orange
¼ part Cypress

Use for relaxing and calming after a hard day at work or with difficult people.

Clearance Oil

⅓ part Carnation
⅓ part Lilac
⅓ part Vanilla

An oil for overcoming unseen obstacles.

Clear Thoughts Oil

⅛ part Cajeput
⅛ part Lemon
¼ part Lavender
½ part Siberian Fir

This is not only useful for study but also for whenever you want to drive out negativity and get on with life.

Concentration Oil

⅓ part Mastic
⅓ part Cinnamon
⅓ part Myrrh

Anoint forehead with small amount to aid in solving a problem. Clears the mind, inspires sudden insights into problems.

Cosmic Beauty Oil

¼ part Tea Rose
½ part Orange
¼ part Lavender
Rose Geranium, a few drops

Assists in bringing about a healthy glow and balancing the aura. Pour a few drops into the palm of your hands and inhale deeply. May be used in the bath as well.

Courage Oil

½ part Ginger
¼ part Black Pepper
¼ part Clove

Wear to increase your courage, especially before being introduced to people, prior to public speaking, and other nerve-racking situations.

Courage Oil II
Mix equal parts:
>   Rosemary
>   Five-Finger grass
>   Gardenia petals

Add 2 tablespoons of the above mixture to 2 ounces of oil. Add a small piece of High John the Conqueror Root to each bottle of oil made.

Add 9 drops of this oil to the bathwater when applying for a job or asking the boss for a raise. When used as perfume, anoint the throat, below the heart, and above the navel to replace fears and timidity.

Crucible of Courage Oil
>   ⅛ part Vanilla
>   ¾ part Carnation
>   ⅛ part Violet

Gives great amounts of courage to those who are fearful or timid. Use to anoint purple candles, and wear the oil when confronting frightening or dangerous situations.

Dove's Blood Oil
>   ¾ part Dragon's Blood
>   ⅛ part Rose
>   ⅛ part Bay

A special blend of incense designed to bring peace of mind and happiness.

Dove's Heart Oil
>   ½ part Lavender
>   ¼ part Rose
>   ¼ part Wisteria
>   Lilac, a few drops

Soothes ruffled feelings and calms restless spirits; aids in any workings of the heart.

Dove's Heart Oil II
>   ½ part Honeysuckle
>   ½ part Vanilla
>   1 drop Peach

Settles quarrels and softens a hard heart.

Dragon's Mist Oil

1 sprig of Scotch Broom
1 piece Irish Moss
2 pinches Vervain
¼ teaspoon Sea Salt
1 part Heather
1 part Oak Moss
3 part Witch Hazel
1 part Pine

Warm all ingredients in an enamel pan on low heat.

Allow to cool and place in a pretty clear bottle. Brings peace, protection, and calm to the wearer.

Easy Life Oil

¼ part Cloves
¼ part Ginger
¼ part Lemon
¼ part Cassia
Orange, a few drops

Will help the wearer relax while others take care of business for him or her. Helps you dominate the thoughts of others, so they they'll help you without complaint.

Easy Life Oil II

⅓ part Coconut fragrance oil
⅓ part Sandalwood
⅓ part Opium fragrance oil

Apply with gentle strokes on the shoulders, neckline, and arms to attract the good life with health, blessings, abundance, great fortune, happiness, and a comfortable old age.

Elf Fire Oil

⅛ part Lavender
⅛ part Cardamom
⅛ part Cinnamon
⅛ part Musk
¼ part Frankincense
¼ part Strawberry

Brings happiness by whatever means is most needed by the user. This oil has a very strange quality: when used in attainment of goals, it brings what you need, instead of what you want. Improves the standard of living.

Enchanted Spiritual Oil

¼ part Frankincense

¼ part Myrrh

¼ part Heliotrope

¼ part Cinnamon

This oil is for protection from all harm. Use this as an anointing oil to protect you from the harmful thoughts of others and to remove all negative magic that is trying to cling to you.

Erzulie Femme Blanche Oil

½ part Gardenia

¼ part Magnolia

¼ part Lily of the Valley

For clearing up difficulties in your life.

Erzulie Love Oil

¼ part Gardenia

¼ part Jasmine

⅛ part Vetiver

⅛ part Strawberry

⅛ part Neroli

⅛ part Rose

To help you in all matters of the heart.

Forgiveness Oil

Equal amounts of each:

Frankincense	Rosewood
Sandalwood	Geranium
Lavender	Lemon
Melissa	Palmarosa
Angelica	Ylang-Ylang
Helichrysum`	Bergamot
Rose	Roman Chamomile Jasmine

To help with forgiving, forgetting, and letting go.

Forgiveness Oil II

½ part Frangipani
½ part Ylang-Ylang
Sweet Pea or Lily of the Valley, a few drops

To heal quarrels between lovers and friends.

Friendly Nature Spirit Oil

⅓ part Lime
⅓ part Carnation
⅓ part Gardenia
Wintergreen, just a drop or two

To invoke and work with plant devas.

Garden Delight Perfume

⅔ part Grapefruit
⅓ part Lavender
A few drops Vanilla

A walk through springtime to help you with fresh starts in any area of your life.

Get Away Oil

1 part Red Pepper
1 part Black Pepper
1 part Patchouli leaves
1 part Ginger (powdered)
1 root of High John the Conqueror
½ cup base oil (see carrier oils section to find appropriate oil for your intentions)

Helps to be protected against all the night phantoms and nightmares you may run across. Anoint a white candle and burn for fifteen minutes before retiring. Also anoint windowsills and doorknobs. May anoint a cotton ball and place under the bed if desired; also anoint dream catchers. *Do not wear.*

Glow of Health Oil

¼ part Orange
¼ part Peach
¼ part Lavender
¼ part Carnation

This oil is for healing and prevention of illness, especially during the change of seasons and trying, emotional times.

Golden Tara Oil
¼ part Carnation
¼ part Peach
¼ part Gardenia
¼ part Frangipani

The Buddhist Tara's name literally means "she who saves." The Buddhist Tara has twenty-one aspects, all of them revolving around compassion. Use this blend when petitioning for her golden offers, rare chances to get ahead.

Green Tara Oil
¼ part Sandalwood
¼ part Jasmine
¼ part Peach
¼ part Lotus

For all sorrowful situations, especially when the proverbial wolves are closing in and you feel hopeless.

Grief Relief Oil
¼ part Lavender
¼ part Chamomile
¼ part Rose
¼ part Ylang-Ylang

Helps in situations of loss and recovery.

Guardian Oil
½ part Lemon
⅛ part Clove
⅛ part Rosewood
⅛ part Patchouli
⅛ part Pennyroyal

Used for protection. Increases the strength of the aura to help against psychic attack.

Happiness Oil
½ part Basil
¼ part Orange
⅛ part Patchouli
⅛ part Rose
Rosemary, a few drops

Sprinkle liberally around the room or use in a diffuser to change luck and reverse ill fortune. It also helps eliminate poverty.

Happy Heart Oil
2 ounces Sweet Almond carrier oil
2 tablespoons Wisteria flowers

Cover flowers with oil and let sit in a dark place for two weeks. Shake daily. Strain the liquid, then bottle. Anoint to attract happiness and good vibrations.

Healing Oil
¾ part Rosemary
¼ part Juniper
Sandalwood, a few drops

Wear to speed healing.

Healing Oil II
½ part Eucalyptus
¼ part Neroli
⅛ part Palmarosa
⅛ part Spearmint

Increases health and endurance, and assists in amplifying life force.

Healing Oil III
½ part Sandalwood
¼ part Carnation
¼ part Violet

Promotes healing of mind, body, and spirit.

Healing Oil IV

⅓ part Rose
⅓ part Carnation
⅓ part Frankincense
Add a few pieces of the Life Everlasting herb to the bottle, if available

Said to be vitalizing when used by convalescents. Dispels fatigue and tiredness in all wearers.

Health Attracting Oil

Use 2 drops in 2 ounces of oil of any of the following scents:
Rose
Carnation
Gardenia
Grated Lemon Peel or Lemon Flowers

This oil is usually anointed on the forehead of the ill.

Health Oil

½ part Rose
¼ part Carnation
⅛ part Citron
⅛ part Gardenia

Use to anoint candles, talismans, or anything pertinent to healing rituals.

Heart Chakra Oil—luxurious!

¼ part Bergamot
¼ part Lavender
⅛ part Melissa
⅛ part Neroli
¼ part Ylang-Ylang
Rose, a few drops

Forgiveness, compassion, and love abound. Use this blend for quiet contemplation, prayer, and forgiveness work. You won't be sorry when you treat yourself to a blend like this. Use it sparingly. Keep it undiluted and just enjoy the aroma, or blend it with 1 ounce Jojoba Oil in a dark glass bottle.

Heart Healing Oil

⅓ part Jasmine

⅓ part Ylang-Ylang
⅓ part Dragon's Blood

Opens a heart closed by pain and/or stress to accept new beneficial associations and opportunities.

Heart Song Oil
⅓ part Orange
⅓ part Vanilla
⅓ part Frankincense
Ambergris Bouquet, a few drops

To bring about childlike feelings of joy, or that feeling when you first fall in love. Great in diffuser to brighten a room.

Helping Hand Oil
½ part Vanilla
½ part Lily of the Valley
Cinnamon, a few drops
Almond fragrance oil, a few drops

Brings harmony to a stormy marriage.

Hygeia Oil
½ part Carnation
¼ part Cucumber
¼ part Rose
Jasmine, a few drops

A blend designed to help women with any chronic problems they may have with uterine area. This includes lower back pain, and emotional stress and discomfort.

Inner Child Oil (victims of abuse, emotional balance)
Equal parts of each:
Orange
Tangerine
Jasmine
Ylang-Ylang
Spruce
Sandalwood
Lemongrass

Neroli

This oil can help to bring out, focus, and amplify your best qualities so healing can take place. Use in a diffuser.

Inner Peace Oil
½ part Rose
¼ part Gardenia
¼ part Magnolia

To help calm the mind and become more relaxed; also assists in helping you with acquiring inner strength and courage.

Innocence Oil
¾ part Rose
¼ part Vanilla

Opens a heart closed by pain and/or stress to accept new beneficial associations and opportunities.

Joy Oil
⅓ part Jasmine
⅓ part Neroli
⅓ part Gardenia
Vanilla, a few drops
Sandalwood, a few drops

This essence brings out the best in the wearer: talents are increased, thoughts become more optimistic, and the body attracts pleasure. If you are depressed and lonely, this can change your whole attitude, and hence your entire life.

Kindly Spirit Oil
½ part Lily of the Valley
½ part Hyacinth
Lemon, a few drops

Will cause others to like you and be sympathetic toward you under all circumstances. Use in a ritual to aid in overcoming loneliness, or when you need a sympathetic ear.

Kindly Spirit Oil II
⅓ part Frangipani

⅓ part Carnation
⅓ part Musk
Clove or Allspice, a few drops (optional)

To summon an unearthly being to your side for aid in accomplishing your tasks. Write your requirement on paper and place the petition beneath a pink candle that you have anointed with this oil.

Knowledge Oil

Sandalwood
Clove, a few drops
Add a few grains of Frankincense to each bottle

To be able to understand and put to use all that is heard or read, apply a drop to the temples and back of the neck each morning after your bath or shower.

Kwan Yin Oil

½ part Lemon
½ part Rose
Lilac, a few drops

Used to worship or invoke the ancient Chinese goddess of compassion.

Lakshmi Oil

½ part Sandalwood
¼ part Lotus
⅛ part Jasmine
⅛ part Gardenia

Lakshmi is an Indian goddess who can instantly resolve all troubles in life. Wear this oil as a perfume to attract Lakshmi, and to honor her presence in your life.

Laughter of the Muses Oil

½ part Rose
½ part Wisteria
Lavender, a few drops
Freesia, a few drops

This blend will chase away the blues, leaving you happy and refreshed.

Liban's Touch Oil

⅛ part Lime
⅛ part Rose

¼ part Sandalwood

¼ part Dragon's Blood

⅛ part Rose Geranium

⅛ part Lavender

Liban is a Celtic goddess of healing and also a mermaid. Use this recipe to speed recovery from illness, especially colds and flu.

Lotus Bouquet

¼ part Rose

¼ part Jasmine

¼ part White or Light Musk

¼ part Ylang-Ylang

Mix until the scent is heavy, floral, and warm. Can use this when a Lotus oil is called for in a recipe.

Love Healing Oil

½ part White Musk

¼ part Gardenia

⅛ part Magnolia or Camellia

⅛ part Carnation

Cinnamon, a few drops

Helps heal conflicts and arguments; helps promote communication.

Memory Drops Oil

¼ part Rosemary

¼ part Vanilla

¼ part Cinnamon

¼ part Clove

Honey, a few drops

Improves mental processes. Great for students and people working with a large population. Can assist you in remembering names, numbers, and locations.

Memory Oil

¼ part Clove

¼ part Coriander

¼ part Rosemary
¼ part Sage

To increase focus, clarity, and retention.

Mystic Wand Oil

½ part Heliotrope
½ part Violet
Sandalwood, a few drops

This oil helps you to draw extra energy and life force.

New-Mown Hay Bouquet

½ part Woodruff
¼ part Tonka
⅛ part Lavender
⅛ part Bergamot
Oak Moss, a few drops

Add a few drops of the bouquet to transformative oils, especially those designed to break negative habits and addictions. Also, anoint the body in the spring with this bouquet (diluted, of course) to welcome the turning of the seasons.

Night Queen Oil

½ part Sandalwood
¼ part Rose
¼ part Jasmine

For peace and tranquility.

Obeah Perfume Oil

¼ part Myrrh
¼ part Patchouli
¼ part Galangal
¼ part Jasmine
Lemon, a few drops

Used to bless an area—a prayer room, Circle, or temple, for example. Protect against evil in all forms when used on a white candle, or in the bath. Banishes bad vibrations, and helps the wearer to gain support for magical agents.

Orange Mist Lace Oil

½ part Bergamot
¼ part Orange

⅛ part Neroli
⅛ part Cinnamon

Light and ethereal, this oil causes a higher vibration of energy in yourself or your environment.

Peace and Protection Oil

¼ part Lavender
¼ part Rosemary
¼ part Basil
¼ part Carnation
Mint, a few drops

This strong blend will release all of the negative energies that others have been sending out to you.

Peace Oil

⅓ part Ylang-Ylang
⅓ part Lavender
⅓ part Chamomile
Rose, a few drops

Wear when nervous or upset to calm you down. Stand before a mirror, and while looking in your eyes, anoint your body.

Peace Oil II

⅓ part Violet
⅓ part Lavender
⅓ part Vanilla

Apply to your person or sprinkle about the house to bring quiet and tranquility into your life.

Peace, Protection, Blessings Oil

⅓ part Heather
⅓ part Lemon
⅓ part Peppermint

A extremely potent blend for house cleansings, and any other area that might need peace and quiet.

Performing Arts Success Oil

¼ part Magnolia

¼ part High John
¼ part Vanilla
⅛ part Ylang-Ylang
⅛ part Sage

Float some pieces of John the Conqueror root in master bottle. Helps the musician's instrument be in tune. Assists the artist to have the best attributes to perform.

Persephone Oil
¼ part Wisteria
¼ part Jasmine
¼ part Amirage fragrance oil
(Substitute Lilac if you cannot find Amirage)
¼ part Vetiver

Used to invoke or worship the goddess; aids in creativity. Activates the "maiden" aspect of the lunar goddess.

Phoenix Oil
⅓ part Lemon
⅓ part Lavender
⅓ part Bay

For healing from emotional or physical trauma.

Purification Oil
¾ part Eucalyptus
¼ part Camphor
Lemon, a few drops

Add to bathwater to be rid of negativity or illness. With this blend, make sure you don't stay in the bath for more than twenty minutes. This works in a way similar to vapor rub—in the tub!

Purifying Oil
½ part Juniper
½ part Pine
Geranium, a few drops

This oil helps to clear out the negative energy brought on by disease or injury.

Rainbow Oil
⅓ part Lilac

⅓ part Rain
⅓ part Carnation
Peach 2 to 3 drops

This oil is for joy, resurrection, and healing. It can give wealth and success, recognition for a job well done, and sparkle to your life when it has been too dreary.

Return to Me Oil

¼ part Rose
¾ part Magnolia
Lotus, a few drops

For pursuits of romantic love, especially long-term—but be careful what you ask for! This oil is very effective at bringing back someone who has gone from you.

Rhiannon Oil

¼ part Carnation
¼ part Frankincense
½ part Jasmine
Rose, a couple of drops
Strip of Willow (optional)

For working with or invoking the Goddess. Rub this oil on your pulse points and chakras to relax your mind and alleviate anxiety.

Sacred Heart Oil

¾ part Rose
⅛ part Lemon
⅛ part Heliotrope

This oil can be used for healing, uncrossing, and spiritual cleansing and blessings.

Sacred Love Oil

¾ part Rain
¼ part Amirage (substitute Lilac if you need to)
Violet, a few drops

Wear this oil and find sacred love for yourself.

Sacred Wood Oil

½ part Juniper

½ part Bergamot
Lemon, a few drops

To draw friendship, good feelings, and fellowship.

San Cypriano Oil

⅓ part Gardenia
⅓ part Ambergris
⅓ part Musk
1 to 2 drops of Civet

To bring reconciliation with a lover, or anyone with whom you are having problems.

Snake Oil

Snake Root extract
Galangal Root

Combine extract with root and let sit in a dark place for two weeks. Shake daily. Used to anoint candles. Protects and lends healing energy to the healer.

Soothing Waters Oil

⅓ part Sandalwood
⅓ part Chamomile
⅓ part Clary Sage
Lilac, a few drops

This oil is intended to be a calming agent. Wear or place a drop on fabric, a cotton ball, etc., and sniff when needed, but don't overdo it.

Sprite Music Oil

⅓ part Rose or Carnation
⅓ part Violet
⅓ part Sandalwood

This oil gains favor from the Faerie folk. Assists with learning or playing music, and the arts in general.

Swallow's Blood Oil

½ part Dragon's Blood
¼ part Sandalwood

¼ part Rose

Jasmine, a few drops

Orris, a few drops

Designed to bring happiness to those who must travel. Soothes nerves while on the road.

Swallow's Heart Oil

½ part Carnation

½ part Ylang-Ylang

A few drops Peach

Helps soften feelings toward you; brings in kindly spirits who assist in love matters.

Taper Perfume Oil

⅓ part Jasmine

⅓ part Cinnamon

⅓ part Patchouli

Olive Oil

Used to float wicks. Usually no more than perfumed Olive Oil, this is more for decoration than for ritual purposes, but the oils tend to attract love, healing, and positive forces.

Tranquility Oil

¼ part Sage

½ part Rose

¼ part Benzoin

To bring some quiet and tranquil times to any upsetting situation; use in a diffuser.

Trinity Oil

½ part Hyssop

¼ part Olive Oil

¼ part Verbena

This blend will draw blessings to you in every area of life and guarantee success in both material and spiritual undertakings. Use sparingly—it's potent.

Turn Over a New Leaf Oil

¼ part Woodruff

¼ part Tonka
¼ part Lavender
¼ part Bergamot
Oak Moss, a few drops

Used in rituals designed to "turn over a new leaf," and for new beginnings and fresh starts. This oil is said to resemble the smell of freshly mown hay.

Voluptuous Venus Oil
Equal amounts of the following:

Rose

Musk

Orris

Sandalwood

Lilac

Cinnamon

Magnolia

Hibiscus

Use this blend to highlight your own beauty and indulge in the luxuries you deserve.

Weight Loss Oil
½ part Honeysuckle
¼ part Musk
¼ part Hyacinth

Helps you stick to that diet or exercise program.

White Wisdom Oil
½ part Lavender
½ part Sage
Camphor, a few drops

This oil is to help give you clear vision with wisdom, insight, and knowledge. The fresh, clean scent helps with clearing the mind and putting things in perspective. This is a great oil for spiritual cleansing, as it rids you of negative spiritual values and superstitions.

Wise Woman Oil

½ part Lavender
¼ part Mandarin
¼ part Lemongrass
Bergamot, a few drops

Use for mood swings and stress relief: calming, balancing, and uplifting.

Wise Woman Oil II

¼ part Basil
¼ part Lime
¼ part Coriander
¼ part Spearmint

Menopause oil blend that assists with mental clarity, fatigue, and increasing energy.

Wisdom Oil

¼ part Cinnamon
½ part Myrrh
¼ part Lavender

Designed to assist you in gaining true insight and wisdom.

Wisteria Perfume

10 drops Wisteria
2 ounces carrier oil (see carrier oil section in Part Three to see which oil would be best used in your particular situation)

Occultists, metaphysicians, healers, and voudounists alike all praise this oil. When worn as a perfume, it attracts good vibrations.

Wolf's Blood Oil

½ part Dragon's Blood
½ part Myrrh

Gives courage when under great pressure. Helps overcome all fear of death. A good formula for those who are in business or the arts and need strength to push their careers further.

Wood Song Oil

⅓ part Violet
⅓ part Honeysuckle
⅓ part Mint

An Elfin fragrance that brings peaceful and happy vibrations. It is also said to aid one in communicating with the Faeries.

Worry Away Oil

¼ part Siberian Fir
1 part Cajuput
1 part Lemon
1 part Lavender
2 ounces Almond Oil base

Often encompassed by difficult times, we find our thoughts muddled with indecision and lack the ability to think clearly. This is a wonderful candle-anointing oil to use for those rites when clear vision and focus are needed. A little goes a long way, so use sparingly but often. Use essential oils for this blend.

XYZ Oil

⅓ part Frankincense
⅓ part Myrrh
⅓ part Clove

To increase happiness and zest in daily activities. This is a three-purpose blend that brings extra benefits: youthful thoughts and feelings, and zest for life.

Yemaya Oil

½ part Lavender
½ part Lily of the Valley
Cucumber, a few drops

Yemaya is the great Ocean Mother. She blesses your home, calms arguments, and brings wealth and blessings.

Zawba Oil

½ part Vanilla
½ part Thyme
Wintergreen, a few drops
Almond, a few drops

To increase happiness and zest in your daily activities.

Zen Oil

⅓ part Lavender
⅓ part Clove
⅓ part Ylang-Ylang

This oil is useful in meditation or for inducing a sense of peace.

Chakras

In the spiritual movement, the word *chakra* (pronounced "shock-ra") often pops up. That's fine if you know what chakra means, but is confusing if you don't. The following is a short explanation of what the chakra system is about.

The human energy field, or aura, is an energetic, multidimensional field that surrounds, penetrates, and is the human body. It has rivers of energy called meridians that nourish every organ and cell in our bodies. These rivers are supplied by seven cone-shaped, spinning energy vortexes called chakras. These chakras, in turn, collect energy from the universal energy field that is all around us.

The seven chakras carry the colors of the rainbow spectrum. The root chakra, located at the base of the spine, carries the color red. The sacral chakra, our creative center, vibrates to the color orange. The solar plexus chakra, our self-centeredness, carries the color yellow. The heart chakra, our feeling center, resonates with the color green. The throat chakra, responsible for our expression, carries the color blue. The brow chakra, responsible for our dreams and questioning of spiritual things, radiates indigo. And the crown chakra, the highest vibrational rate in the spectrum, radiates a violet or white.

When things get out of whack, try this massage technique, which may help.

Blend the oils listed after the description of each chakra as follows:

Using essential oils: 3 drops per oil in a 10-ounces bottle of carrier oil (apricot or grape seed oil are best). Massage chakra area for at least twenty minutes before moving to the next chakra.

7th Chakra—Crown

This chakra is located at the top of the head, slightly to the back. It is associated with our feeling of "oneness" with the universe, our spiritual wisdom, a final understanding, and alignment with our true inner spirit. Physically, this chakra is linked to the pineal gland, the upper brain, and the right eye. This chakra is said to be your own place of connection to God/Christ/Buddha. A weak crown chakra can cause a feeling of disconnection with the vital flow of life, feeling uninspired, feeling misunderstood, and practicing self-denial. When overactive, the crown chakra may cause a disconnection with the earthly plane, being impractical, feeling disconnected with reality, over-imaginative.

½ part Myrrh

¼ part Lotus

¼ part Frankincense

A few drops Camphor

6th Chakra—Third Eye

This chakra is located just above your eyes, and at the center of your forehead. This chakra is used to question the spiritual nature of life. Our inner vision is contained here—inner dreams, gifts of clairvoyance, wisdom, and perception. The dreams of your life are held in this chakra. In order for the head chakra to work at its best, the heart chakra must also be strong and balanced. Physically, this chakra is linked to the nervous system, lower brain, left eye, ears, nose, and pituitary gland. When weak, this center may cause headaches, self-doubt, forgetfulness, or an inability to trust your instincts. If overactive, you may be oversensitive, spaced out, and experience psychic overload.

½ part Carnation

¼ part Lavender

¼ part Rosemary

5th Chakra—Throat

This chakra is located on the spine in the throat area, and is associated with our communication and expression abilities, right side of brain, speech, and hearing. Physically, it is linked to the throat, vocal cords, esophagus, mouth, teeth, thyroid and parathyroid glands, and upper lungs. When this chakra is weak, it may cause communication problems, an inability to express feelings and ideas, a tendency to withhold words and surrender to others. An overactive throat chakra may result in negative speech, criticizing, domineering words, hyperactive attitude, overreacting, and stubborn beliefs.

¼ part Cedarwood

¼ part Mimosa

¼ part Rosemary

¼ part Clove

4th Chakra—Heart

Located on the spine, in the area of the heart. This chakra is associated with our ability to give and receive love, to feel compassion, to reach out to others. The Asians say this is the house of the soul. It is the center of the chakras and can balance the activities of the seven energy centers. Physically, it is linked to the heart, lower lung area, circulatory system, thymus gland, and immune system. An important chakra for healing, when it is too weak, you may feel closed to others, experience low self-esteem, insecurity, jealousy, feel unloved, have a "poor me" attitude, and be self-doubting. When the heart chakra is overactive, you may experience the "martyr" syndrome, giving too much of yourself, and feeling overconfident, jealousy, and stingy.

½ part Violet
¼ part Vanilla
¼ part Ylang-Ylang
A few drops Eucalyptus

3rd Chakra—Solar Plexus

Located at the spine and just above the naval, this chakra is associated with the intellect and thinking process, personal power, anger, strength, and with the ability to take action. Your sensitivity is stored here. It is the seat of your emotional living. This is an important psychic center and where we experience "gut feelings" about someone or something. It is where emotional baggage gets stored. Physically, it is linked to the digestive system (pancreas, stomach, liver, and gall bladder). It helps the body assimilate nutrients. A weak solar plexus chakra can mean a mental slump, lethargy, feeling isolated and overcautious. When the solar plexus chakra is overactive, it can cause nervousness, mental bullying or unrest, digestion problems, mental overload, and a general feeling of disharmony.

¼ part Frankincense
¼ part Honeysuckle
¼ part Galangal
¼ part Lemon Verbena

2nd Chakra—Sacrum

This chakra is located on the spine in the lower abdomen, between the naval and the base of the spine. It is associated with sexuality, creativity, emotions, desire, and the ability to sense things on a psychic level. Physically, it is linked to the reproductive system and the gonads (endocrine gland). If this chakra is weak, you may feel unresponsive sexually and emotionally, antisocial, unoriginal, repressed. When overactive, it can make one feel lustful, selfish, arrogant, and overburdened by too many vibes and impressions received from others.

⅓ part Orange
⅓ part Oak Moss
⅓ part Sandalwood

1st Chakra—Root

This center chakra is located at the base of the spine. It's the chakra closest to the earth, and it represents earthly grounding. Fear is felt in this chakra; it controls your sense of survival, or your fight-or-flight response. Physically, it influences the supra-renal glands, as well as the legs, feet, kidneys, bladder, and spine. When this chakra is weak, you may feel very tired, overly cautious, afraid of change, and cold from poor circulation. You may need someone to light a fire under you. When it is over-energized, you may feel aggressive, oversexed, reckless, too impulsive, or belligerent.

⅛ part Civet
⅛ part Muguet
¼ part Ambergris
¼ part Cinnamon
¼ part Musk

Chakra Balancing Oil

¼ part Lemon
¼ part Orange
¼ part Lavender
¼ part Myrrh
A few drops Clove
Use this oil to balance any of your chakras or whenever you feel out of sorts.

Psychic and Spiritual

Magical oil blends can assist you in acquiring the everlasting wisdom of our Guides and Ascended Masters for making your life abundant, prosperous, and fulfilling. Visualization is the art of creating mental images. Pictures—not words—are involved. Form a mental image in your mind of what you desire; what is necessary for the needed change. Hold that image until you live that image through your five senses. This makes the image real. Record any messages or visions you receive in a journal, so you don't forget them. The oils gathered in this section are for dream work, meditation, astral travel, and working on your clairvoyance.

AC/DC Oil

¼ part Jasmine
¼ part Rose
¼ part Frankincense
¼ part Cinnamon
2 to 3 drops Lemon

The formula for this is a closely guarded secret by those who know it, but a few occult shops do carry it. While it obviously has connotations of heterosexual and homosexual love variations, it can be used by anyone who is facing a decision of choice. Apply to the forehead just before going to sleep, and a dream or vision may help you decide which way to move in your situation.

African Ju-Ju Oil

9 drops Galangal
½ ounce carrier oil (see carrier oils to find which one resonates with your intent)
Piece of Galangal Root in bottle

When applied to the brow area, facilitates and enhances psychic experiences and makes the wearer more intuitive; can be used as a crossing oil.

Ancient Shrines Oil

¼ part Sandalwood
¼ part Frankincense
¼ part Lotus
¼ part Narcissus
A few drops Cinnamon

A traditional mixture. Helps to clarify muddled thinking and promote telepathic faculties. Rub on the forehead during any ritual to protect against counter forces.

Arabian Bouquet

¼ part Sandalwood
¼ part Musk
¼ part Myrrh
¼ part Allspice

A special oil designed to cleanse the spirit before calling on the good spirits. This oil will also protect against hexes.

Astral Projection Oil

½ part Sweet Orange
½ part Anise
5 drops Jasmine
5 drops Eucalyptus
5 drops Wintergreen
⅛ cup Sweet Almond oil as a carrier oil

Facilitates astral projection.

Astral Travel Oil

¼ part Frankincense
¼ part Myrrh
¼ part Cypress
¼ part Jasmine

Assists in facilitating astral travel.

Astral Travel Oil II

½ part Patchouli
½ part Sandalwood
Cinnamon, a few drops

Anoint the stomach, wrists, back of the neck, and forehead. Lie down and visualize yourself astral projecting.

Astral Travel Oil III

1 part Lime
1 part Frankincense
1 part Myrrh

Travel the realms and visit the past and future; unfold the greatest mysteries of all time.

Astral Travel Oil IV

¾ part Sandalwood
⅛ part Ylang-Ylang
⅛ part Cinnamon

Anoint the body prior to an astral projection session.

Astral Travel Oil V

¼ part Orange
¼ part Lemon
¼ part Frankincense
¼ part Myrrh

Anoint the stomach, wrists, back of the neck, and forehead. Lie down and visualize yourself astral projecting.

Astral Voyage Oil

¾ part Sandalwood
⅛ part Ylang-Ylang
⅛ part Cinnamon

Facilitates astral travel and assists in out-of-body experiences. Very good for lucid dreaming exercises.

Aum Oil

¼ part Sandalwood
¼ part Orris
¼ part Mastic
¼ part Cinnamon

A special mixture designed to give off vibrations necessary for meditation and other spiritual work.

Black Star Oil

⅓ part Opium fragrance oil
⅓ part Musk
⅓ part Narcissus

For psychic revelation and, yes, for seduction too.

Blue Angel Oil

½ part Lavender
½ part Sandalwood
Holy Water, a few drops
Spring Water, a few drops

For love and invoking Spirit's aid. Use the oil with pink candles to attract friendship; anoint your astral candle or personal protection.

Clairvoyance Oil

¼ part Heliotrope
¼ part Honeysuckle
½ part Sandalwood
Wisteria, a few drops

A powerful blend for stimulating inner sight and clairvoyance.

Conjure Oil

¾ part Frankincense
⅛ part Myrrh
⅛ part Clove
Ambergris, a few drops

Spirits find this fragrance very appealing. Anoint candles before lighting them to attract those spirits necessary to accomplish the intention you seek.

Conjure Oil II

⅓ part Frankincense
⅓ part Sandalwood
⅓ part Lotus

Works like a genie in a bottle. This oil will help manifest anything you need into reality. Creative visualization is vital when using this oil.

Crystal Temple Oil

⅛ part Frankincense
⅛ part Orris
¼ part Sandalwood
¼ part Lotus

Used for meditation and yoga.

Crystal Woodlands Oil

¼ part Fir
⅛ part Pine
¼ part Juniper

Communication with astral/animals. Assists in helping you find totem or spirit animals and guides.

Déjà Vu Oil

½ part Sandalwood
¼ part Orris
¼ part Cinnamon
Mastic, a drop or two

Used to remember past lives and/or to become more aware of them.

Divination Oil

¼ part Musk
¼ part Ambergris
¼ part Vetiver
¼ part Violet
Lilac, a few drops

Divination oil is intended to open up the psychic facilities for clarity and increased eyesight. It is often used to anoint the forehead (third eye) and the temples.

Divination Oil II
½ part Camphor
¼ part Orange
¼ part Clove

An oil to open the Eye of Sight and see that which is cast in shadow. Whether you are using Tarot cards, runes, tea leaves, or witch balls, this oil is created to assist in seeing the patterns of what was, is, and will be.

Divination Oil III
½ part Lotus
⅛ part Clove
⅛ part Orange
¼ Sandalwood

This oil makes the perfect aid for rituals and spells if you are seeking information. Whether you're using it to anoint tools and candles for rituals or drip into a scrying bowl, it is designed to enhance and empower spells when you seek to divine the future, seek out lost information, or otherwise improve your wisdom concerning the world around you.

Divination Oil IV
⅓ part Myrrh
⅓ part Sandalwood
⅓ part Bay

This oil is used to anoint and consecrate a tarot deck or other divination tools before using them for divination. It can also be used to anoint the diviner's third eye before the divination tools are consulted and read.

Divination Oil for the Full Moon
⅓ part Myrrh
⅓ part Lotus
⅓ part Jasmine

Wear to increase and deepen your psychic powers during a Full Moon.

Divine Oil

¾ part Sandalwood
¼ part Orange

Wear to increase accuracy and perception during the divination process.

Divine Protection Oil

½ part Rose
¼ part Lavender
⅛ part Hibiscus
⅛ part Mint

This oil is for warding off evil. Wear the oil when you feel in any kind of danger, physical or spiritual.

Dragons Oil

¼ part Opium fragrance oil
¼ part Allspice
¼ part Cinnamon
¼ part Amber

To help invoke dragons for good luck, wealth, protection, and other positive uses.

Dream Oil

½ part Rose
¼ part Jasmine
⅛ part Chamomile
⅛ part Violet

To cause a prophetic or instructional dream.

Dream Oil II

¼ part Marjoram
¼ part Mugwort
¼ part Chamomile
¼ part Sandalwood
Add a sodalite stone to the bottle
½ ounce carrier oil (see carrier oils to find which one suits your intent)

Use to cause a prophetic or instructional dream. Use essential oils only for this blend.

Dream Chaser Oil

⅓ part Lavender
⅓ part Violet
⅓ part Sandalwood or Rosewood
Lemon, a few drops
Lemongrass, a few drops

Helps with achieving lucid dreaming and keeping negative forms out of the dream state.

Dreamer Oil

½ part Rose
¼ part Jasmine
¼ part Chamomile

Prepare this blend by pouring the oils in a 10-ounce bottle and then adding organic vegetable oil to fill. Anoint the third eye, sacrum, and solar plexus. Pour a few drops into the palm of your hand and inhale deeply; may use in the bath as well.

Dream Potion

½ part Jasmine
½ part Nutmeg
Clary Sage, a few drops

Not for internal use. Anoint dream pillows and/or third eye upon retiring for bed.

Dreamtime Oil

⅓ part Carnation
⅓ part Sandalwood
⅓ part Vanilla

This oil is for peaceful, healing sleep and creative dreaming. Use it in a diffuser, or make it into incense.

Dreams/Visualization Oil

Equal amounts of all:

Sandalwood	Blue Tansy
Bergamot	Tangerine
Ylang-Ylang	Black Pepper
Juniper	Anise

Use for prophetic and divinatory dreams. Write your special wish on a candle before you retire; burn the candle for fifteen minutes nightly for seven nights.

Energy Oil

⅓ part Vanilla
⅓ part Musk
⅓ part Lemon Verbena

To increase emotional and physical energy and endurance.

Energy Oil II

½ part Orange
¼ part Lime
¼ part Cardamom

Wear when feeling depleted, when ill, or just to strengthen your own energy reserves. Especially useful after magical rituals to recharge your bodily batteries.

Faerie Enchantment Oil

⅔ part Rose
⅓ part Thyme
Evening Primrose in master bottle

This oil will aid in opening up your third eye so that you may view the Savage Garden (the Faerie Realm). If the Fae permit it, that is.

Faerie Fire Oil

1 Garnet crushed
1 part Dragon's Blood
1 part Coriander
Coriander Seeds

For seeing the Faerie Realm and working with them. A fabulous oil for learning art and creative divination techniques.

Faerie Fire Oil II

½ part Peach
¼ part Ylang-Ylang
⅛ part New Mown Hay
⅛ part Dark Musk
⅛ part Chamomile
⅛ part Poppy
Dragon's Blood, a few drops
Garnet in the master bottle

Useful in contacting Faeries connected with the Fire element: Will o' the Wisps, Flame Dancers, etc.

Faerie Flower Oil

½ part Elder Flower
½ part Lavender
Dried Rosebuds

For working with flower devas, and for learning how to listen to the messages that different plants and their devas offer you.

Faerie Magic Oil

⅛ part Lemon
¼ part Gardenia
⅛ part Jasmine
¼ part Violet
$\frac{1}{16}$ part Lavender
$\frac{1}{16}$ part Lemongrass
$\frac{1}{16}$ part Rose geranium
$\frac{1}{16}$ part Ylang-Ylang

Useful for working with Faerie magic. Wear it on Midsummer's Eve to increase chances of Fae encounters.

Faerie Oil (Elemental Water)

½ part Camphor
¼ part Lavender
¼ part Lemon
Primrose, a few drops
Rose Geranium, a few drops

Use this oil when contacting Faeries connected to the Water element, such as Undines, Naiads, Sirens, etc.

Faerie Spirit Oil

¼ part Oak Moss
¼ part Rosemary
¼ part Cypress
¼ part Patchouli

To use when working with the Fae.

Faeries Oil

⅛ part Mimosa

⅛ part Lily of the Valley

¼ part Vanilla

¼ part Peach

This recipe is for the sweet, beguiling Faeries that charm and enchant all who come within their realm. If you wish to create a magical, enchanted Faerie atmosphere in your home, use this oil in a diffuser.

Faerie Ring Oil

¼ part Elderflower

¼ part Lavender

¼ part Musk

⅛ part Lilac

⅛ part Frankincense

Myrrh, a few drops

For use in Faerie Circles.

Grant me your favors, Fair Ones I pray
Your tales I shall tell, your songs I shall play!
With harm to none, no secrets betray,
Lend me the might of your talents today!
So Mote It Be!—author unknown

To enhance beauty and musical/artistic skill. Beware of its enchantment!

Far-Sight Oil

⅓ part Acacia

⅓ part Cassia

⅓ part Anise

Bergamot, a few drops

Wear to aid in seeing your past lives. (Caution: rest this oil first; it may irritate your skin.)

Fire of Azrael Oil

⅓ part Sandalwood

⅓ part Cedar

⅓ part Juniper

Bergamot, a few drops

A scrying oil based on a 500-year-old recipe from ancient England.

Flower Faerie's Fancy

⅔ part Rose

⅓ part Clary Sage

Jasmine, a few drops

Flying Oil

You will need at least a 1- or 2-ounce bottle to blend this oil, as there are many ingredients.

Use equal parts of the following:

Calamus

Musk

Juniper

Sandalwood

Bayberry

Anise

Cinnamon

Clove

Allspice

Flying oil was designed to assist and protect during astral travel. After blending the oil, wrap in a dark cloth, and hide it in a secret place for nine days. Unwrap it and let sit in the moonlight for thirteen nights. Best to start twenty-four hours after the New Moon so it will be finished right before the Full Moon. You can put it out under the Full Moon's light for the intuitive blessings of Mother Moon. Then it will be ready for the astral projection of your choice.

God Fire Oil

⅓ part Pine

⅓ part Musk

⅓ part Cinnamon

Awakens the higher spiritual aspect of the earth gods.

Good Luck Mystic Oil

½ part Sandalwood
¼ part Musk
¼ part Gardenia

This oil is designed to attract mystic guides for further psychic development.

Gypsy Magic Oil

¾ part Peppermint
¼ part Thyme
½ ounce Borage Seed carrier oil

Simple yet effective divination oil. Use this oil to anoint your third eye prior to any divination or spellwork.

Heather Oil

¼ part Mastic
¼ part Frankincense
¼ part Cinnamon
¼ part Lavender
Bay, a few drops

Helps to bring forth psychic power. Wonderful for clairvoyance. Anoint forehead while in ritual. Use in your bath before retiring to secure prophetic dreaming.

Hindu Grass Oil

¼ part Cinnamon
¼ part Coriander
¼ part Sage
¼ part Patchouli
Curry, a pinch

A special oil designed to heighten psychic, clairvoyant, and meditation powers.

Holy Trinity Oil

⅓ part Rose
⅓ part Gardenia
⅓ part Lotus

This oil is for powerful guidance, spiritual resources, and protection.

Indian Spirit Guide Oil

½ part Neroli
¼ part Bayberry
¼ part Cedarwood
Calamus, a few drops (if available) or Calamus herb (optional)

This oil blend is great for psychics, mediums, and those who just need some spiritual guidance.

Inner Journey Oil

½ part Frankincense
¼ part Cedar
¼ part Lemon

Great for meditation and past-life regressions.

Invocation Oil

¼ part Jasmine
¼ part Rose
¼ part Myrrh
¼ part Frangipani

An all-purpose invoking essence that is nice to always have on hand.

Kindly Spirit Oil

⅓ part Frangipani
⅓ part Carnation
⅓ part Musk
Clove or Allspice, a few drops (optional)

To summon an unearthly being to your side for aid in accomplishing your tasks, write your requirement on paper and place the petition beneath a pink candle, which has been anointed with this oil.

Kundalini Oil

¼ part Saturnian

¼ part Ambergris

¼ part French Musk

⅛ part Civet

½ part Valerian

Cinnamon, a drop or two

Raises the energy of the kundalini. Place oil at the heart, throat, and behind the ears.

Lucid Dreaming Oil

½ part Valerian

½ part Lavender

Clary Sage, a few drops

To cause a prophetic or instructional dream.

Lucky Mystic Oil

⅓ part Basil

⅓ part Lavender

⅓ part Orange

Silver glitter (optional)

Attracts good spirits and aids in honing clairvoyant skills.

Lucky Prophet Oil

¼ part Frankincense

¼ part Juniper

¼ part Sandalwood

¼ part Rose

This is a formula that can activate inborn clairvoyant powers so this gift can be developed to its full potential.

Maa-Isa Oil

⅛ part Myrrh
⅛ part Vetiver
½ part Frankincense
⅛ part Civet
⅛ part Styrax
Myrtle, a few drops
Orange rind, in master bottle

Ancient Egyptian blend which means "the truth of Isis." Used by the Priestesses of Isis to aid in counsel, to seek the truth in a matter, or for works of divination.

Magnolia Bouquet

¼ part Neroli
½ part Jasmine
⅛ part Rose
⅛ part Sandalwood

Just as with Lotus oil, no genuine Magnolia oil exists. An excellent addition to meditation and psychic awareness oils, as well as love mixtures. Use compound Magnolia oil or make your own. Try to have a fresh flower nearby so that while mixing you can try to duplicate the scent. You can use this mixture whenever a recipe calls for Magnolia. And remember, it's okay to use fragrance oils, too.

Meditation Oil

¼ part Frankincense
¼ part Cedarwood
¼ part Tangerine
¼ part Chamomile

Facilitates meditative work, also tends to be very good at attracting spirits. Use in protected environment.

Meditation Oil II

½ part Sandalwood
¼ part Orris
¼ part Mastic
Cinnamon, a few drops

A special mixture designed to give off vibrations necessary for meditation or other spiritual work. Especially good for psychic endeavors. A strong Spirit attractant tends to add success to any ritual.

Meditation Oil III

½ part Frangipani
¼ part Musk
¼ part Narcissus

This carries a strong mystical aura and should be used only while meditating, praying, or doing psychic work.

Merddin Bath Oil

¼ part Lilac
¼ part Violet
¼ part Narcissus
⅛ part Wisteria
⅛ part Ambergris

Use to aid your prophetic spells. Place 6 drops in bathwater and soak for twenty minutes.

Mimosa Magic Oil

⅓ part Acacia
⅓ part Yellow Rose
⅓ part Lilac
Bay, a few drops

Rub all over the body before sleep to produces prophetic dream. Anoint a blue or white candle for the same effect, or use in the bath or bed to permit good—and only good—dreams to come true.

Moon Oil

½ part Jasmine
½ part Sandalwood

Wear to induce psychic dreams, to speed healing, to facilitate sleep, to increase fertility, and for all other lunar influences. Also wear at the time of the Full Moon to attune with its vibrations.

Moon Oil (Planetary)

¼ part Nutmeg
¼ part Myrrh
⅛ part Anise
⅛ part Clary Sage
⅛ part Wintergreen
⅛ part Eucalyptus

For any work with lunar intention. Intensifies clairvoyance and psychic vision.

Moonlight Grove Oil

¾ part Jasmine
⅛ part Lemon
⅛ part Frankincense

A lunar oil with romance in mind. Brings psychic visions of those you love and wish to be with.

Moses Oil

⅓ part Solomon's seal
⅓ part Hyssop
⅓ part Rose

Usually called the Oil of Moses, this is a holy oil, used during séances by those attempting to talk to the spirits in the other worlds, and for consecrating altars, utensils, and tools.

Mystic Hermit Oil

⅛ part Allspice
½ part Ylang-Ylang
⅛ part Cinnamon
¼ part Galangal

For spiritual growth, looking inward, and being able to listen to the "voice within."

Mystic Veil Oil

⅛ part Cinnamon
½ part Sandalwood
⅛ part Clove
¼ part Myrrh

This is used for pathworking, psychic endeavors, or to break through the astral plane.

Nirvana Oil

¼ part Coriander
¼ part Sage
¼ part Patchouli
¼ part Cinnamon

Used in the pursuit of deep meditation. Soothes emotional states so that mental work can take place.

Olympian Oracle Oil

⅛ part Cinnamon

¼ part Myrrh

½ part Vetiver

⅛ part Clove

This oil helps to open the spirit to vibrations from other planes so they can communicate with this plane.

Oracle Oil

¼ part Cinnamon

¼ part Sandalwood

¼ part Clove

Myrrh, a few drops

Use to aid in prophetic magic.

Orange Mist Lace Oil

½ part Bergamot

¼ part Orange

⅛ part Neroli

⅛ part Cinnamon

This light, ethereal oil helps to cause a higher vibration of energy in yourself or your environment.

Papyrus Oil

½ part Sandalwood

¼ part Orris

¼ part Mastic

Cinnamon, a few drops

To aid in meditation.

Past Lives Oil

⅓ part Clove

⅓ part Sandalwood

⅓ part Orange

Aids in past life meditations; helps recall past lifetimes clearly and without emotional entanglement.

Peaceful Thoughts Oil

⅓ part Lavender

⅓ part Rosemary

⅓ part Wintergreen

Anoint forehead and temples with this oil before meditating.

Prayers Oil

½ part Frankincense

½ part Myrrh

Vanilla, a few drops

For help with prayer and spellwork; great for meditation, too.

Prophetic Dream Oil

½ cup Olive Oil

Pinch of Cinnamon

Pinch of Nutmeg

1 teaspoon Anise

Put herbs in Olive Oil and heat until warm, but not hot. Strain herbs and then bottle. Store bottle in a dark place. Write the question you want answered on a piece of paper and place under your pillow. Apply oil to forehead and temples before sleep. Do this for three nights in a row.

Psychic Attack Protection Oil

¼ part Bergamot

¼ part Dragon's Blood

¼ part Rue

¼ part Frankincense

Piece of High John Root

Activates and increases the wearer's psychic abilities.

Psychic Oil

¾ part Lemongrass

¼ part Yarrow

Wear to increase psychic powers, especially when working with rune stones, quartz crystal spheres, and other such tools.

Psychon Oil

¼ part Cinnamon
¼ part Galangal
¼ part Cedar
¼ part Orris
Myrrh, a few drops

Helps the wearer to open up the third eye.

Purple Wisdom Oil

¼ part Violet
¼ part Vanilla
¼ part Lilac
¼ part Lotus

This oil can help you open the doorways to your intuition that may be lurking within you. It can also help you gain wisdom and psychic insight.

Quieting Oil

⅓ part Lemon
⅓ part Lavender
⅓ part Balm of Gilead
Sugar, a few grains
Salt, a few grains

An intoxicating voudoun mixture that helps to induce a deep meditative state before rituals or other meditation work.

Sacred Light Oil

¾ part Sandalwood
⅛ part Nutmeg
⅛ part Cinnamon

Use to safely assist the spirit in letting go of the body to travel to other planes.

Serenity Oil

½ part Cucumber
½ part Lavender
5 drops Cinnamon

Calm, soothing, quiet tranquility, and peace can be had when using this oil. Wonderful oil for meditation and massage work.

Seven Chakras Oil

1 part of each oil:

    Rose (base)

    Bergamot (sacral)

    Lemon (belly)

    Benzoin (heart)

    German Chamomile (throat)

    St. John's Wort (head)

    Lavender (crown)

    ½ ounce base oil (select a carrier oil from the list that will best suit your intent)

An oil designed to assist in balancing the chakras and aura. Perfect for massage, or to have in a diffuser.

Sleep Oil

    ¾ part Rose

    ¼ part Mace

Anoint the temples, neck, pulse of both wrists, and soles of the feet. It brings on natural sleep. Essential oils are recommended, but not mandatory. If you do decide to use essentials, place in 1 cup of carrier oil.

Sleep Oil II

    ½ part Rose

    ¼ part Jasmine

    ¼ part Chamomile

Anoint the temples, neck, pulse of both wrists, soles of the feet. It brings on natural sleep.

Smudge Blend Oil

    ½ part Sage

    ¼ part Lavender

    ¼ part Amber

This oil is like having a liquid smudge stick at your disposal. When the smoke from a smudge stick is too much for people, just place a few drops of this in your diffuser.

Song of the Elder Gods Oil

⅓ part Sandalwood
⅓ part Musk
⅓ part Wisteria

This oil is for communicating with your own personal muse for any work that requires inspiration and creativity.

Spirit Oil

¼ part Sandalwood
¼ part Violet
¼ part Crocus
¼ part Gardenia

Assists in communicating with deceased friends and relatives. Sprinkle on ground or use as incense or to anoint white candles. Never wear the oil on your body.

Spiritual Healing Oil

⅛ part Frankincense
⅛ part Orris
¼ part Sandalwood
½ part Lotus

To cause a higher vibration of energy in yourself in order to perform healing sessions. Great oil for chakra work.

Spiritual Vibration Oil

½ part Sandalwood
¼ part Heliotrope
⅛ part Magnolia
⅛ part Frankincense

An enchanting oil designed to strengthen and enhance the individual's power for spellwork and psychic ability.

Star Daughter Oil

½ part Rose
½ part Lilac
Verbena, a few drops

A beautiful blend designed to help you request a personal spirit guide and establish sensitivity to communications with your guide.

Sweet Repose Oil

½ part Rose
¼ part Lavender
¼ part Magnolia

This is a relaxing, sleep-inducing blend which helps to develop inner peace and tranquility.

The Phoenix Oil

⅓ part Lemon
⅓ part Lavender
⅓ part Bay

A blend to safely assist the Spirit in letting go of the body to travel to other planes.

Tiger Perfume

Wintergreen, a few drops
¼ part Gardenia
¼ part Rose
¼ part Peppermint
¼ part Bay

A voudoun recipe that awakens psychic power and clairvoyance.

Vibrance Oil

½ part Orange
½ part Ginger
Spanish Moss, a few drops

Vibrance Oil brings about a sense of well-being while working on cleansing the aura.

Vision Oil

¼ part Magnolia
¼ part Rose
½ part Apple Blossom

Anoint yourself with this oil before any psychic workings.

Vision Oil II

¼ part Bay
¾ part Lemongrass
Nutmeg, just a few drops

Anoint forehead to produce psychic awareness. Very good for tarot readers.

Vision Seeker Oil

¼ part Vanilla
¼ part Gardenia
½ part Violet

This blend assists you in opening up your psychic awareness.

Visionary Dreams Oil

⅓ part Patchouli
⅓ part Lavender
⅓ part Ylang-Ylang

Use this oil to increase the depth and perception of your dreams.

Wishbone Oil

½ part Patchouli
¼ part Musk
¼ part Jasmine

This oil can bring luck, grant wishes, and aid in psychic development. Place a few drops of this oil in a water bowl before you retire for the night, and pray to receive psychic information through your dreams, or pray over the water to have your wishes granted. In the morning, just dispose of the water down the drain.

Zorba Perfume

⅛ part Mastic
¼ part Frankincense
¼ part Cinnamon
⅛ part Lavender
⅛ part Bay

Helps to bring forth psychic power; wonderful for clairvoyance. Anoint forehead while in ritual. Use in your bath before retiring to secure prophetic dreams.

Home

Protection for the home is a common goal of magical workings. Of course, these aren't replacements for commonsense things, like locking your doors and getting a house alarm if needed, but magical working certainly supports those mundane solutions.

A very simple way to protect the home is to anoint the doors and windows with one of the oils below in a five-spot pattern (like a pentagram). Put a little oil on your fingers, touch each corner of the door and the middle while praying Psalm 23 or praying in your own words. This will literally drive your enemies away from your home and reflect anything they throw at you back with a vengeance.

Air Freshener Oil
½ part Lime
¼ part Geranium
¼ part Sandalwood

Dilute 6 to 8 drops of blend with carrier oil and use in a potpourri burner.

Angel or Archangel Oil
½ part Lavender
½ part Sandalwood
Holy Water, a few drops
Spring Water, a few drops

Used in angelic invocation and to create a peaceful atmosphere; use with pink candle to attract friends, or with a white candle to calm a troubled home.

Apartment Hunting Oil

⅓ part Honeysuckle
⅓ part Jasmine
⅓ part Heliotrope

Use this oil when in search of a new dwelling. Anoint a piece of paper on which you have drawn or listed what you desire. Include price, utilities, pets etc. Be as detailed as you can. Come back to the list, in an hour or so, read over it, and add or delete as needed. Anoint each of the four corners of the paper, fold it, and take it with you on your search. When you find the place you desire, leave the paper on the premises (out of view, of course).

Bathroom Oil

⅛ part Bergamot
¼ part Lavender
⅛ part Thyme
¼ part Lemon
¼ part Orange

Dilute with 2 cups water and use as a spray for surfaces, or dilute 6 to 8 drops with water and use in a burner. Alternative oils: Citronella, Sage, Oregano (be careful around wooden furniture; test surfaces first).

Bedroom Oil

¾ part Rose
¼ part Ylang-Ylang
2 drops Clary Sage

Dilute with water and place in a burner. Alternative oils: Roman Chamomile, Nutmeg.

Citrus Purification Oil

⅓ part Orange (sweet)
⅓ part Lemongrass
⅓ Lemon
1 drop Lime
⅛ cup carrier oil such as Olive, Almond, Sunflower, or Jojoba

Blend these essential oils and then add dried zest of orange, lemon, or lime. Also add one of the following to enhance the power of the oil: Aquamarine, Blue Calcite, or Salt. Anoint white candles with this oil and burn in the home to purify it. *DO NOT wear or go out into sunlight with this oil in your skin, since it can burn skin quite badly.*

Cleansing Oil

¼ part Lotus

¼ part Frankincense

¼ part Amber

¼ part Cedarwood

This is a general-purpose, purifying blend. Used in incense or water, it is intended to cleanse the premises of any negative or unwanted energy.

Dragon Shield Oil

½ part Patchouli

½ part Sandalwood

Lilac, a few drops

This blend is for protection against physical, mental, and emotional attacks.

Durga Oil

¼ part Patchouli

¼ part Musk

¼ part Vetiver

¼ part Amber

This oil is for protection from all harm.

Flying Devil Oil

½ part Lavender

½ part Frankincense

This blend was created to get negativity out of your house, whether in the form of imps or demons, or simply bad influences that will not leave you alone. Use this oil to anoint your front door with the aid of either a cross or Pentagram. Purchase a new broom that will be used only to perform this spell. Take a large pail or bowl of water and add a few drops of the oil. Place it in the center of the room, dip the broom into the water, and, using sweeping motions, brush the water across the floor and toward the door.

General Protection Oil

¼ part Basil

¼ part Geranium

¼ part Pine

¼ part Vetiver

Wear for protection against all kinds of attacks. Also anoint windows, doors, and all other parts of the house to guard it.

General Protection Oil II

⅛ cup carrier oil

1 part Patchouli

1 part Frankincense

1 part Myrrh

1 teaspoon broken Mandrake

3 heaping teaspoons Sea Salt

Pout ⅛ of a cup of carrier oil into a clean sterilized jar and add the oils as listed above. Swirl to mix and label. Let it sit for two weeks, shaking it daily. Then strain, place in dark bottle, and store in refrigerator.

Wear for protection against all kinds of attacks. Also anoint windows, doors, and all other parts of the house to guard it.

Gypsy Blood Oil

2 parts Patchouli leaves

1 part Guinea Pepper

2 tablespoons carrier oil

Said to make troublesome neighbors uproot and move when sprinkled on their door-knobs.

Happy Home Oil

¼ part Geranium

¼ part Dragon's Blood

$\frac{1}{16}$ part Tonka

$\frac{1}{16}$ part Violet

$\frac{1}{16}$ part New Mown Hay

$\frac{1}{16}$ part Thyme

⅛ part High John the Conqueror

⅛ part Bergamot

A few drops of each:

Dill

Earth Oil

Lilac

Jasmine

To ensure your living quarters are blessed and protected.

Happy Times Oil

⅓ part Orange
⅓ part Vanilla
⅓ part Violet

Changes luck and reverses unfortunate circumstances. It also assists in eliminating poverty.

Home Blessing Oil

⅛ part Juniper
⅛ part Basil
¾ part Jasmine

To anoint candles when moving into a new home.

Home Protection Oil

Use equal parts of the following:
Five Finger Grass
Sandalwood
Gardenia Petals
Purslane
Add to 2 tablespoons of carrier oil
Add one pinch of blessed salt

Anoint charms designed to protect the home from evil. Sprinkle around the home to keep evil and harm away.

House Blessing Oil

½ part Lavender
¼ part Jasmine
⅛ part Cucumber
⅛ part Frangipani

Use House Blessing oil to clear a home's negative vibrations.

Louisiana VanVan Oil

¼ cup extra virgin Olive Oil
1 ounce Lemongrass herb
Pinch of salt

Place in a jar, cover, and steep in dark place for three weeks. Shake the jar daily, and visualize power pouring into the oil. Strain out the herb; add more herb, and repeat until the oil is strongly scented with the herb. When it is to your liking, strain out the herb, bottle, and store in dark place. Use to anoint candles, doorways, and amulets for extra power.

Mint Bouquet Oil

⅓ part Pennyroyal
⅓ part Mint
⅓ part Lemon

Removes bad spells; particularly loved by good spirits. When invoking the aid of voudoun gods, place this oil in a dish as an offering to gain their assistance.

Mistress of the House Oil

2 tablespoons Calamus
2 ounces Olive Oil

A small piece of Devil's Shoestring is added to each bottle of oil made. This oil is used by women who want to be the boss of the house. Sprinkle on mate or love's shoes or clothing to gain control over his actions.

Moving Oil

½ part Rose
½ part Lemon
Cinnamon, a few drops

Encourages troublesome neighbors to move somewhere else quietly and quickly.

Peaceful Home Oil

⅓ part Lemon
⅓ part Rose
⅓ part Lilac

Ensure a serene and tranquil domestic life. Each week, add Peaceful Home Oil to a bowl of water that is placed in the center of the home. It will clear the premises of all baneful vibrations. To enhance the calm atmosphere of the premises, apply a drop of this oil to one or several small cotton balls and place them at strategic points so that they waft their soothing odor over the entire home.

Protection Against Thieves Oil

¼ part Caraway
¼ part Rosemary
¼ part Juniper
¼ part Elder
Bergamot, a few drops

Protects your property from being stolen.

Protection Oil

½ part Basil
¼ part Geranium
¼ part Pine
Vetiver, a few drops

Wear for protection against all kinds of attacks. Also anoint the windows, doors, and other parts of the house to guard it.

Protection Oil II

½ part Sandalwood
½ part Lily

Same as above.

Protection Oil III

½ part Rosemary
½ part Frankincense
Lavender, a few drops

Use to strengthen, restore, and cleanse yourself. Visualize a spiritual wall being restored around yourself for protection.

Purification Oil

½ part Orange
¼ part Lemongrass
¼ part Lemon
Lime, 2 to 3 drops

Anoint white candles and use in a diffuser to purify the home.

Purifying Oil

½ part Sage
½ part Rosemary
Clove, 2 to 3 drops

This blend is designed to be used before blessing a space, object, or person to be certain no negativity remains.

Run Devil Run Oil
⅓ part Dark Musk
⅓ part Sandalwood
⅓ part Myrrh

Evil simply cannot abide this scent and will not tarry in the vicinity where it is used. Sprinkle it outside on all windowsills and doorways so that no evil spirits can gain entry into the home. Renew once a week, preferably on a Saturday.

Sacred Shield Oil
½ part Dragon's Blood
½ part Bergamot
Myrrh, a few drops
Cedar, 2 to 3 drops

To rid a place or person of all negativity and blocked energy regardless of the source.

Sorceress Oil
½ part Patchouli
½ part Galangal

Use to aid you in protection spells. When mixing these oils, imagine a strong wall being built around you, only allowing good things to pass through it.

Stay at Home Oil
¼ part Patchouli
¼ part Lavender
¼ part Cedarwood
¼ part Pine
Camphor, a few drops

Encourages lover to stay at home by emphasizing the qualities of comfort and stability as well as arousing feelings of loyalty and passion toward the lover or spouse.

Stay at Home Oil II
⅓ part Patchouli
⅓ part Musk
⅓ part Angel Perfume fragrance oil

This oil inspires wayward loves to stay with you, whether it be the family cat who won't come back in or the kids who stay out too late.

Stone Circle Power Oil

¼ part Rosemary
½ part Frankincense
¼ part Vetiver

Use this blend for banishing and protection from physical and spiritual danger.

Sword of the Ancients Oil

½ part Frankincense
½ part Sandalwood
Amber, a drop or two

Use to aid you in protection spells. When mixing these oils, imagine a strong wall being built around you allowing only good things to pass through it.

Thief Oil

½ part Frankincense
½ part Carnation
Cinnamon, a few drops

This oil will help you retrieve lost or stolen items. Specifically, it can be used to help you catch a thief and have what is stolen returned to you. Or sometimes, what is stolen returns to you in other ways.

Vesta Oil

¼ part Rose
¼ part Lily
¼ part Lavender
Peppermint, a few drops

An oil that inspires domestic activity and cleanliness; an everyday banishing mixture.

Yemaya Oil

½ part Lavender
½ part Lily of the Valley
Cucumber, a few drops

Yemaya is the great Ocean Mother. She blesses your home, calms down arguments, and brings wealth and blessings.

Money Oils

I have always enjoyed crafting money and prosperity oils. They bring about a feeling of abundance and light that cannot be duplicated at any other time. Working with the Law of Attraction when preparing these blends can also assist you in giving your potion an energy that is conducive to bringing you what you desire.

The Law of Attraction is pretty simple. It is the thought that *Like Attracts Like*. While making money oils—or any magical working, for that matter—the Law of Attraction can be the difference between failure and an extremely potent potion!

Simply think about what you desire your blend to do for you while crafting it. Block out all negative thinking. If you have to, stop working and come back to your work later if negative thinking is creeping into your work.

Believe in yourself, and the infinite possibilities that you can create by just keeping a positive outlook, and you will be able to make it a reality.

Here is a situation that will help you understand how the Law of Attraction will work for you:

You place a pot of water on the stove to boil. You have enough water in the pot and the heating element is turned on. You can then walk away, knowing the pot on the stove will boil. Again, you know it will boil. It may take time, but it *will* happen.

Magic is that simple too! Believe in yourself and what you are doing. Make your intent known to the universe; it will work, and you know it will.

The oils that follow will assist you in manifesting what you need. Remember that nothing is written in stone. If you need to adapt an oil to suit your situation, feel free to do so. Just remember to write it down, so if it works for you, you can make it again the next time you need it.

Abundance Oil

⅛ part Spruce
⅛ part Myrrh
⅛ part Patchouli
⅛ part Cassia
⅛ part Orange
⅛ part Clove
⅛ part Ginger
⅛ part Frankincense

To draw plenty and riches of all sorts.

As You Please Oil

⅓ part Neroli
⅓ part Musk
⅓ part Cinnamon

The use of this oil will bring success in almost any endeavor, as it is formulated to overcome the objections of others to your plans. Just before you present your idea or plan, apply this oil to the fingertips, soles of the feet, and the throat, and others will be willing to go along with your proposal.

Astral Bank Oil

¼ part Neroli
¼ part Sandalwood
¼ part Tonka
¼ part Honeysuckle

Use when you need to make a withdrawal from the "Astral Bank" to make ends meet.

Bankrupt Oil

2 tablespoons powdered Devil's Shoestring
2 ounces Olive Oil
Optional: add one small piece of Devil's Shoestring to each bottle of oil made

Said to force an enemy to go broke, it is used in rituals designed to force someone to spend their money. This oil can be anointed on charms made to bring bad luck, and placed in a business to make the business go bankrupt.

Bayberry Oil
22 drops Bayberry fragrance oil

2 ounces carrier oil

Attracts spirits of prosperity and will aid the wearer in claiming debts owed.

Bayberry Blessing Oil
¾ part Bayberry

⅛ part Orange

⅛ part Cinnamon

Brings money to the pockets and blessings to the home of those who daily anoint their wrists with this legendary scent.

Bergamot Mint Bouquet
½ part Lemon

½ part Lemongrass

Peppermint, a few drops

Bergamot has a minty-lemony fragrance, and it is used in money and prosperity oils. There are a great many synthesized versions out there that should not be used. Instead, make this bouquet.

Calling Abundance Oil
⅓ part Chamomile

⅓ part Cedar

⅓ part Patchouli

Clove, a few drops

You can use this oil to anoint candles. Place a small amount on the right-hand corner of dollar bills and place them in your wallet. Or keep a stone anointed with the oil to bring abundance into your life.

Cavern Treasure Prosperity Oil
½ part Sandalwood

½ part Myrrh

Allspice, a few drops

Cinnamon, a few drops

Not quite a "money draw" oil, this helps the wearer to have a sense of well-being and wealth. It also decreases anxiety over money matters and one's lifestyle.

Collect Debts Oil

¾ part Bayberry

⅛ part Vetiver

⅛ part Apricot

To get help returned to you from those you have helped before.

Commanding Oil

⅛ part Patchouli

⅛ part Myrrh

¾ Sandalwood

Commanding Oil is dabbed on uncounted coins, which are then left in the light of a Full Moon as a statement that money is required.

Compelling Oil

4 ounces clear base

Add equal parts of the following:

Verbena

Jasmine

Rose

Lilac

Myrrh

Lavender

Violet

Honeysuckle

Gain power for yourself. Use this oil to change things so they go in your favor. It will compel others to give in to your desires. To induce someone to pay you money that is owed to you, write the name of the debtor and the amount of money due on a piece of parchment. Place it beneath a purple candle, which you have dressed with Compelling Oil. Burn the candle for 15 minutes daily until the debt is repaid.

Crown of Success Oil

⅓ part Sunflower carrier oil

⅓ part Orange

⅓ part Allspice

Ambergris, a few drops

Gold glitter added to bottle

Used to attract the favor of the gods and their aid in all aspects of your life.

Crown of Success Oil II

⅓ part Sandalwood

⅓ part Neroli

$\frac{1}{16}$ part Orange

$\frac{1}{16}$ part Honeysuckle

5 drops Clove

Stops vicious gossip and envy and brings the user the success he or she seeks.

Customer Attraction Oil

¼ part Rose

¼ part Patchouli

¼ part Cedarwood

¼ part Orange

Elderberries added to bottle

Used both to bring customers and to stabilize business. Anoint green candles and burn in the place of business. Or make an incense, spray mist, or floor wash from the scent.

Easy Times Oil

⅔ part Lilac

⅓ part Clove

Piece of cut-up one-dollar bill in master bottle.

Will aid the wearer in getting anything desired more easily, whether it be money, material goods, affection, or _____?

Fast Money Oil

¼ part Patchouli

¼ part Cedarwood

¼ part Vetiver

¼ part Ginger

Wear, rub on the hands, or anoint green candles to bring money. Also, anoint money before spending to ensure its return!

Fast Money Oil II

½ part Basil
¼ part Ginger
¼ part Tonka

Use the same as directed above.

Fast Money Oil III

¼ part Oakmoss
¼ part Cedarwood
¼ part Patchouli
¼ part Ginger

This is a Scott Cunningham recipe. It's amazing; it smells like money! You can anoint candles with it and concentrate on your need for money or resources, or you can anoint cash before spending it, or in a charm to have money return to you.

Fast Money Oil IV

½ part Honeysuckle
¼ part Mint
¼ part Vervain
Rub this on your hands or your money to attract financial prosperity!

Follow Me Boy Oil

½ part Jasmine
½ part Rose
Vanilla, a few drops
Piece of coral
Gold glitter

The traditional version of this product also contains a piece of coral and gold glitter. It was favored by New Orleans prostitutes to ensure they would make plenty of money through the appreciation of their passions.

Follow Me Boy Oil II

½ part Jasmine
½ part Opium

A great oil to wear if you work for tips!

Ganesha Oil
½ part Sandalwood
¼ part Coconut
⅛ part Honeysuckle
⅛ part Ambergris

Ganesha is the Hindu god of success and wealth who removes the obstacles that bar your way to attaining your dreams.

Gold and Silver Oil
½ part Honeysuckle
½ part Jasmine
Coconut, a few drops

Use as a daily perfume to entice fun and excitement into your home and life.

Gold Buddha Oil
⅛ part Frankincense
½ part Heliotrope
¼ part Cinnamon
⅛ part Bay

Use to aid you in prosperity spells. When mixing these oils, focus on confidence and success.

Goona-Goona Oil
⅓ part Nutmeg
⅓ part Orris
⅓ part Rose
Patchouli, a few drops

Used to create an atmosphere of trust and understanding, to reduce tensions when dealing with difficult people. It's also good for those working in retail situations.

Has No Hanna Oil
½ part Rose
½ part Gardenia
An open safety pin in a bottle

Used to keep the wearer from losing things, especially love or money.

Has No Hanna Oil II

¼ part Apple Blossom

¼ part Sandalwood

¼ part Cinnamon

This New Orleans voudoun formula for luck has been around for quite a long time.

Hetep Oil

⅓ part Myrrh

⅓ part Allspice

⅓ part Cinnamon

To attract success and prosperity.

High Conquering Oil

High John Root in bottle

½ part Vetiver

½ part Bergamot

A very powerful means of attracting wealth, prestige, love, and health. Use generously when changes are desired. Works rather quickly. One of the best oils for good work.

High John the Conqueror Oil

½ part White musk

¼ part Bayberry

¼ part Sandalwood

Verbena, a few drops

Patchouli, a few drops

Keep a Jalep Root in master bottle. This oil makes you unstoppable and enables you to accomplish anything. It is strong good-luck oil and very effective when gambling. Rub your palms with the oil before engaging in games of chance. To obtain money, love, and health, anoint a green candle with High John the Conqueror Oil and burn it completely. This ritual works best if you start on a Sunday and repeat daily for seven days.

Horn of Plenty Oil

½ part Apple Blossom

¼ part Cherry

⅛ part Vanilla

⅛ part Lime

Khus Khus, a few drops

Rub on forehead and body to force a change of fortune. This oil helps the practitioner overcome poverty and brings him or her much wealth and prestige.

Horn of Plenty Oil (Cornucopia)

½ part Vanilla

⅛ part Anise

⅛ part Apricot

⅛ part Peach

⅛ part Orange

For great wealth and other awards and esteem, carry a design known as the Second Pentacle of Jupiter with you at all times. This is one of the many magical seals of Solomon that can be found in the Greater Key of Solomon. The design is "proper for acquiring glory, honors, dignities, riches, and all kind of good, together with great tranquility of mind." It is also used to discover treasures and chase away the Spirits that preside over them. Anoint the talisman every Sunday to keep its power potent. Protect it by keeping it in a clean white cloth.

I Can, You Can't Oil

¼ part Palma Christi

¼ part Rose

⅛ part Magnolia

⅛ part Narcissus

⅛ part Apple Blossom

⅛ part Wisteria

Use this oil when an enemy is trying to "diminish" you in any way (take away your job, lover, or is spreading gossip about you, etc.). Sprinkle this oil on an object she/ he must touch. After the charm is set, spend no further thought or energy on the problem. It will be taken care of its time and in a way that is to your advantage and benefit.

Inspiration Oil

¼ part Pine

¼ part Lily

¼ part Hyacinth

¼ part Clove

Sprinkle on someone who needs a boost in morale. It builds confidence and inspires someone to do good deeds. It also causes the wearer to become more optimistic and creates a festive atmosphere.

Interview Oil
½ part Ylang-Ylang
½ part Lavender
Rose, a few drops

Wear to interviews of all kinds to calm you. Helps make a favorable impression.

Inspiring Oil
⅓ part Hyacinth
⅓ part Ambergris
⅓ part Vanilla

Are you in need of a mystic muse? Someone to inspire you when you feel your creativity is being blocked? Wear this oil when you're tackling a job that seems overwhelming.

Instigation Oil
¼ part Allspice
¼ part Vanilla
¼ part Orange
¼ part Clove

This oil will aid in causing others to become motivated to begin new projects. It also aids in the accomplishment of difficult endeavors. This oil has mild commanding and compelling qualities have positive effects, but use caution.

Invigorating Oil
¼ part Grapefruit
¼ part Mandarin Orange
¼ part Tangerine
¼ part Geranium

To increase your strength and endurance both emotionally and physically. Helps to bring out, focus, and amplify your best qualities.

Jyoti Oil
½ part Galangal
½ part Patchouli

Nasturtium seeds (powdered)

Use while trying to overcome the hex of an enemy and to gain financially. Purifies and protects when sprinkled or rubbed around the premises.

King Solomon Oil
⅓ part Solomon's Seal
⅓ part Hyssop
⅓ part Rose

Brings forth wisdom and intuitiveness. Makes the user more psychic than before. Draws wealth. Use in a ritual where your faculties are to be called into play.

King Solomon Oil II
Solomon's Seal (a few drops) or herb (1 to 2 leaves)
½ part Rose
½ part Frankincense

This blend is for gaining the wisdom that results in improved wealth.

Millionaire's Dream Oil
⅓ part Sandalwood
⅓ part Bayberry
⅓ part Cinnamon
Peach, a few drops

If you want to be the one—and are willing to take the necessary steps to gain that goal—start with the following prosperity chant each morning and anoint the temples with a drop of oil.

For silver and gold, I now pray,
Send me my needs, do not delay.
More and more, I now request
For this reward I'll do my best.
Piles of money at my feet,
Oh, blessed be, it is so sweet.—Lady Rhea

Money Oil
¼ part Frankincense
⅛ part Heliotrope
⅛ part Bay
⅛ part Orange

⅛ part Cinnamon
¼ part Sandalwood

To use in any financial situation to increase fortune. Use to anoint green candles to bring money into the home.

Money and Luck Oil

¼ ounce Olive Oil
⅓ part Nutmeg
¼ part Oak Moss
¼ part Bergamot
9 drops Earth
9 drops Tonka
6 drops Clove
8 Dill Seeds

Draws money and luck. It is important that this recipe be followed in the order listed. Be sure to have your mind in the right place when formulating this blend.

Money-Drawing Oil

¼ part Patchouli
¼ part Cedar
¼ part Vetiver
¼ part Ginger

This is the classic oil for drawing money to you.

Money-Drawing Oil II

½ part Honeysuckle
¼ part Hyacinth
¼ part Lotus
Sandalwood, a few drops

Rub on the inside of your wallet each day and anoint the four corners of all bills in your possession once a week.

Money-Drawing Oil III

⅓ part Marjoram

⅓ part Lemon

⅓ part Eucalyptus

Gypsies roll their bills rather than keeping then flat. Smearing the outside bill with this oil is believed to attract cash.

Money Fast Oil

½ part Patchouli

¼ part Cedarwood

¼ part Vetiver

Ginger, a few drops

Wear, rub on the hands, or anoint green candles to bring money. Also anoint money before spending to ensure its return.

Money Fast Oil II

½ part Basil

¼ part Ginger

¼ part Tonka Bouquet

An oil to assist in drawing ready cash when you need it quickly for a necessity.

Money House Blessing Oil

¾ part Sandalwood

¼ part Neroli

Cinnamon, a few drops

To be rewarded with enrichments aplenty before the day is done, recite this small rhyme as you apply the oil to the nape of your neck and your wrists each morning after your bath or shower:

Fruit in the cupboard,
Bread in the house,
Money in the pocket,
Love and friends hereabout. ~Lady Rhea

Money Magnet Oil

½ part Patchouli

¼ part Pine

¼ part Bay

Use to aid you in prosperity spells. When mixing these oils, focus on confidence and success.

Money Mist Oil

¼ part Frankincense
¼ part Neroli
¼ part Sandalwood
$\frac{1}{16}$ part Vetiver
$\frac{1}{16}$ part Bay
Nutmeg, a few drops

Rub on your wallet to attract fantastic amounts of money and to protect the cash you do have on hand.

More Money Oil

¼ part Prosperity Oil (page 153)
¼ part Money-Drawing Oil (page 150)
¼ part Road Opener Oil (page 174)
¼ part Success Oil (page 162)

This is an all-purpose oil to wear when job hunting, gambling, or making decisions about important purchases. Use it to anoint your palms before work or a job interview. Also anoint your credit cards, lottery tickets, etc. Try to think of uses for it that will bring you money. And put a drop of the oil on each business letter you send.

Nine Indian Fruits Oil

Equal parts of the following:

Watermelon
Cherry
Orange
Coconut
Vanilla
Strawberry
Almond
Apple
Kiwi (or Lime)

This oil brings networking, prosperity, harmony, and new partnerships.

Oak Moss Bouquet

¾ part Vetiver
¼ part Cinnamon

Use to attract money. Dilute and wear or rub into cash before spending.

Pentacles Oil

¼ part Sandalwood
¼ part Amber
¼ part Clove
¼ part Lotus

In the Tarot, Pentacles stand for the material plane, money, possessions, and situations of satisfaction. This oil represents the wealth of the Earth. Use this oil to obtain unusual treasures and wealth.

Positive Energy Oil

½ part Dragon's Blood
½ part Sandalwood
Frankincense, a few drops
A bit of Saffron

Used to increase energy in any situation. It also negates any bad influences from the area.

Prosperity Oil

⅓ part Frankincense
⅓ part Sandalwood
⅓ part Myrrh
Allspice Berries added to the bottle

This oil is designed to bring ready cash.

Prosperity Oil II

¼ part Almond Fragrance Oil
¼ part Honeysuckle
¼ part Bayberry
¼ part Mint

Use this oil to anoint your wallet or purse.

Prosperity Oil III

⅓ Almond fragrance oil
⅓ part Bergamot
⅓ part Pine

Brings abundance, wealth, and success in whatever venture you wish.

Prosperity Oil IV

¾ part Heliotrope
⅛ part Cinnamon
⅛ part Bay

This oil draws riches and abundance on all levels.

Shaman Oil

⅓ part Lemon Verbena
⅔ part Rose
Cedar, a few drops

Use to aid you in prosperity spells. When mixing these fragrances, focus on confidence and success. Use in working shamanic magic.

Shi Shi Oil

⅓ part Clove
⅓ part Bay
⅓ part Angelica

Draws wealth and overcomes poverty. Alleged to work very quickly. Very helpful to those who need a stroke of fortune. Anoint a green candle and burn for seven nights for fifteen minutes. Can also anoint a dollar bill and keep it folded in your wallet.

Shi Shi Oil II

¾ part Carnation
¼ part Peppermint

Gives fast results in spells to overcome poverty or increase wealth; also can help uncross or draw things to you.

Showers of Gold Oil

¼ part Bay
¼ part Sandalwood

¼ part Frankincense
¼ part Myrrh
Cinnamon, a few drops
Benzoin, a few drops

Use when long-term wealth is desired.

Thrifty Oil

¾ part Lavender
¼ part Basil

Should you require the generosity of friends, relatives, or complete strangers, their willingness to part with their money can be increased if this oil is rubbed surreptitiously onto the back of their hands.

Tonka Bouquet

Benzoin
A few drops Vanilla tincture (extract)

This has been used for a long time in creating artificial vanilla, which was widely sold in the United States until it was determined that it was a health hazard. This warm, vanilla-like scent can be included in money recipes. Try creating your own scent with the above recipe.

Three Kings Oil

½ part Frankincense
¼ part Rose
⅛ part Myrrh
⅛ part Cinnamon

Many talents, endowments, and favors may come to those who use this perfume. Apply it to the temples for wisdom, to the throat so that you speak only kindly and with truth, and to the wrists so that the hands will be helpful to those in need.

Job & Financial

Arabka Soudagar Oil

¾ part Frankincense
¼ part Tonka
Frankincense tear in bottle

Use whenever business is bad. It is said to bring luck and financial gain.

As You Please Oil

⅓ part Neroli
⅓ part Musk
⅓ part Cinnamon

Use this to bring success in almost any endeavor. It is formulated to overcome the objections of others to your plans. Apply it to the fingertips, soles of the feet, and throat just before you present your ideas or plans, and others will be willing to go along with your proposals.

Binding Job Oil

¼ part Heliotrope
¼ part Musk
¼ part Patchouli
¼ part Ambergris
Civet, a few drops

Especially developed for bringing final resolution to job-hunting efforts. Used on application or resume to secure an interview. Worn as a personal oil for the interview, it may result in an offer of employment.

Black Panther Oil

½ part Orris
¼ part Vanilla
⅛ part Clove
⅛ part Lavender

Bestows confidence in your own abilities. This oil is especially good for a salesperson.

Blue Indian Oil

½ part Sandalwood
⅛ part Cinnamon
⅛ part Benzoin
⅛ part Lavender
⅛ part Neroli

Helps with cash flow.

Boss Fix Oil

10 drops Musk
Chili Powder, a pinch
Tobacco, a pinch
Pulverized Newsprint
Enough oil to cover (I use sunflower)

Let jar sit in a dark place for seven days. Shake every other day. Strain. Sprinkle around your boss's office at work and your own work area to get him or her to leave you alone to work. It helps stop harassment and, when used in private life, it will cause others to treat the wearer with more consideration.

Business Success Oil

¾ part Bergamot or Mint Bouquet
⅛ part Basil
⅛ part Patchouli
1 pinch of ground Cinnamon

Mix the oils, then add the pinch of Cinnamon. Anoint the hands, the cash register, business cards, or the front door of the place of business to increase cash flow.

Chango Macho Oil

¼ part Frankincense

¼ part Coconut fragrance oil

⅓ part Musk

¼ part Cinnamon

⅛ part Apple Blossom (optional)

An exhilarating fragrance specially formulated to draw wealth. This blend was created to honor the powerful Santerian god Chango. His specialties are business, dancing, romancing, and finances.

Employment Potion Oil

Equal parts of all:

Sandalwood

Patchouli

Clove

Frankincense

Nutmeg

Anoint wrists, palms, and soles of feet before an interview. *Not for internal consumption.*

Employment Pyramid Oil

¼ part Honeysuckle

¼ part Gardenia

¼ part Musk

5 drops Cinnamon

This oil is designed to help you find a new job or get a promotion. It is also great for freelancers and the self-employed who are seeking work, clients, business partners, contacts, and so on.

Empowerment Oil

½ ounce carrier oil (choose one from the list of carrier oils)

1 pinch Purple Basil

1 pinch Myrrh

1 pinch Cinnamon

Place the herbs in the carrier oil and let it sit in a dark place for two weeks beginning at the New Moon. Shake daily. On the Full Moon, strain through a coffee filter into a clean bottle. Place the herbs in a compost or in the garden. Designed to promote personal empowerment.

Flame of Desire Oil

⅓ part Cinnamon
⅓ part Galangal
⅓ part Bay

Use to become irresistible, or to make anybody want anything. Good for a salesperson.

Gypsy Gold Oil

½ part Musk
½ part Lily of the Valley
Magnolia, a few drops
Honeysuckle, a few drops

Helps to promote steady work for freelancers, or to remedy employment problems.

Job Interview Oil

½ part Ylang-Ylang
½ part Lavender
Rose, 2 to 3 drops

Wear to interviews to calm you and make a favorable impression.

Job Oil

⅓ part Heliotrope
⅓ part Hyacinth
⅓ part Patchouli
Cinnamon, a few drops

A personal-anointing or ritual-anointing oil used to speed up the job-hunting process and ensure its success.

Ju Ju Oil

¼ part Myrrh
¼ part Mimosa
¼ part Jasmine
¼ part Patchouli

An extremely powerful oil used to cross enemies and uncross clients. A very protective item. Also, when worn, will make the wearer alluring, bewitching, and seductive. It is a protective oil that helps guard the wearer from hexes.

Master Oil

½ part Bayberry
½ part Musk
A few grains of Dragon's Blood Powder

A man's oil for love and luck. Popular conjuring oil used in all love matters, also brings luck and power. Anoint a brown candle with a drop or two of the oil. Or rub the oil on the palms of your hands when going to important business meetings or any other situation where you must be self-possessed and confident.

Memory Oil
¼ part Clove
¼ part Coriander
¼ part Rosemary
¼ part Sage

To increase focus, clarity, and retention.

Memory Drops Oil
¼ part Rosemary
¼ part Vanilla
¼ part Cinnamon
¼ part Clove
Honey, a few drops

Improves the mental processes, great for students and people working with a large population. Assists in remembering names, numbers, and locations.

Nine Mysteries Oil
⅔ part Orange
⅓ part Violet
Wintergreen, a few drops

Excellent for overcoming all domestic or business troubles. Sprinkle around a business or a home as a blessing. Burn as a blessing or attractant incense, or anoint candles with the oil to bring a speedy change in fortune.

Nuada Oil
¼ part Frankincense

⅛ part Cinnamon
½ part Jasmine
⅛ part Lily of the Valley
Clove, a few drops
Rose, a few drops
Strip of Willow Bark in bottle (optional)

Used to worship or invoke the God. It is used in money magic to bring prosperity. This oil is an all-purpose Solar blend with old Celtic energy.

Success Oil

¾ part Bergamot Mint Bouquet
⅛ part Basil
⅛ part Patchouli
1 pinch ground Cinnamon

Anoint the hands, the cash register, business cards, or the front door of the place of business to increase cash flow.

Success Oil II

¼ part Orange
¼ part Vanilla
¼ part Peach
¼ part Rose
Allspice, a few drops

The God of Victory should smile on anyone who rubs this oil on currency, coins, and money containers. Wear it as a perfume so that your undertakings in all areas of your life will thrive, flourish, and bear fruit.

Sweet Success Oil

Use equal parts of the following oils:

Neroli	Jasmine
Frankincense	Bayberry
Gardenia	Bay
Sandalwood	Nutmeg

To assist you in getting the job done and succeeding in any venture you wish.

Wall Street Oil

½ part Sandalwood

¼ part Musk
⅛ part Vetiver
⅛ part Rose

This oil is to help would-be investors achieve their dreams. It assists you in making the right decisions.

Wealthy Way Oil

¾ part Tonka Bouquet
¼ part Vetiver

Wear to attract wealth in all forms. Also anoint candles and burn while visualizing the abundance you seek.

Wealthy Way Oil II

⅓ part Jasmine
⅓ part Vanilla
⅓ part Lotus
Frankincense, 3 drops
Nutmeg, 3 drops
Allspice, 3 drops
Cinnamon, 3 drops

This oil is worn to attract riches, especially when worn to bingo games or the race track, or while indulging in any games of chance.

Luck & Legal

Chinese Luck Oil
⅓ part Neroli
⅓ part Jasmine
⅓ part Ylang-Ylang
Rain perfume oil, a few drops (optional)

Chinese Luck Oil is a favorite blend for improved luck, wealth, and harmony.

Court Case Oil
½ part Hyacinth
½ part Lily of the Valley
Lavender, a few drops

This blend is designed to protect the user against the wrath of the court and to obtain judgment that is favorable. It is used as a anointing oil for candles, or worn as a perfume.

Court Oil
Safflower Oil carrier oil
¾ part Bergamot
¼ Allspice
Piece of High John the Conqueror Root

Believed to carry you through legal proceedings with serenity and back into the free world when they are concluded. Pure anointing oil for external use only.

Day in Court Oil

⅓ part Cinnamon
⅓ part Anise
⅓ part Sandalwood
Carnation Petals, in master bottle
Galangal Root, in master bottle

To ensure a fair and impartial hearing.

Dragon's Hoard Oil

⅛ part Clove
⅛ part Patchouli
½ part Frankincense
⅛ part Pine
⅛ part Bergamot

Helps you find opportunity and resources.

Drawing Oil

½ part Lavender
¼ part Bayberry
⅛ part Rose
⅛ part Lemon
Almond, a few drops

To draw anything toward you.

Drawing Oil II

½ part Orange
¼ part Frankincense
⅛ part Bay
⅛ part Myrrh

A powerful force for bringing money, luck, or love to the one who wears this as a perfume.

Elegua Oil

¼ part Honeysuckle
¼ part Coconut fragrance oil

¼ part Cinnamon

⅛ part Sandalwood

⅛ part Vetiver

Elegua is the ruler of our paths in life. He is the keeper of the keys to the gates of destiny. He opens roads and gives great success where it is warranted. He is a protector of your path. If your road is closed, then use this oil on white candles to open your path or tell you why it is closed so that you may learn the lesson and grow from your experience.

Fast Luck Oil

½ part Patchouli Oil

¼ part Carnation

¼ part Mimosa

Use to turn bad luck to good luck in a hurry.

Fast Luck Oil II

½ part Patchouli

½ part Rose

Juniper, a few drops

Use to aid you in prosperity spells. When mixing these oils, focus on confidence and success.

Friendly Judge Oil

½ part Carnation

¼ part Anise

¼ part Cinnamon

Use when dealing with courts and lawyers. Add to bathwater for three days before a court date. Rub on arms, bosom, and throat on the court date. Rub on fingers before signing legal papers.

Get Out of Jail Oil

¼ part Dragon's Blood

½ part Coconut fragrance oil

¼ part Nutmeg

Have the person working with you place this oil on all paperwork that has to be signed. Just a little dab on the finger and then touching all the paperwork will do.

Good Luck Oil

1 tablespoon dried Wormwood

3 teaspoons ground Nutmeg

½ teaspoon powdered Mandrake Root

13 drops Pine fragrance oil

¼ cup Olive Oil

Brings good luck, especially in any psychic working, astral travel or divination.

Good Luck Mystic Oil

¼ part High John the Conqueror

¼ part Galangal

¼ part Cinnamon

¼ part Squill

A highly spiritual blend that helps you receive prophetic dreams.

Happy Times Oil

⅓ part Orange

⅓ part Vanilla

⅓ part Violet

Changes luck and reverses unfortunate circumstances. Also assists in eliminating poverty.

Helping Hand Oil

½ part Vanilla

¼ part Wintergreen

⅛ part Jasmine

⅛ part Oleander

Narcissus, a few drops

Used in court situations. It will bring peace to a stormy marriage or aid in any kind of domestic or household troubles.

High John the Conqueror Oil

½ part Violet

½ part Lavender

3 drops Juniper

3 drops Heliotrope

Brings about favorable results in all your undertakings.

Hoodoo Just Judge Oil

½ part Carnation
¼ part Anise
¼ part Cinnamon

Use 2 tablespoons of this mixture to 2 ounces carrier oil. Add a piece of Galangal Root to each bottle. Put some in your bathwater before any confrontations. Also use as a perfume on your pulse points. Carry a Galangal Root, John the Conqueror Root, with Snake Root or Indian Tobacco in a small bag anointed in the oil. Give this oil added punch with Van Van Oil. I would also carry a Horse Chestnut dressed in Van Van Oil.

Jockey Club Oil

½ part Bergamot
¼ part Coconut fragrance oil
⅛ part Clover
⅛ part Ylang-Ylang
Heather, a few drops

Used to anoint talismans of luck or letters before mailing them. Also used to uncross.

Jury Winning Oil

½ part Hydrangea
¼ part High John
¼ part Galangal
Asafetida, just a pinch

A traditional oil to be sprinkled on a judge's feet or in the jury box to help in a court case. Anoint a purple candle with this to help in issues of law.

Jury Winning Oil II

¼ part Frankincense
¼ part Cinnamon
¼ part Myrrh
¼ part Benzoin
Heliotrope, a few drops

When faced with court proceedings, it can be advantageous to copy Psalm 20 with Dove's Blood ink onto parchment paper. Take the talisman to court each day, anointing the corners with this blend just before court begins to turn the wheels of justice to your favor.

Just-Judge Oil

Violet Leaf in bottle
¼ part Myrrh
¼ part Patchouli
½ part Rosewood

This is worn to court when justice is in the balance and mercy is needed to tip the scales in your favor.

Just-Judge Oil II

¼ part Patchouli
¼ part Sandalwood
¼ part Hyacinth
¼ part Dragon's Blood

Another preparation to protect against negative results in court cases. It is said to guarantee favor, compassion, and fairness from the magistrate's bench.

Lady Luck Oil

½ part Frangipani
½ part Musk
Vanilla, a few drops
Carnation, a few drops
Cinnamon, a few drops

For good fortune to smile on your cards, numbers, or horse, be sure the money you wager is rubbed with this oil before placing the bet. It can also be used as a perfume or rubbed on the back of the hands when playing games of chance.

Law-Stay-Away Oil (Espanta Policia)

To 2 ounces of carrier oil add contents of one vitamin E capsule and equal parts of the following herbs:

Anise
Dragon's Blood
Licorice Sticks (not the candy)
Deer's Horn Powder

Let sit for several weeks and shake daily. Strain through cheesecloth and bottle. Assists in helping you become invisible to the law.

Lodestone Oil
½ part Rose
¼ part Frankincense
⅛ part Myrrh
⅛ part Cinnamon
Add iron filings and a small lodestone to the bottle

For anointing magnetic lodestones, or wear to develop good fortune and change bad luck to good.

Luck Around Business Oil
⅓ part Honeysuckle
⅓ part Dark Musk
⅓ part Neroli

Place a green candle near the entrance to your shop, anoint it with the oil, and burn during business hours.

Luck Oil
⅓ part Basil
⅓ part Bayberry
⅓ part Vervain

This oil helps you turn bad luck to good. Be sure to wear it when going out for any game of chance. May be worn as a daily perfume as well.

Lucky Bingo Gold Oil
⅓ part Jasmine
⅓ part Ambergris
⅓ part Orange

Dress all the lucky charms you like to carry with this oil.

Lucky Dog Oil
¼ part Vanilla
¼ part Cinnamon
¼ part Strawberry
¼ part Watermelon

A favorite of gamblers who believe it attracts favorable vibrations. Used to anoint Southern John Roots—7 drops once a week is said to keep them healthy and active.

Lucky Job Oil

¼ part Honeysuckle

¼ part Jasmine

⅛ part Amber

¹⁄₁₆ part Clove

¹⁄₁₆ part Allspice

Cinnamon, a few drops

Assists you in being at the right place at the right time when it comes to employment.

Lucky Life Oil

½ part Cinnamon

¼ part Chamomile

¼ part Peony

Add a Tonka to each bottle

To gain favor from the Faerie folk and to give you help in any game of chance.

Lucky Lodestone Oil

½ part Cinnamon

½ part Lavender

Lodestone in bottle

Excellent all-around oil for developing good fortune and changing bad luck to good.

Lucky Lottery Oil

¼ part Neroli

¼ part Rose

¼ part Jasmine

¼ part Musk

A specially prepared scent for anointing tickets to increase their chance of winning.

Lucky Nine Oil (Nine Mystery)

Equal amounts of all:

Musk	Bergamot
Rose Geranium	Citrus (orange, lemon)
Sandalwood	Allspice
Frankincense	Vervain
Myrrh	

Bless your business or home to overcome domestic and business troubles. Also works as an attractant. Or, anoint candles with this for success, to bring speedy change in fortunes.

Lucky Number Oil

½ part Neroli
½ part Musk

When purchasing lottery tickets, choosing a bingo card, or selecting a number of any kind for gambling purposes, anoint the fingertips of both hands before the ticket, card, or number is chosen.

Lucky Oil

½ part Olive Oil
¼ part Myrrh
¼ part Jasmine

Anoint the feet before putting on shoes.

Lucky Oil II

⅓ part Thyme
⅓ part Anise
⅓ part Mint
Olive Oil, a few drops

Add a sprig of mint to the bottle for extra effectiveness.

Lucky Root Oil

⅓ part Cinnamon
⅓ part Benzoin
⅓ part Vetiver
Vetiver Root herb, whole

This is a luck oil that is especially effective when added to an herbal charm bag.

Lucky Thirteen Oil

½ part Coconut fragrance oil
¼ part Almond fragrance oil
¼ part Sandalwood

Take away all the unfavorable implications of thirteen with this oil. It also eliminates the negative and accentuates the positive aspects of your life.

Madama Oil

½ part Jasmine
¼ part Peach
¼ part Rose

Madama's job is to set everything right, to furnish protection, to keep away all harm, and to provide wealth and good luck in the home. The Spirit of Madama is a fierce protector of all her charges.

Magnet Oil

¼ part Cinnamon
¼ part Rose
½ part Rose Geranium
A lodestone in master bottle with iron filings

Similar to Lodestone Oil, this blend attracts all kinds of good fortune to the wearer.

Red Fast Luck Oil

¼ part Cinnamon
¾ part Vanilla
Wintergreen, a few drops

To bring luck in any situation; it works extremely well with changing bad luck to good very quickly.

Road Opener Oil

⅓ part Sandalwood
⅓ part Honeysuckle
⅓ part Vanilla
Gardenia, a few drops

This oil removes problems and obstacles in your path. Opens the road to success and improves your luck in everyday affairs. A good standard oil to have on hand.

Road Opener Oil II

⅓ part Sandalwood
⅓ part Honeysuckle
⅓ part Vanilla
Carnation, a few drops

The goal of this oil is to be objective and to give a miracle or extra luck when needed.

Seven Knots Candle Wish Oil

⅓ part Lilac
⅓ part Vanilla
⅓ part Lily of the Valley

This oil is for making wishes come true. It was created for the candles that have seven knots or balls in order to make a specific wish on each knot. To use, anoint each knot with this oil, light the candle, allow it to burn down one knot, and then extinguish it. Repeat this action each day/night until your candle is finished.

Special Favors Oil

¼ part Lime
¼ part Carnation
¼ part Gardenia
¼ part Wintergreen

Attracts friendly nature spirits. Anoint altar or room for best of luck and success.

Special Oil #20

⅓ part Gardenia
⅓ part Jasmine
⅓ part Lily of the Valley

When your luck really "sucks," you need Special Oil #20!

Success Oil

2 parts powdered Sandalwood
2 parts Five Finger Grass (Cinquefoil)
2 parts Frankincense Tears
1 part powdered Cinnamon
1 part grated Lemon Peel or Lemon Flowers

Use 2 tablespoons of this mixture in 2 ounces of oil.

Optional: Add a small piece of High John Conqueror Root to each bottle of oil made. Brings success in whatever venture you wish. Let the root steep in the oil for two weeks beginning at the New Moon. At the Full Moon strain it into a clean bottle through a coffee filter. Keep in a cool, dark place.

Van Van Oil

¼ part Vanilla
¼ part Vetiver
½ part Lemon
Rose, a few drops

Brings luck (whether love or money) quickly to any work.

Van Van Oil II

¼ cup Olive Oil
1 ounce Lemongrass
Pinch of salt

Use to anoint candles, doorways, and amulets for extra power. Let lemongrass soak in the Olive Oil for six weeks. Shake every other day. Strain through a coffee filter into a clean glass bottle, label, and store in a dark place.

Van Van Oil III

¾ part Vanilla
¼ part Rose
Almond fragrance oil, a few drops

Many, many uses for this oil. Anoint charms, seals, or talismans with it to increase their powers. Dress candles with it for more potency, particularly the Seven-Knob Wishing Candles under which you have placed your secret desire written on parchment paper. Worn on the arms and shoulders, the oil attracts interest and love. For uncrossing, use 7 drops in the bath for seven consecutive days.

Win at Court Oil

⅓ part Frankincense
⅓ part Heliotrope
⅓ part Musk

Ease your way through the justice system by wearing this as your perfume whenever you are consulting with attorneys or going into court before the judge or jury.

Gambling

Algiers Oil
⅓ part Vanilla
⅓ part Patchouli
⅓ part Cinnamon

To attract romance, and luck in gambling.

Beneficial Dream Oil
¾ part Lavender
¼ part Ylang-Ylang
Musk, a few drops

This oil is designed to assist you in playing the lottery. Place 7 drops in a container filled with water, and place it on the nightstand before you go to bed. Ask your Guides or Spirit Guides to help you find your lucky numbers while you sleep.

Chypre Oil
¾ part Vanilla
¼ part Cinnamon
Frankincense, a few drops

Rub on hands before gambling for luck and guaranteed winning. Also brings other financial gain. This is most effective when your hands actually come into contact with the gambling materials (dice, cards, etc.).

Fortuna Oil

¼ part Frankincense
¼ part Lemon
½ part Lavender
Citronella, a few drops

Fortuna Oil is especially good for anointing lucky charms, and yellow and orange lucky candles. It is also said to disperse the energies of luck in your favor when rubbed on the palms of the hands before playing games of chance. A typical Puerto Rican practice is to buy a lottery ticket and place it beneath a candlestick holding a dripless yellow candle anointed with this oil. The candles should be held in the hand and anointed from the middle of the shaft to the top and then from the middle to the base, as this symbolically addresses the wish for luck to Heaven and to the energies manifesting on Earth.

Gambler's Luck Oil

½ part Cinnamon
¼ part Carnation
¼ part Anise

Place a small piece of High John the Conqueror Root in each bottle of oil. Anoint charms designed to bring luck in gambling. Or rub it on the palms before gambling. Anoint each corner of your bingo card before the game begins. Anoint your shoes before you go to the race track.

Gambler's Oil

½ part Lily of the Valley
¼ part Sandalwood
⅛ part Mimosa
⅛ part Cinnamon
Rose, a few drops

Use to aid you in prosperity spells. When mixing these oils, focus on confidence and success.

Gambler's Lucky Charm Oil

½ part Rose
¼ part Carnation
¼ part Apricot

Use a one-ounce or larger bottle when blending this oil, as you will need extra room to add these additional ingredients: Marigold Flowers, Vetiver Root, Chamomile Flowers, gold glitter, one penny, a pinch of iron filings, and a paper dollar bill (optional). Rub on hands and use to anoint all lucky charms.

Gypsy Gold Oil

½ part Orris
¼ part Frankincense
⅛ part Vetiver
⅛ part Sandalwood
Bergamot, a few drops
Gold glitter

For fast luck in finances or gambling.

Haitian Gambler Oil

⅓ part Patchouli
⅓ part Lemon
⅓ part Jasmine

Use to banish a stream of even the worst luck. Very good for anointing talismans, seals, Ouanga bags (used in Voudoun), playing cards, etc.

Haitian Gambler Oil II

¾ part Jasmine
¼ part Vanilla
3 drops Strawberry

The Haitian voudoun practitioners are reputed to have great powers when it comes to gambler's luck, and this oil invokes that luck.

Herb Oil

½ part Basil
½ part Oregano
¼ part Sage
⅛ part Thyme
⅛ part Lemon

Brings good luck in gambling and will increase the memory of anyone who wears it. Also commonly used as a health oil.

Jamaica Bush Oil

⅓ part Patchouli
⅓ part Vetiver
⅓ part Lemon
Jasmine, a few drops

Can help the wearer in any gambling or investments. It attracts good fortune in all areas of life. Use with caution.

Mad Oil

¼ part Capsicum (Cayenne pepper works well)
¼ part Ammonia Crystals
¼ part Coriander
¼ part Pine

Brings luck and success to the user. Clears channels for success. Use sparingly, as this can be used to hex others by driving them to insanity. Use on talismans, poppets, candles, and so forth. *Do not* wear.

Prosperity Oil

¼ part Sandalwood
¼ part Lotus
¼ part Dark Musk
¼ part Carnation
Lotus, a few drops

Very similar to Wealthy Way Oil. It attracts and draws luck and success in business deals and in gambling.

Sure to Win Oil

⅓ part Vetiver
⅓ part Lotus
⅓ part Musk

Rub on hands before playing cards, dice, or roulette, or anoint one's bingo card, lottery ticket, or any other gambling paraphernalia to sway luck in your direction.

Ten Silvers Oil

⅓ part Clove
⅓ part Pine
⅓ part Lilac
½ ounce carrier oil

To attract the things one needs, also good for gamblers; to bring raise in salary.

Three Jacks Oil

¼ part Galangal
¼ part Vetiver
¼ part Patchouli
¼ part Cardamom

Anoint the palms, the forehead, and a candle with this before any gambling venture.

Three Jacks Oil II
⅓ part Clove
⅓ part Vetiver
⅓ part Cinnamon

The luckiest of all the good-luck oils. New Orleans gamblers always rub it on their hands before opening a deck.

Three Knaves Oil
Same as Three Jacks Oil.

Winner's Circle Oil
¼ part Vanilla
¼ part Musk
¼ part Gardenia
¼ part Narcissus

This oil was designed more than just for games of the chance gambler. This blend is for the person who has a dream of walking to his or her own beat and hitting it big.

Winner's Circle Perfume
¼ part Sandalwood
¼ part Orris
¼ part Allspice
¼ part Musk
Deer's Tongue, a few drops

This blend is sometimes simply called Winner's Oil. This blend assists acquiring riches in gambling ventures.

Gods & Goddesses

In modern Pagan religions, people feel drawn toward many of the ancient gods. While this is by no means a complete list, it's a good place to start. Other gods and goddesses are sprinkled throughout the book, according to their powers.

Anubis Oil

¼ part Cinnamon
¼ part Low John
¼ part Cedar
¼ part Orris
Myrrh, a few drops

To invoke or worship the Egyptian god of the Underworld; to get rid of unwanted things. Also for protection of canine companions and their place and belongings; helps in any undertakings involving travel to the Underworld.

Arianrhod Oil

⅓ part Cedar
⅓ part Grape Seed
⅓ part Honeysuckle
Silver glitter

Warm all ingredients (except the glitter) in an enamel pan on low heat. Allow to cool; add the glitter and place in a pretty clear bottle. Arianrhod is the Welsh goddess of reincarnation, and the goddess of the astral skies. Use this oil to anoint your third eye when traveling in the Astral Realm.

Artemis Oil

¼ part Lemon
¼ part Rose
⅛ part Violet
⅛ part Narcissus
¼ part Ylang-Ylang
Carnation, a few drops

To worship or invoke the goddess. Use to attain goals, and for luck in sports, especially for female athletes.

Astarte Oil

¼ part Sandalwood
¼ part Rose
⅛ part Orange
⅛ part Jasmine

To invoke or worship the Phoenician goddess. For works of fertility, love, or war.

Athena Oil

¼ part Honeysuckle
¼ part Carnation
¼ part Neroli
¼ part Musk

To invoke or worship the Phoenician goddess. Use to civilize a situation and to achieve goals.

Baphomet Oil

½ part Vetiver
¼ part Cypress
¼ part Patchouli

Rub this ritual-spell oil on items relating to Baphomet.

Blodeuwedd Oil

⅓ part Lily of the Valley
⅓ part Violet
⅓ part Honeysuckle
Lemon Balm herb in bottle

To invoke or worship the goddess. Use to civilize a situation and achieve goals.

Cerridwen Oil

¼ part Sandalwood
¼ part Rose
⅛ part Jasmine
⅛ part Orange
⅛ part Patchouli
⅛ part Civet
Camphor, a few drops

To invoke or worship the goddess. This oil induces inspiration, aids in shape shifting and acquiring occult knowledge.

Danu Oil

½ part Dragon's Blood
½ part Vervain

Danu is the principle of birth and beginnings, of generation and fertility. Danu is the prime mover, she who came before everything else. As an aspect of the Great Mother, she encompasses both light and dark, both giving and receiving. Use this oil to help wash away discord and bring back balance into your life.

Dark Huntress Oil

½ part Jasmine
¼ part Verbena
¼ part Dragon's Blood

Use to aid you in binding spells.

Demeter Oil

½ part Myrrh
¼ part Vetiver
¼ part Oak Moss Bouquet

Anoint candles or other items to attract money and for the successful completion of your protections and dreams. Also wear when planting, tending, harvesting, or working with herbs and plants to ensure a fruitful yield. Helps you tune into the energies of the Earth.

Diana Oil

Equal amounts of all:

Nutmeg

Benzoin

Vanilla

Patchouli

Cinnamon

Vetiver

Myrrh

Bay

To invoke or worship the goddess; used in accomplishment of goals. This is a good all-purpose lunar ritual oil. It is also good for anyone working with animals.

Egyptian Oracle Oil

⅛ part Acacia

¼ part Sandalwood

¼ part Patchouli

⅛ part Cinnamon

Authentic 2,000-year-old recipe very typical of its time. It is used to raise vibrations.

Egyptian Protection Oil

⅓ part Amber

⅓ part Civet

⅓ part Frankincense

Juniper, a few drops

Ambergris, a few drops

Use this blend for daily protection, especially when doing magic pertaining to Ra, the Sun God.

Egyptian Temple Oil

¼ part Myrrh

¼ part Frankincense

¼ part Lotus

⅛ part Mimosa

⅛ part Ambergris

This is an exotic blend especially for use as an anointing oil or as an incense for practitioners of the Egyptian magical arts.

Elegua Oil

¼ part Honeysuckle

¼ part Coconut

¼ part Cinnamon

⅛ part Sandalwood

⅛ part Vetiver

Elegua is the ruler of our paths in life. He is the keeper of the keys to the gates of destiny. He opens roads and gives great success where it is warranted. He is a protector of your path. If your road is closed, then use this oil on white candles to open your path or tell you why it is closed so that you may learn the lesson and grow from your experience.

Forest Lord Oil

¼ part Patchouli

¼ part Cedar

¼ part Dark Musk

¼ part Violet

Lemongrass, a few drops

Sandalwood, a few drops

For working with the Dark Lord and The Hunt.

Goddess of Evil Oil

Iron filings

22 drops Galangal

Pinch of Black Horsehair

2 ounces carrier oil

Let this sit from one New Moon to the next New Moon (approximately twenty-eight days). Strain and bottle. Protects the wearer from all bad spells and allows him or her to cast hexes on others; use on a voudoun doll for bad intentions.

Green Man Oil

¼ part Cedar

¼ part Citronella

¼ part Spruce

⅛ part Patchouli

⅛ part Vetiver

Cinnamon, a few drops

Orange, a few drops

To invoke and work with the Lord of the Forest.

Hecate Oil
¾ part Myrrh
¼ part Cypress
Patchouli, a few drops
1 dried Mint leaf

Mix the essential oils in a base of sesame oil. Add the dried mint leaf to the blend. Wear during rituals of defensive magic. Also wear during the Waning Moon in honor of Hecate, goddess of the fading crescent.

Hecate Oil II
⅛ part Rose
¼ part Myrrh
½ part Patchouli
⅛ Lotus

Use to worship or invoke the goddess, or to work in any of her attributes

Hecate Oil III
½ part Vetiver
½ part Jasmine
Myrrh, a few drops

She is the mother of the Underworld, goddess of magic and mystery. Invoke her powers for counsel and wise wisdom. When there is a problem that is too difficult for you to handle, ask her guidance and protection from harm.

Heka Oil
¼ part Musk
¼ part Myrrh
⅛ part Olibanum
⅛ part Benzoin
⅛ part Balm of Gilead
⅛ part Cassia
Lotus, a few drops

Used to invoke or worship the magical and holy aspect of the goddess Hecate.

Hermes Oil

⅓ part Lavender

⅓ part Mastic

⅓ part Cinnamon

Use to invoke or worship the god. It aids in the development of concentration and creativity.

Hermes Oil II

½ part Sandalwood

¼ part Cinnamon

¼ part Rose

Other names for Hermes are Mercury, Thoth, Ganesha, Elegua, and Eshu. He is the god of merchants and new inventions.

Horned God Oil

¼ part Frankincense

¼ part Cinnamon

⅛ part Bay

⅛ part Rosemary

¼ part Musk

Wear to invoke and worship the Horned God.

Horus Oil

⅓ part Frankincense

⅓ part Myrrh

⅓ part Heliotrope

Lotus, a few drops

Orange, a few drops

Used to invoke or worship the god; brings qualities of radical change.

Ishtar Oil

¼ part Sandalwood

¼ part Rose

¼ part Orange

¼ part Jasmine

Wear to honor the goddess during rituals.

Ishtar Love Oil

¼ part Sesame Seed

¾ part Sandalwood

To invoke or worship the goddess, or work with the qualities of love and war combined.

Isis Oil

¼ part Lotus

¼ part Cypress

¼ part Frankincense

¼ part Rose Geranium

Helps increase determination, will power, and the ability to concentrate.

Isis Oil II

¼ part Lotus

¼ part Frangipani

¼ part Musk

¼ part Black Narcissus fragrance oil

The purpose of this oil is to invoke the goddess Isis in Circle.

Jezebel Oil

⅓ part Ylang-Ylang

⅓ part Jasmine

⅓ part Rose

Rose Petals, in bottle

Red Jasper, in bottle

Used by a woman to control a man. It can cause people to offer you things that you need.

Jezebel Oil II

⅓ part Frankincense

⅓ part Frangipani

⅓ part Heliotrope

A secret formula used by women who wish to have their way with any man, as it can cause males to do their bidding without question.

Jezebel Oil (Do as I Say/Man Tamer)

½ part Palma Christi

¼ part Bergamot

¼ part Ginger Blossom

Dark Musk, a few drops

Like Jezebel Oil II, this oil is used by women to ensure men do their bidding.

Kali Ma Oil

⅓ part Patchouli

⅓ part Musk

⅓ part Amber

Or

⅓ part Lotus

⅓ part Patchouli

⅓ part Musk

Optional ingredients (small pinches may be added to individual bottles): cemetery dirt, grains of paradise (Guinea pepper), Black Pepper, Dragon's Blood, a few drops of red wine, and sulfur.

Goddess Kali Ma is known as the "slayer of demons." Petition Kali Ma in times of danger, when all other attempts at protection have brought no results. She will defend you against all harms and crush the evil in your life and those who would strongly oppose your ability to live freely. She is the great mother of wisdom and the slayer of the ego. It is said that she will slay those whose egos unjustly oppose yours.

Lilith Oil

⅓ part Lily of the Valley

⅓ part Jasmine

⅓ part Lotus

Used to invoke or worship the goddess, or kick your enemy's butt from here to kingdom come.

Merlin Oil

¼ part Vetiver
¼ part Pine
¼ part Green Forest
¼ part Oak Moss Bouquet
Cypress, 5 to 6 drops
Rose Geranium, 5 to 6 drops
Clove, 2 to 3 drops

For wisdom and clarity when working in the magical realms. Helps with understanding and working with sigils.

Merlyn's Might Oil

½ part Dragon's Blood
¼ part Vanilla
¼ part Ginger

To boost your magical powers and protection in all magical endeavors.

Morrigan Oil

½ part Lavender
¼ part Cypress
¼ part Apple Blossom
Pinch of Dragon's Blood Resin
1 hawthorn berry

Used to invoke or worship the goddess. Morrigan can aid you in battle, overcoming enemies, prophetic efforts, and Waning Moon and banishing magic.

Obeah Oil

⅓ part Jasmine
⅓ part Violet
⅓ part Orange
Wintergreen, a few drops

Much prized by sorcerers and voudounists, who use it in magical rites and rituals. To remove any evil spirit, have the bewitched one wear a piece of Burdock Root in a bag around the neck. As you place the necklace on the person, anoint the crown of the head with the Obeah Oil and have the jinxed one count from 50 to 1. As the jinxed one is counting backwards, you count from 1 to 50 in the usual order. This spell should banish any curse, and its effectiveness should last for 50 days, after which it can be repeated if necessary.

Obitzu Oil

⅓ part Jasmine

⅓ part Violet

⅓ part Citronella

Use to keep away evil. This general protective oil is made according to an ancient and very secret recipe. Use the oil in a sub-ritual within a major uncrossing ritual to add efficacy.

Oshun Oil

½ part Jasmine

¼ part Rose

¼ part Neroli

5 drops Cinnamon

5 drops Anise

(Honeysuckle can be substituted for any one of the oils above)

The number five is the sacred number of the goddess Oshun, the Santerian goddess of love and marriage. She is the African Aphrodite. This blend celebrates beauty, pleasure, and dancing.

Osiris Oil

¼ part Lavender

¼ part Lemon

¼ part Violet

⅛ part Orris

⅛ part Cardamom

Used to worship or invoke the god. Brings luck; helps those involved in agriculture of any kind; enhances the understanding of resurrection and rebirth.

Pan and Astarte Oil

¼ part Bayberry

¼ part Musk

¼ part Rose

¼ part Ylang-Ylang

Fertility oil; perfect to wear to your favorite rites of spring.

Pan Oil

⅔ part Patchouli

⅓ part Juniper
Pine, a few drops
Oak Moss Bouquet, a few drops
Cedarwood, 2 to 4 drops

Wear to be infused with the spirit of Pan. Ideal for magical or ritual dancing, music making, singing, and so on. Also for attuning with the Earth.

Pomona Oil

⅓ part Frankincense
⅓ part Strawberry
⅓ part Cardamom
Tangerine, a few drops

To invoke or worship the goddess of cultivation. It helps the wearer to see plans to fruition and will provide a priest to anyone who invokes this goddess.

Rhiannon Oil

½ part Dragon's Blood
½ part Rue
1 pinch Paprika
Piece of Rose Quartz

For working with the goddess of the magical arts, birds, and the Underworld.

Rites of Isis Oil

½ part Rose
¼ part Camphor
¼ part Blue Hyacinth
Tincture of Myrrh, a few drops

Blend the oils of Rose, Camphor, and Blue Hyacinth during the Waxing Moon. Bottle and keep till the Moon wanes. Add the Myrrh at that time.

Sekmet Oil

¼ part Verbena

¼ part Galangal

¼ part Peppermint

¼ part Rue

Cinnamon, a few drops

To worship or invoke the goddess while protecting the wearer.

Seven African Powers Oil

Equal amounts of all:

Rose

Orris

Frankincense

Vetiver

Bay

Lavender

Lemon

Traditional voudoun mixture; invokes the seven archetypal forces of African mythology.

Star of the Sea Oil

⅓ part Rose

⅓ part Lily of the Valley

¼ part Ambergris

To honor and invoke the goddess of the sea, Aphrodite.

Strega Oil

½ part Vetiver

¼ part Juniper

¼ part Lavender

Honey, a few drops

This ancient oil is from an authentic Italian recipe and is used in witchcraft. It represents matriarchal power and strength.

Saints & Angels

The saints information would not exist if it wasn't for the assistance of the most incredible witch, Lady Maeve Rhea and her book *The Enchanted Formulary.* (Citadel Press, 2006) and the amazing store Magickal Realms (Enchanted Candle Shoppe Inc.) Thank you and may your lives be blessed!

I'm sure you've seen the glass-encased, seven-day candles with pictures of the saints on them that are sold at many supermarkets and botanicas. These candles can be lit in the honor of your chosen saint, in an appeal for help and guidance from him or her. The following recipes can be used to anoint to the tops of these candles. They can also be used in incense and placed on an altar next to a picture or statue of a saint or added to diffusers on an altar or dressed on any candle or part of the body as a blessing oil.

All Saints' Oil
To 2 ounces base oil, add equal parts:

> Cinnamon
> Tonka
> Patchouli
> Vanilla
> Lavender
> Gardenia
> Vetiver

Anoint candles in rituals to bring added success. This is an African-inspired classic and is a powerful anointing oil for uncrossing rituals, healing success, and where the cooperation of the highest spiritual planes is desired. Each of the seven African deities is represented by an herbal oil. It is both loving and powerful in the effect it has when used on white, yellow, or blue candles.

Angel Blessing Oil
> ¼ part Lavender
> ¼ part Rose
> ¼ part Ylang-Ylang
> ¼ part Frangipani

Removes negative vibrations and energies and increases your ability to draw to you what you need and want.

Angel Brilliance Oil
¾ part Bergamot
¼ part Neroli
Rose, a few drops
Cinnamon, a few drops

Brings light and energy into your life. Works best on yellow candles. Prepare this blend by pouring the oils in a 10-ounce bottle and then adding organic vegetable oil to fill. Anoint the third eye, sacrum, and solar plexus. Pour a few drops into the palm of your hands and inhale deeply. May use in the bath as well.

Faith, Hope, and Charity Oil
⅓ part Honeysuckle
⅓ part Wisteria
⅓ part Lily of the Valley

These three goddesses give us the light we need when times seem really dark. You can call on them for any purpose, at any time.

Four Angels Oil
Mix equal parts of the following:
Michael—Cinnamon
Raphael—Carnation
Gabriel—Lavender
Uriel—Musk

This oil can be blended together to represent the power of the four angels united, or the oils can be used individually to represent the power for that specific angel.

Gran Poder Oil
½ part Honeysuckle
½ part Lily of the Valley

Rose, 3 drops

The name means "Great Power." This oil is for overcoming great troubles, often to remove curses, jinxes, and hexes.

Guardian Angel Oil

½ part Rose
½ part Lilac
Vanilla, 10 drops

You can anoint yourself with this oil during times of prayer, during meditation for guidance, and in times of stress when you need something to calm you.

Justice Judge Oil (Justo Juez)

¼ part Rose
¼ part Carnation
¼ part Lily of the Valley
⅛ part Camphor
⅛ part Sandalwood

In Santeria, the Justice Judge is often called Olofi, Earth's guardian, one of the aspects of God. Since Jesus is believed to be a guardian of the people, Olofi was associated with the crucifixion, and so Justice Judge candles have an image of the crucifixion on them. He protects you from earthly harm, gives justice to one's enemies, and is used as a shield from evildoers. Very often he is prescribed in unfair court cases and triumphs for the underdog. Use this oil for justice spells, especially in court cases.

La Candelaria Oil

½ part Jasmine
½ part Gardenia
Strawberry, 5 drops

La Candelaria is one of the guises of the Santerian goddess Oya. This is Our Lady of Conflagration. She is fiery in her aspect and is often depicted holding a candle. Her birthday is February 2, which is also the Wiccan holiday Candlemas, Imbolc, or Lady Day. It is the day that marks the warming of the Earth. In Brazil, her name is Yansa, and she is considered a woeful adversary to all enemies of her devotees. In Ireland, she is Brid, or Brigit, and is a goddess of creativity and of the forge.

You can use this oil for any Fire spell, or for transformation and creativity. Great in a diffuser or burned as an incense, and of course, perfect for anointing candles.

Madonna Loretto Oil
½ part Magnolia
½ part Frangipani
Cedarwood, 3 drops

This Mother goddess helps all who ask her find a home. Her image is often depicted in one of two ways: as a virgin with no arms or as a woman seated on top of a house. Use her oil on seven-day Madonna Loretto candles. If you keep an altar, anoint this oil on a small figure of a house, or a photograph or drawing of one.

Mercedes Oil
⅓ part Frangipani
⅓ part Ylang-Ylang
⅓ part Ambergris
Or
¼ part Magnolia
¼ part Lavender
¼ part Lily of the Valley
¼ part Lilac

The Virgin Mercedes is associated with the Santerian god Obatala. This father god calms and protects. He helps clear the mind and sharpen the senses. His female counterpart is Our Lady Mercedes. She is a Blessed Virgin and is often invoked to protect people from prison and other desperate situations. She is a goddess of mercy and is compassionate to all who seek help. She clears the mind when it is clouded and confused. Use this oil for clarity in confusing situations and for mercy in times of desperation.

Milagrosa Oil
⅓ part Lotus
⅓ part Rose
⅓ part Lily

Milagrosa means "Miraculous Mother." She is also known as the Virgin Mary. If you need a miracle, pray to Milagrosa and ask for guidance. Anoint a blue or white candle with the oil, and place your petition below the candle holder. (Safety first.)

Ocean Mother Oil
½ part Ambergris
¼ part Lotus

⅛ part Opium fragrance oil
⅛ part Lily
Sandalwood, a few drops

This oil is for devotional use for all water deities. The Santerian goddess Yemaya is a water goddesses and is also known as the Virgin Regla. Water is a great psychic conductor. Many psychics can see the future with a bowl of water rather than a crystal ball. This oil is for opening up your psychic intuition, and it will help you tap into a similar process, especially if you gravitate toward this aspect of the Great Mother.

Our Lady of Fatima Oil

½ part Rose
½ part Sandalwood

Our Lady of Fatima is the Queen of the Holy Rosary, Mother of Peace. She is a miracle maker and answers those who pray to her with sincere devotion. Use this oil on seven-day Fatima candles, and anoint all talismans and rosary beads for prayer and healing.

Our Lady of Lourdes Oil

½ part Rose
½ part Lily of the Valley

Our Lady of Lourdes is the goddess of a miraculous grotto where countless pilgrims come to be saved, witness miracles, and be healed of all calamities that affect the body and soul. This oil can be used for healing and easing suffering of all sorts.

Our Lady of Mount Carmel Oil

⅓ part Sandalwood
⅓ part Carnation
⅓ part Lily of the Valley

Our Lady of Mount Carmel is an aspect of the Santerian goddess Oya. She has great powers to remove obstacles and to protect from harm all who worship her. This oil is especially powerful as an uncrossing oil to be used in times of desperation.

Sacred Heart Oil

¾ part Rose
⅛ part Lemon
⅛ part Heliotrope

The Sacred Heart is the miraculous, all-healing Son of God (or in Pagan belief systems, Sun God). People use this blend to help heal sickness, whether physical or those of the heart and mind. A wonderful oil for anointing the stones you carry.

Saint Alex Oil (An Alejo)

⅓ part Cinnamon
⅓ part Allspice
⅓ part Frankincense

This saint is known for chasing away all evils, demons, and wrongdoers. Invoke his presence to protect you from people who would cause you harm. For example, this formula will help squelch malicious gossip, hide you from bullies, and keep you and your loved ones safe. It can also be used for cleansing and healing when someone has already done you harm.

Saint Anna Oil

½ part Rose
¼ part Violet
⅛ part Lavender
⅛ part Sandalwood

This saint is the mother of Mary and the grandmother of Jesus Christ. She is for all grandmothers who want to make prayers on behalf of their grandchildren. We also pray to her for help in learning and education, as she was an excellent teacher to her daughter Mary. Anoint seven-day candles for guidance. Dab on books, or your computer, or whatever tools you use for educating yourself. Anoint a charm to give to a grandchild for protection.

Saint Anthony Oil

½ part Sandalwood
¼ part Ylang-Ylang
¼ part Musk
Carnation, a few drops
Patchouli, a few drops

Saint Anthony is the miracle worker. If you have lost something, he can help you find it. He restores wealth to the needy and intercedes on behalf of the poor in financial and legal matters. He is associated with the Santerian god Elegua. Saint Anthony is the patron saint of marriage and lost things and is also know for helping sick animals. Anoint a green candle and ask for his guidance to help an ailing pet. Dab some on your paper money before you spend it to have it returned to you.

Saint Barbara Oil

¼ part Coconut fragrance oil
¼ part Honeysuckle
¼ part Cinnamon
¼ part Sandalwood

This saint is often associated with the Santerian god Chango, and they have many similarities. He holds a two-headed axe; she holds a double-edged sword. One of his symbols is a tower; she is also often depicted with a tower. They both wear a crown. She is associated with lightning; he is the god who sends lightning down from the heavens. If you have a need for protection in business affairs, this is a great oil to work with.

Saint Christopher Oil

½ part Vanilla
½ part Carnation
5 drops Opium fragrance oil

Saint Christopher is the patron saint of travelers. Although the Catholic Church no longer recognizes Saint Christopher as a canonized saint, that doesn't stop longtime practitioners from invoking his aid in travel. Use the oil to anoint yourself or a talisman or charm for protection during travel, whether it is a daily route or a long voyage. Dab some on the dashboard of your car. You can also use it on yourself as a protection from any danger.

Saint Clara Oil

⅓ part Rose
⅓ part Lilac
⅓ part Carnation

Or

⅓ part Carnation
⅓ part Vanilla
⅓ part Wisteria

Many people turn to Saint Clara when someone they care about is blinded by anger or high emotion, and that person cannot see clearly. She is prayed to for her abilities to calm down angry husbands, wives, children, and sweethearts. She brings peace and clarity to stressful situations. This is a great oil to make incense with or to use in a diffuser to infuse your home when emotions are running high.

Saint Elijah Oil

½ part Heliotrope
¼ part Neroli
⅛ part Sandalwood
⅛ part Vetiver

Saint Elijah is called Baron Del Cementario, "Baron of the Cemetery," in Santeria. This powerful saint is invoked for the destruction of enemies. In Spanish, he is San Elias. He is called on during times of need where dangers abound in life and well-being has been threatened. He removes all black magic and the dark energies that come from a psychic attack, defeats all enemies, and works wonders in setting things right.

You can anoint this oil on your front door if you feel that unseen forces are attacking you. Or dab some on a talisman and wear until the problem is resolved.

Saint Expedito Oil

¼ part Allspice
¼ part Sandalwood
¼ part Honeysuckle
¼ part Ambergris

This oil is for pushing things forward and making them happen quickly. It is also for general luck, especially in gambling. Saint Expedito is associated with Elegua. He is very popular in New Orleans, where practitioners leave offerings associated with gambling (such as small sets of dice and playing cards) at his statue. Use this oil when you need something to happen quickly. It is a great supplement oil to any spell.

Saint Francis of Assisi Oil

⅓ part Sandalwood
⅓ part Apple Blossom

⅓ part Musk

Saint Francis of Assisi is known for his love of all humankind, and he is also associated with the god Orunla, who rules divination in the Santerian belief system. He assumed an attitude of martyrdom and deprivation to expound on his acts of kindness towards others. I recommend this blend for healing any sick animal, pet, or human loved one. This is also a great oil to use for finding a new pet. Soon the animal you are looking for may just show up at your door. This oil can be used for divination work of any kind: Tarot, scrying, runes, and so on.

Saint Helena Oil
⅓ part Apple Blossom
⅓ part Orange Blossom
⅓ part Peach

Saint Helena is often prayed to in order to aid in returning straying lovers. The sweet allure of these intoxicating florals is what makes this blend work so well. Drunk on the scent of the perfume, she uses her seductive powers to get your lover to come back. No man can resist the call of Helena! Anoint pink figure candles facing each other with this oil. Keep them lit for fifteen minutes per day and gradually move them closer. Repeat the process until both the candles have finished burning and the male candle has reached the female candle.

Saint Joseph Oil
½ part Frankincense
¼ part Sandalwood
¼ part Lily of the Valley
Olive Oil, a few drops

Saint Joseph was the earthly father of Jesus, the husband of Mary, and a simple carpenter. He is the original family man and will send counsel to those who are having trouble keeping the family together. He is also very well known for helping sell one's property. Bury a statue of Saint Joseph upside down in your back yard while you are trying to sell your house. I suggest you anoint the statue with the oil first! Then when the property is sold, dig the statue up, clean it, and give it a place of honor in your new home.

Saint Jude Oil
⅓ part Bayberry
⅓ part Cinnamon
⅓ part Jasmine

Saint Jude is the saint of impossible causes. He cures the incurable, grants the impossible, and favors the needy. All he asks in return is that you make public notice of his answered prayers. You may have seen dollar bills posted on walls with "Thank you, Saint Jude, for answering my prayers" written on the money. Or maybe you've seen public thank-yous posted on bulletin boards, or notices in the newspaper, offering praise and thanks. I often refer my clients to this saint when they have told me that everything they have tried has failed. Anoint green or white candles with the oil.

Saint Lazarus Oil

½ part Sandalwood
¼ part Musk
⅛ part Lavender
Vetiver, a few drops
Patchouli, a few drops

This saint is invoked often and is dearly loved for his work in healing the sick, giving money to the poor, cleansing both spiritual and physical wounds, and being a great protector of his followers from spiritual harm. This saint is associated with the Santerian god Babalu Aye. He rules over all health matters, cleansings, and wealth matters. Use this oil on a seven-day novena Saint Lazarus candle, or any candle in yellow, purple, or gold.

Saint Lucy Oil

⅓ part Lavender
⅓ part Gardenia
⅓ part Rose
Basil, a few drops
Violet, a few drops

Saint Lucy is the patron saint of Sicily. She is an important saint who settles all disputes, cures all illnesses having to do with the eyes, and removes the evil eye (a very important factor for some Italians). She gives a good harvest and sees to it that you get justice. Look to her for help in legal problems.

Saint Martha Oil

¼ part Gardenia
¼ part Vetiver
¼ part Carnation
¼ part Ambergris

Saint Martha helps separated couples reunite. A fierce protectress of her followers, she shields them from harm and defends them against spiritual attacks. She helps find money and work for the unemployed and needy. This oil can be used to bring back a straying lover, defeat all who would stop you from success, help provide you with work, and, most of all, lend you the strength to change and accept what you cannot change.

Saint Martin Oil

½ part Frankincense
½ part Rose
Orange, a few drops

This is the first black American saint. He is from Peru and was born in poverty, but he never rejected it. Instead, he used it to help himself and countless others. He is known as the healer of the sick and one of the first veterinarians. Anoint this oil on a seven-day Saint Martin novena candle, and ask for his help. You can also use purple, white, or green candles.

Saint Michael Oil

½ part Musk
¼ part Frangipani
¼ part Carnation
Cinnamon, a few drops

Saint Michael is a fierce protector of all that is righteous and good. But this is not his only purpose. The following is a meditation practice Lady Rhea has written to invoke the guidance of Saint Michael—or any angel or guide.

Anoint this oil on your temples, on the sides of your neck, inside your wrists and on the soles of your feet. Choose a red taper candle and dress it with the oil. Place it on a low table so that you are more or less at eye level with your candle when you are seated on the floor. Shut out all the lights, and sit in a cross-legged position, comfortably as you can manage on the floor. Take a deep breath, hold for at least ten seconds, and then exhale. Repeat this several times until you are relaxed and the candle has begun to change its image. It may move in and out of your vision. The candle may flicker intensely. Call on Michael to descend and communicate with you. Ask for guidance and it shall come to you. Feel the glow surround you as his guiding light engulfs your being. Listen to what he has to say. Perhaps he will not use words, but rather he will make you feel something instead. When this feeling has passed, allow the candle to continue to burn until it is finished as an offering to Saint Michael.

Saint Peter Oil

⅓ part Frankincense
⅓ part Myrrh
⅓ part Sandalwood

Saint Peter is the keeper of the gate and the keys to the Kingdom of Heaven. He was bestowed the gift of binding and loosening—he has the powers to stop something or to set something free. This saint is associated with Elegua, who is the keeper of the keys that open and close the doors of life. You can invoke Saint Peter when you want to close or open a doorway in your life. For instance, if you want to close the doors on ill fortune, anoint a candle with this oil and say, "O Saint Peter, lend me your golden key, open the lock and unleash all manner of blessings upon me." Use this oil on all seven-day saint candles for Saint Peter and Elegua.

Saint Teresa Oil

¾ part Rose
¼ part Lilac

Saint Teresa does great acts in small, humble ways for those who are devoted to her. It is said that if you make a sincere prayer to her, sometimes right before she answers you someone will give you a rose or a flower. So you know your answer is on the way. Use this oil to produce small miracles in your life, or someone else's. She is equated in Santeria with an aspect of Oya. Candle colors are pink and white.

Seven African Powers Oil

Equal amounts of the following:

Frankincense: Olofi—Justo Juez
Coconut: Chango—Saint Barbara
Sandalwood: Elegua—Saint Anthony
Magnolia: Obatala—Virgin Mercedes
Cinnamon: Oshun—Caridad Del Cobre
Ambergris: Yemaya—Virgin Regla
Lotus: Orunla—Saint Francis
Myrrh: Ogun—Saint John the Baptist

Pour each ingredient very slowly, or use a dropper, when blending this oil. It is best to mix this by the ounce, or more, to get the measurement right. The famous "Seven African Powers" are the seven orishas (deities) that make up the pantheon of Santeria. Special seven-day novena candles are available in seven different colors with a picture of the orishas in their saint aspects painted on the glass. This family of powers is very popular, as you have all the realms of life covered here. Each power covers a specific area in life. Use this blend to anoint any seven colored candles, or a Seven African Powers candle to bring balance into your life.

Nine African Powers Oil

Add the following oils to the Seven African Powers Oil:

> Vetiver: Oya—Saint Martha
> Lavender: Babalu Aye—Saint Lazarus

Use it as you would use the Seven African Powers Oil, to bring balance to all aspects of your life.

Virgin Guadalupe

> ½ part Rose
> ¼ part Jasmine
> ¼ part Vanilla
> Carnation, a few drops

The Virgin Guadalupe—the Holy Mother of Mexico—answers the prayers of her people and followers. She is considered one of the Miraculous Mothers of the world and has millions of followers of many different faiths. She is a good one to turn to in times of illness, hunger, and desperate need. If you are suffering financial difficulties, ask for her blessing when using her oil. Anoint this oil on a seven-day Virgin Guadalupe novena candle for blessings. Green, blue, and yellow candles will work also.

Hexing, Banishing & Uncrossing

The witches of old were often in demand for their ability to hex and curse murderers, rapists, child molesters, and other unsavory sorts. Witches and "root-workers" were often the only healers to be found in the villages of old. Their knowledge of herbs, roots, minerals, and other natural remedies was legendary. Use these oils when all else fails and justice must be done. Curses don't have to be the dark deeds of magical villains. They can be the common negative energy that ordinary psychic vampires bombard us with daily. Here I have a list of oils that should do the trick if you should have to do a little work on the "dark" side.

Agarbatti Chandan Oil
½ part Lavender
½ part Hyssop

To overcome adversity, hexes, and bad luck.

Banishing Oil
½ part Frankincense
⅛ part Rosemary
⅛ part Bay Laurel
⅛ part Angelica
⅛ part Basil

To banish anything unwanted in your life.

Banishing Oil II

⅓ part Carnation
⅓ part Basil
⅓ part Rue

Should you have unwanted visitors from time to time, and your cool reception has not discouraged them, write their names on a small square of parchment paper. Anoint each corner of the paper with this oil and bury the charm on the pathway to your doorway. Those whose names are scribed on the talisman will soon cease their unwelcome visits.

Banishing/Exorcism Oil

3 whole Cloves
2 cloves Garlic
¼ Basil mixed with carrier oil

This works wonderfully on neighbors whom you would like to move. Just rub some of the oil on their doorknobs. If neighbors are of the spiritual nature, place dabs of oil on all mirrors in the home. Let the cloves of garlic sit in the carrier oil for six weeks. Shake the mixture every few days. Strain through a coffee filter and bottle tightly.

Bat's Blood Oil

¾ part Magnolia
¼ part Peppermint

Used in practice of black arts to create discord, tension, and havoc; used on voudoun fetishes.

Bat's Eye Oil

⅓ part Myrrh
⅓ part Dragon's Blood
⅓ part Bayberry

Use with a real bat's eye when working with evil spirits to hex someone who has wronged you; highly dangerous to the operator. *Use with caution.*

Bend Over Oil

½ part Rose
¼ part Frankincense
¼ part Honeysuckle
Vetiver, a few drops

Makes other people do your bidding. Use to break any hexes and to order evil spirits to return to their sender. Said to be extremely potent.

Black Arts Oil

¼ part Myrrh

¼ part Patchouli

⅛ part Cinnamon

⅛ part Gum Mastic

⅛ part Galangal

⅛ part Vetiver

Sage, a few drops

Special crossing oil used only for placing hexes on hated competitors. *Use with extreme care.*

Black Arts Oil II

One double boiler

Grape Seed or Olive Oil

2 teaspoons Mullein Herb

1 teaspoon Wormwood Herb

1 tablespoon Patchouli Herb

3 Blackberry Leaves

1 teaspoon Mandrake

1 tablespoon Myrrh Resin

Graveyard Dirt (optional)

Put water in the bottom part of the double boiler and the herbs and about a cup of oil in the top part of the boiler. Boil the water and let the herbs steep in the oil for approximately ten minutes. When the oil is well scented with the herbs, strain thoroughly and put in a bottle or jar. Add 9 drops of 190-proof alcohol (Everclear) to the brew to preserve it. *Note: You can use the above direction to make any type of oil from herbs.*

Black Arts Oil III

½ part Patchouli

½ part Black Pepper fragrance oil

Pinch of Valerian Root

Pinch of black poodle dog hair

Pinch of Black Mustard seeds

Pinch of Spanish Moss

Pinch of Mullein

Pinch of powdered Sulphur

9 whole Black Peppercorns

Blend into ½ ounce carrier oil, such as Almond. For all works of hexing, banishing, and cursing. Works extremely well to rid yourself of a person or situation that you cannot rid yourself of in any other way.

Black Devil Oil

¼ part Bay
¼ part Frangipani
¼ part Lavender
¼ part Cinnamon
Pinch of Sugar or Salt

Mixed with sugar and salt to stop a married man or woman from playing around. It should be carefully sprinkled on their undergarments while they sleep.

Compelling Oil

⅓ part Clary Sage
⅓ part Lavender
⅓ part Pine
3 Calamus Roots or use (Marigold leaves) in master bottle

Optional: Roll a candle in Mugwort and/or Nutmeg blend; swirl and anoint candle in spell. Wear near the person from whom you want the truth. They do not stand a chance of lying.

Confusion Oil

To 2 ounces of base oil, add contents of one vitamin E capsule and:

½ part Coconut
¼ part Lavender
¼ part Violet
¼ part Black Pepper
2 drops Ginseng

Will help to confuse others who are working against the wearer or user; an aid in breaking hexes, it will work better when a hex is "fresh," but will also work for older curses.

Confusion Oil II

2 parts Rue Herb
1 part Guinea Pepper

Add 2 tablespoons of this to 2 ounces of oil and steep for a few weeks in a dark place, or over low heat for about an hour. Then cool and strain through cheesecloth.

Conquering Glory Oil

¼ part Sandalwood

¼ part Bayberry

¼ part Tonka

¼ part Orange

To kick ass in any contest and gain power over others, no matter what the purpose.

Conquering Glory Oil II

¼ part Sandalwood

¼ part Bayberry

¼ part Tonka

¼ part Orange

To gain power over others, write their names on parchment and place the paper beneath a purple candle that you have anointed with the oil. Light the candle and repeat this little chant seven times quickly:

(Name), (Name), do as I say,

For I know what's best for you.

(Name), (Name), this I pray,

Follow me to Timbuktu.

Controlling Oil

¼ part Clove

¾ part Vetiver

1 part Calamus Root in master bottle

Keep a piece of licorice root in a master bottle for the energies this blend needs. Use to anoint all spell items.

Controlling Oil II

⅓ part Clove

⅓ part Vetiver

⅓ part Storax

Particularly useful with love rituals. Use on a red male figure candle. Also effective when mixed with voudoun doll stuffing herbs.

Controlling Oil III

2 tablespoons Calamus
2 ounces Olive Oil

Place three drops of this oil on another's shoe. To have better control over a situation or person, write the situation or the person's name on a piece of paper, place the paper under a purple candle dressed with this oil. Burn daily until the candle is consumed, and your dominance over the situation or person should be established.

Crossing Oil

Mix equal parts:
Wormwood
Pepperwort

Put 2 tablespoons of mixture into 2 ounces of Olive Oil. You may add a small piece of Ivy Root to each bottle of oil to enhance its power. Use on candles or charms used in rituals designed to curse another.

Curse-Breaker Oil

¾ part Sandalwood
⅛ part Bay
⅛ part Bergamot

Anoint a black candle and burn for seven nights during the Waning Moon to assist you in breaking a curse.

Do as I Say Oil

⅓ part Patchouli
⅓ part Musk
⅓ part Lotus

For self-control, self-mastery, and self-confidence, one should wear this daily. It imparts assuredness that others bend to the will of the wearer without even being aware they are under another's spell.

Domination Oil

½ part Patchouli
¼ part Vetiver
⅛ part Lime
⅛ part Frankincense

Keep a piece of Calamus Root in the master bottle. Use in all ways of domination. Anoint seals, mojo bags, candles, etc.

Domination Oil II

½ part Cinnamon
¼ part Allspice
¼ part Vanilla

Anoint your body with this oil to make others do as you wish. You will have the ability to dominate a situation with power and confidence.

Double-Cross Oil

¼ part Myrrh
¼ part Mimosa
¼ part Jasmine
¼ part Patchouli
Clove, a few drops

A magical blend that spans the disciplines of different traditions of folk magic. Double-Cross Oil was created to turn back any negative magic and undo the hex of an adversary practitioner.

Double XX (Hexing Oil)

Lemon Oil
Plus all other odds and ends from spent bottles of blended formulae

Confuses enemies. Wear behind your knees and ankles, and inside your elbows. Use at business meetings with unethical people; it will turn the situation in your favor.

Dragon Protection Oil

¼ part Amber
¼ part Dark Musk (plain Musk may be substituted)
¼ part Rue
¼ part Almond

Mix oils, then add 1 pinch of sea salt and 1 or 2 small pieces of Dragon's Blood Resin and a small piece of Amber. Wear as a personal oil to enhance your powers and to call on the dragon's power, protection, and wisdom.

Dragon's Blood Oil

½ part Musk
½ part Myrrh
Dragon's Blood Resin (optional), a few grains

This oil is for getting rid of evil and dark magic.

Druid's Curse Oil

⅛ part Dill
¼ part Galangal
¼ part Anise
¼ part Myrrh
Hyssop, a few drops

To kick ass in any contest and gain power over others, no matter what the purpose.

Escaping Oil

⅓ part Cedarwood
⅓ part Cypress
⅓ part Rosemary

To get anything to go away or to get out of a negative situation, no matter what. When used on a doll to represent a person, it will remove that person from your life.

Espanta Muerta Oil

½ part Peppermint
½ part Lavender

The name means "ghost chaser" in Spanish. If you are experiencing a haunting, try this blend. It gets rid of negative magic, which many believe is brought about by evil spirits, demons, or malefic ghosts who are condemned to roam the Earth. The cleansing properties of the mint and lavender combination is awesome.

Evil Eye Oil

⅓ part Rose
⅓ part Heliotrope
⅓ part Musk

Used to get rid of a hex or curse, or put the "evil eye" on someone else. Aids the user in averting evil when rubbed on the hands for seven days; the protection can last up to a year.

Excalibur Oil

¼ part Lemon
⅛ part Orange
⅛ part Thyme
⅛ part Ginger
⅛ part Rose Geranium

¼ part Lavender

Will force others to do your bidding without question. Use with care.

Exodus Oil

2 ounces Safflower Base
1 ounce Patchouli
½ part Myrrh
½ part Narcissus

Keep Devil's Shoestring Root in master bottle. Anoint a white candle and burn to receive help from the Holy Spirit. Anoint a doll representing the person you want out of your life with the oil to make them go away. Write the person's name on a white piece of paper. Also write the following: "We both go to our higher good separately, in different directions, through divine power." On a Sunday, wrap the doll in the paper. Every Sunday thereafter, take the doll out and anoint it once again. Continue until your nemesis finds fit to get out of your life.

Exorcism Oil

Take equal amounts of these oils:
Hyssop
Clover
Lavender
Controlling
Keep Hyssop Herb in the master bottle

Use to purge and banish any evil or negative energies in a place or surrounding a person.

Exorcism Oil II

¼ part Healing Oil
¼ part Blessing Oil
¼ part Sandalwood
⅛ part Bergamot
⅛ part Myrrh
Frankincense, a few drops
Lemon Verbena, a few drops

Use same as above.

Fast Action Oil

⅓ part Dragon's Blood
⅓ part Lemon
⅓ part Rosemary
Cinnamon, a few drops

Add to any other oil to speed its effects.

Fiery Command Oil

¼ part Dragon's Blood
¼ part Frankincense
¼ part Myrrh
¼ part Cinnamon

Will force others to do your bidding without question. Use with care.

Fiery Wall of Protection Oil

⅓ part Dragon's Blood
⅓ part Frankincense
⅓ part Myrrh
Salt, a few grains in bottle

The added element of Fire, or Dragon's Blood, will protect you even from a very strong attack.

Fiery Wall of Protection Oil II

⅓ part Amber
⅓ part Cinnamon
⅓ part Frankincense

While similar to Protection Oil, and used for the same objectives, this is an especially effective formula for instances when one feels unduly pressured by another person.

Flying Devil Oil

Black Pepper, a pinch
½ part Dragon's Blood Oil
¼ part Cassia
¼ part Patchouli

A special voudoun uncrossing oil used to overcome the power of a strong Ouanga or hex. Very dependable and is said to work very quickly. *Not to be worn.*

Go Away Evil Oil

⅓ part Lilac
⅓ part Rose
⅓ part Ambergris fragrance oil

This is a deep-toned fragrance designed to drive away evil by its sheer power of wholesomeness, rather than making you smell overpowering as many Go Away Evil blends do. This oil repels negativity through grace, subtlety, and positive light.

Graveyard Oil/Goofer Oil

Patchouli Leaves
½ part Mullein
½ part Vetiver

You can use ordinary herbs/dust with this oil to create "graveyard dust," a maximum healing mixture.

Gris-Gris Oil

½ teaspoon Sandalwood
½ teaspoon Bay
Asafetida, a pinch
Dill Seed, a pinch
¼ teaspoon Uncrossing Oil
2 teaspoon tincture of Benzoin

A voudoun recipe for all-purpose power. Use in any situation when added energy is needed.

Hell's Devil Oil

¾ Capsicum
¼ Mustard
Black Peppercorns

One of the best oils for placing a hex on someone. Dress black candles to strengthen the hex's power to cause harm. *Use with caution. Not to be worn.*

Hindu Oil

See Van Van Oil on page 176.

Hot Foot Oil

Chili Powder, a pinch
½ Red Sandalwood
Black Pepper, a pinch
½ part Cinnamon
Pinch of Sulfur

A hexing oil used when you wish to make an enemy uncomfortable. It doesn't hurt anyone permanently and just causes temporary suffering. *Not to be worn.*

I Can, You Can't Oil

¼ part Palma Christi
¼ part Rose
⅛ part Magnolia
⅛ part Narcissus
⅛ part Apple Blossom
⅛ part Wisteria

Use this oil when an enemy is trying to "diminish" you in any way (take away your job or lover, spread gossip about you, etc.). Sprinkle this oil upon an object she or he must touch. After the charm is set, spend no further thought or energy on the problem. It will be taken care of in its time and in a way that will be to your advantage and benefit.

I Tame My Straying Animal Oil

⅔ part Peppermint
⅓ part Clove
Onion Oil (optional, can be found in some botanicas)

This preparation, which originates in Mexico, is intended in keeping a wandering lover at home.

Inflammatory Confusion Oil

1 part Rue Herb
1 part Guinea Pepper
1 part Poppy Seeds
1 part Black Mustard Seeds
4 drops Capsicum Oil
½ ounce carrier oil

Use to cause confusion between lovers who are cheating. Stops infidelity when sprinkled on the altar, or a figure candle representing the one who is straying.

Jinx-Killer Oil

½ part Lavender
¼ part Frankincense
⅛ part Rose
⅛ part Rue

This formula brings luck when one become convinced that a destructive force has descended on his or her home or person.

Jinx Oil

⅔ part Clove
⅓ part Cyclamen

There are different varieties of this oil: Black Jinx is used to ward off evil and break hexes, to purify an altar, or for any ritual of cursing; Green Jinx is used to gain financial wealth and success in any endeavor; Purple Jinx increases clairvoyant powers and makes the wearer more deeply psychic; Red Jinx is used to attract potential marriage partners and new lovers.

Jinx-Removing Oil

½ part Carnation
½ part Sandalwood
Myrrh, a few drops

Powerful in overcoming ill effects from the most horrible curses. For all those in a crossed condition, rub on the temples every day until the situation is improved.

Jockey Club Perfume

¼ part Cinnamon
¼ part Carnation
¼ part Clove
¼ part Bay
Piece of tanned leather in bottle

A strong hex breaker. Used only for uncrossing purposes. Can be depended upon to protect against all evil-doings.

Lost and Away Oil

½ part Mistletoe fragrance oil
¼ part Orris
¼ part Sage

One of the most powerful recipes for getting rid of an unwanted person or enemy.

Love-Breaker Oil

⅓ part Vetiver
⅓ part Patchouli
⅓ part Lemongrass

To spoil any love affair or marriage. To be used in a spell against one's own mate to cause a split if desired, or to rid oneself of undesired attention.

Magus Oil

⅓ part Lemon
⅓ part Orange
⅓ part Frankincense
Sandalwood, a few drops
Vetiver, a few drops

For protection and power. Anoint a purple candle with this mixture.

Mandrake Perfume

⅓ part Galangal
⅓ part Hyssop
⅓ part Dill
Licorice, a few drops
Musk, a few drops
Piece of Mandrake in the bottle

Combines a hexing and protection formula. Seldom used except by the very experienced, as it tends to be highly reversible. The ingredients invoke elementals and must be used with extreme caution.

Mint Bouquet Oil

¾ part Rose
¼ part Mint
¼ part Rain fragrance oil

A love uncrossing oil. Also helps to change one's luck.

Mogra Oil (Sheik)

⅓ part Sweet Pea
Then add equal amounts of each:
Jasmine
Lotus

Narcissus

Rose

Orange

Heliotrope

Musk, a few drops

An old authentic Persian mixture used to command others to do your will. Most Powerful Hand Oil

½ part Sandalwood

⅛ part Lily of the Valley

⅛ part Jasmine

⅛ part Mimosa

⅛ part Musk

Use this oil against the dark arts and for judgment against those who would do you harm.

Pentatruck Oil

¼ part Myrrh

¼ part Bay

¼ part Clove

¼ part Cinnamon

An uncrossing and protection blend from New Orleans.

Purification Oil

½ part Frankincense

½ part Myrrh

Sandalwood, a few drops

This oil can be placed in a diffuser or worn to help negativity and bad influences stay away. Very nice blend for Circle work.

Purification Oil II

¾ part Rose

¼ part Rosemary

Frankincense, a few drops

This oil purifies an object, place, or person.

Quitting Oil

½ part Nutmeg

½ part Cinnamon

½ ounce Apricot

Will cause a married member of the opposite sex to leave the wearer alone and can be used to stop others from hexing the wearer.

Reveal Truth Oil

¼ part Patchouli

¼ part Honeysuckle

¼ part Sage

¼ part Balm of Gilead

This oil assists in removing the veil of deceit and illusion so the truth can be known.

Reversing Oil

½ part Eucalyptus

½ part Lemongrass

Rock Salt in bottle

Helps reverse the effects of a spell that you have done in error, or that another has done against you. Use essential oils for best results.

Reversing Oil II

⅓ part Lavender

⅓ part Rose

⅓ part Cinnamon

This oil can protect against attack and return it to sender.

Root Oil

½ part High John

½ part Galangal

Adam and Eve Oil, 8 drops

A general-purpose, hex-breaking blend.

Separation Oil

⅓ part Vetiver

⅓ part Sandalwood

⅓ part Black Pepper
Clove, a few drops

Causes a couple or partnership to separate. Use to liberate yourself from a bad situation.

Seven-Day Uncrossing Oil

⅓ part Hyssop
⅓ part Verbena
⅓ part Pine
Basil, a few drops
Clove, a few drops

An excellent blend to use in overcoming a particularly strong curse. Must be sprinkled on the hexed person's head for seven days. (I place some of the blend in a bottle of shampoo.)

Shut Up Oil (Tapa Boca)

⅓ part Vetiver
⅓ part Patchouli
⅓ part Bay
Lime Oil, 3 drops

In Spanish, *tapa boca* means "shut up." This is a great blend that stops gossip, back stabbers, and people mumbling vicious spells against you.

Spell Breaker Oil

½ part Lavender
½ part Rose
Garden Mint, a few drops
Orange, a few drops

To break a spell, whether your own or someone else's.

Spell Weaver Oil

½ part Dragon's Blood
¼ part Myrrh
⅛ part Pine

To confirm and anchor magical workings.

Spider Oil

½ part Egyptian Musk

¼ part Rose Geranium

¼ part Rose

A dark essence used in workings of destruction or binding. Helps in situations calling for manipulation.

Squint Drops

⅛ part Clove

⅛ part Allspice

¼ part Mullein

¼ part Sage

Deer's Tongue herb in the bottle

Will help the wearer to discover if a partner has been unfaithful.

Stray No More Oil

Mix 2 parts Spikenard

1 part Lavender Flowers

1 part Herba Mate

2 tablespoons to 2 ounces carrier oil

Optional: A small piece of Magnolia Root is put in each bottle of oil made

Said to keep a lover or spouse faithful. Use in your mate's bathwater, anoint on soles of your lover's shoes, or sprinkle on bed sheets.

Tar Perfume (not to be worn)

½ part Molasses

¼ part Castor

¼ part Turpentine

Pinch Bitter Aloes

Creosote in bottle

Specially designed to create strife. Use only when you wish to cause problems for others. A blend that borders on the very negative. *Think carefully before using.*

Tipareth Oil

¼ part Pine

¼ part Myrrh

¼ part Dragon's Blood

¼ part Patchouli

Can be used for good or evil purpose, either to break or cast a curse or hex. Also can draw Solar good fortune or health.

Truth Oil
2-dram clean Amber or Cobalt vial
Sweet Almond Oil
½ part Violet Leaf
¼ part Lemon
¼ part Rosewood
1 drop Heliotrope
1 drop Patchouli

Add the essential oils to the bottle and swirl them gently in order to blend. Add any crystals (make sure they are clean) and then add your base oil to top the bottle off.

Unbinding Oil
¾ part Peach
¼ part Cucumber

This oil was created to release one who is bound to another, or is obsessive over something that seems unreasonable. Wear this blend as anointing oil whenever you are stressing over your given situation.

Uncrossing Oil
⅓ part Lemon
⅓ part Rose
⅓ part Lily
Bay, a few drops

Rids the wearer/user of bad luck and hexes.

Uncrossing Oil II
¼ part Cedarwood
¼ part Clove
½ part Vetiver

Same as above.

Uncrossing Oil III
½ part Rose
¼ part Bay

¼ part Clove

Carnation, a few drops

This is a very powerful uncrossing blend that will remove any hex or spell.

Uncrossing Oil IV

⅓ part Sandalwood

⅓ part Patchouli Leaves

⅓ part Myrrh

Pinch of Five Finger Grass (Cinquefoil)

Add 2 tablespoons of this to 2 ounces Olive Oil. Put a pinch of blessed salt and 8 drops household ammonia in each 1-ounce bottle of oil made. Shake well before use.

Uncrossing Oil V

¼ part Wisteria

¼ part Lilac

¼ part Verbena

¼ part Rose Geranium

Keep an amethyst in the master bottle.

This oil removes hexes and curses.

Uncrossing Oil VI

⅓ part Rose

⅓ part Lily of the Valley

⅓ part Lavender

To remove all types of hexes, curses, and crossed conditions, add nine drops to the bathwater for nine consecutive days.

Unfaithful Oil

⅓ part Garden Mint

⅓ part Rose

⅓ part Nutmeg

Sprinkle on an unfaithful partner to stop him or her from playing around. On the other hand, if you wear it, it could encourage your partner to be unfaithful, if that is what you desire.

Witchbane Oil

½ part Palma Christi

¼ part Verbena
¼ part Pine
Few drops Frankincense
Saint John's Wort in master bottle
2 ounces carrier oil

Primarily used to break a hex, this blend can be used for banishing, or to reflect and return magic. Oil is enhanced when used during the Waning Moon.

X-Hex Oil

⅓ part Sandalwood
⅓ part Patchouli
⅓ part Myrrh
Few pinches of Cinquefoil
2 ounces Olive Oil
1 pinch Salt
16 drops of Ammonia

Combine dry ingredients and grind to a fine powder. Mix all of them together thoroughly. Add 2 tablespoons of powder to the oil and mix. Add salt and blend. Add ammonia and shake well. Divide contents between 1-ounce dark bottles for storing. Use remaining herb mix as incense in combination with oil if you desire.

Yuza Yuza Oil

½ part Myrrh
½ part Cypress

A dreaded mystical oil blend used for calling the spirits of the dead. Very dangerous. Never use in jest. Also for causing hexes.

The Mother Moon

There are thirteen Full Moons. Each has a traditional name.

Wolf Moon—January

Storm Moon—February

Chaste Moon—March

Seed Moon—April

Hare Moon—May

Dyad Moon—June

Blue Moon—variable

Mead Moon—July

Wyrt Moon—August

Barley Moon—September

Blood Moon—October

Snow Moon—November

Oak Moon—December

Use for Full Moon workings, charging, empowering, invoking, fulfillment, accomplishing goals, and honoring the Mother Goddess. Anoint candles, use for ritual bath when preparing for ritual, and anoint members as they enter Circle.

January: Full Wolf Moon Oil

¾ part Musk

¼ part Mimosa

February: Full Snow or Storm Moon Oil

¼ part Wisteria

¼ part Heliotrope

¼ part Myrrh

¼ part Sage

March: Full Worm or Chaste Moon Oil

¾ part Honeysuckle

¼ part Apple Blossom

April: Full Pink or Seed Moon Oil

½ part Pine
⅛ part Bay
⅛ part Bergamot
¼ part Patchouli

May: Full Flower or Hare Moon Oil

¾ part Sandalwood
¼ part Rose

June: Full Strawberry or Dyad Moon Oil

½ part Lavender
½ part Lily of the Valley

July: Full Buck or Mead Moon Oil

¾ part Frankincense
¼ part Orris

August: Full Green Corn or Wyrt Moon Oil

½ part Frankincense
½ part Heliotrope

September: Full Harvest or Barley Moon Oil

¾ part Gardenia
¼ part Bergamot

October: Full Hunters or Blood Moon Oil

⅓ part Strawberry
⅓ part Cherry
⅓ part Apple Blossom

November: Full Beaver or Snow Moon Oil

¼ part Cedar
⅛ part Hyacinth
⅛ part Peppermint
¼ part Lemon
¼ part Narcissus

December: Full Cold or Oak Moon Oil

¼ part Patchouli

¼ part Geranium

¼ part Frankincense

¼ part Myrrh

A few drops Lilac

Blue Moon Oil (2nd Full Moon in a Month)

¾ part Lavender

¼ part Sandalwood

A few drops Rosemary

Sabbats & Rituals

There are eight Pagan holidays, or Sabbats, celebrated each year. The word "Sabbat" comes from the French word *s'ebattre,* which means to rejoice, frolic, and revel. That is exactly what these days are for, the joyous celebration of life and nature. Sabbats are determined by nature, not by people. Remember, Washington's and Lincoln's birthdays were combined, and then moved to Monday. You can't get much more arbitrary. The eight Sabbats are determined by the Earth and Sun, and the natural energy created by their relationships to each other. This makes them entirely natural holidays, where the natural energies are at high or low points. These were also important dates to our ancestors, who used them to help determine when to plant and harvest.

So what are these Sabbats?

Once a year in the Northern Hemisphere, we have the longest night of the year, accompanied by the shortest day. We call this day the Winter Solstice. On the exact opposite point on the Wheel of the Year, we have the longest day of the year and the shortest night. This we call the Summer Solstice. Each spring, there comes a day when the hours between sunrise and sunset are exactly equal to the hours between sunset and sunrise. This we call the Vernal Equinox. Each fall, there is another day when the hours of darkness and the hours of daylight are exactly in balance. This we call the Autumnal Equinox. These four days are known as "quarter days," as they divide the year into four equal sections. To Pagans, these are also know as the Lesser Sabbats.

The other four holidays are defined by the first four. These days bisect, or are at the midpoint, of the other four holidays. Hence, they are sometimes called the "cross quarter" days. These Sabbats are considered by some to be the four most important holidays, as they represent turning points in the seasons. Between Winter Solstice and Vernal Equinox is Imbolc. Between the Vernal Equinox and Summer Solstice is Beltane. Between Summer Solstice and Autumnal Equinox is Lughnasadh (Lammas). Between Autumnal Equinox and Winter Solstice is Samhain (Halloween). Samhain is also the turning of the year, and is considered to be the most important and powerful of all the Sabbats.

The oils below can assist you in everything from anointing candles to mixing with incense and anointing individuals as they enter the Circle. Some of the oils are for rituals you may perform at any time of the year, for consecration of tools, and for placing in an atomizer to bring a certain energy into a room.

Abramelin Oil

1 part Myrrh
½ part Cinnamon
½ part Galangal
¼ finest Olive Oil

This oil, used for anointing, is made according to the recipe in Mathers' translation of *The Sacred Magic of Abramelin the Mage*—one part Myrrh, ½ part Cinnamon, ½ part Galangal, and half the total weight in the best Olive Oil. Although many people make this oil from essential oils, which are very convenient, essential oils can concentrate too much of certain aspects of herbs and leave out others This oil is made from large quills of Cinnamon Bark, Tears of Myrrh, and sliced Galangal Root. The ingredients are crushed (a messy process!) and macerated in the oil for one month to take up all the complexities of the herbs used. The herbs are then allowed to settle out, leaving their scent in the oil. This oil will not burn your skin as oils jacked up with Cinnamon essential oil can.

All-Purpose Blessing and Anointing Altar Oil

⅓ part Sandalwood
⅓ part Myrrh
⅓ part Frankincense
Clove, a few drops

Used to anoint the altar and altar tools.

All-Purpose Oil

¾ part Palma Christi (Castor Oil)
⅛ part Heliotrope
⅛ part Lotus
⅛ part Honeysuckle
⅛ part Vetiver, White Musk, or Oak Moss

These blended oils are very powerful. When you are not sure which oil suits your intent best, you can use this oil.

However you need to focus on a specific purpose if you use it in this manner. Use as a scent on a light ring or for candle anointing.

It gives a pleasant feeling to a room.

Good for consecrating ritual tools, candles, altars, and work rooms.

Altar Oil

½ part Frankincense
¼ part Myrrh
Cedar, a few drops

Anoint the altar with this oil at regular intervals and call your deity to watch over it.

Altar Oil II

½ part Frankincense
¼ part Myrrh
⅛ part Galangal
⅛ part Vervain
Ambergris, a few drops

Anoint your altar once a week, especially on a Sunday or another holy day. Place in an open dish in a room to heighten spirituality, call in the assistance of positive spirits, and to create a holy atmosphere.

Ambrosia Oil

½ part Honeysuckle
¼ part Coconut
¼ part Hibiscus
Cinnamon, a few drops

This is a special blend for Sabbats. Perfect for the summer holidays at Midsummer and Lammas.

Anointing Oil

¼ part Patchouli
¼ part Cinnamon
⅛ part Verbena

Bless candles with this oil before they are used in a ceremony. It is said to magnetize the candle or to give it more occult strength. Can be used to wipe down an altar or a worship room. For success: use on candles, add to incense, or to bathwater. Dress curio bags.

Anointing Oil II

¼ part Sandalwood
¼ part Cedarwood
¼ part Orange
¼ part Lemon

Use for general ritual anointing purposes.

Anointing Oil III

⅛ part Rosemary
⅛ part Frankincense
⅛ part Peppermint
⅛ part Sandalwood
Cinnamon, a few drops

Use for general ritual anointing purposes.

Anointing Oil IV

½ part Rose
¼ part Cinnamon
⅛ part Orange
⅛ part Lavender

In general, any oil can be used for anointing, since to anoint simply means to rub over with oil or to apply oil especially for consecration.

Arabian Bouquet Oil

¼ part Sandalwood
¼ part Musk
¼ part Myrrh
¼ part Allspice

A special oil designed to cleanse the spirit before calling on the good spirits. This oil will also protect against hexes.

Arch Druid Oil

¼ part Apple Blossom
¼ part Vanilla
¼ part Cherry
¼ part Olive Oil

For any kind of Druid rite.

Beltane Oil

½ part Lily of the Valley
¼ part Violet
¼ part Honeysuckle
Pinch of Lemon Balm

Mix in bottle. Anoint altar and candles for Beltane celebrations.

Beltane Oil II

⅓ part Rose
⅓ part Dragon's Blood
⅓ part Coriander

To wear on the grand Sabbat of Beltane (May Day).

Bible Oil

½ part Hyssop
½ part Frankincense

For ritual success, anoint all candles on altar, except black ones, with Bible Oil.

Black Moon Oil

¼ part Vanilla
¼ part Calamus
½ part Orchid
A few poppy seeds

A beautiful dark, mysterious scent. Best made with fragrance oils from a reputable dealer. Make during a Waning Moon.

Candlemas/Brid's Oil

½ part Almond fragrance oil
¼ part Sage
¼ part Dragon's Blood

To wear on the grand Sabbat of Candlemas, or to work or invoke the goddess Brid; for works of fertility, love, or war.

Circle Oil

½ part Frankincense

¼ part Myrrh

¼ part Benzoin

4 drops of each the following:

Sandalwood

Cinnamon

Rose

Vervain

Vervain

Bay

Bergamot, a couple of drops—no more

Use when creating a sacred space for your operations of magic.

Conjure Oil

½ part Myrrh

¼ part Patchouli

⅛ part Galangal

⅛ part Jasmine

Lemon, a few drops

Used to anoint candles for general work; brings more power to any operation, especially for making conjure bags.

Consecration Oil

¼ part Lemon

¼ part Vetiver

¼ part Vanilla

¼ part Rose

Use to consecrate magical instruments and candles.

Consecration Oil II

⅓ part Frankincense Oil

⅓ part Myrrh Oil

⅓ part Cinnamon Oil

A bay leaf

½ ounce carrier oil

For the consecration of magical weapons and instruments.

Dark Moon Oil

½ part Jasmine

¼ part Chamomile

¼ part Patchouli

Sandalwood, a drop or two

For working with New Moon energies.

Dressing for Candles

1 drop Rose

1 drop Vanilla

1 part Vetiver

3 part Lemon

A traditional blend used to dress candles before any kind of service or rite.

Enochian Oil

¼ part Frankincense

¼ part Rose

¼ part Hyssop

¼ part Myrrh

For invoking the Enochian entities, or for visiting the Aethyrs.

Esbat Oil

¼ part Mint

¾ part Vervain

Mix equal parts and use during rituals and spells on the Full Moon.

Esbat Oil II

¼ part Frankincense

¼ part Rose

¼ part Lemon

¼ part Jasmine

This general anointing oil may be used for your watchtower candles, as an oil for the Circle, and for you to help personalize yourself for the gods.

Full Moon Oil

¾ part Gardenia
¼ part Lotus
Jasmine, a few drops

Helps in making preparations, blessing items, and making wishes and petitions during this time of generation and emergence.

Full Moon Oil II

½ part Jasmine
¼ part Rose
¼ part Sandalwood
Lemon, a few drops
Add a moonstone to the bottle

Helps to bring any project that needs growth to come to fruition, such as love, fertility, and financial ventures.

Full Moon Oil III

⅔ part Sandalwood
⅓ part Lemon
Rose, a few drops

Another oil to invoke the powers of the Moon when she is round.

Full Moon Oil IV

½ part Jasmine
½ part Sandalwood

Same as above.

Full Moon Oil V

½ part Sandalwood
¼ part Vanilla
⅓ part Jasmine
Rose, just a few drops

Mix prior to a Full Moon. Charge in a clear container or vial in the light of the Full Moon. Use to anoint candles or yourself for Full Moon rituals or just when you feel like you need the Moon's energy.

General Anointing Oil

½ part Frankincense
¼ part Cedarwood
⅛ part Sandalwood
⅛ part Myrrh

A general anointing oil for candles, tools, altar, and yourself when performing magical work.

Gibbous Moon Oil

¼ part Lavender
¼ part Rose
¼ part Patchouli
¼ part Sandalwood

For working with the Waxing Moon with she is three-quarters full. An excellent time for manifestation spells and rituals. I love this oil!

God Oil

¼ part Musk
¼ part Patchouli
⅛ part Ambergris
⅛ part Cinnamon
⅛ part Frankincense
⅛ part Cedarwood
Rose Oil, just a few drops
Add an amber stone to the bottle

To invoke the masculine side of your spiritual self for magical workings.

God Within Oil

⅓ part Cypress
⅓ part Rose Musk
⅓ part Vanilla

For working with the divine masculine in spellwork.

Goddess Oil

½ part Rose
¼ part Tuberose
⅛ part Lemon
⅛ part Palmarosa
Ambergris, a few drops

Make oil in a Waxing Moon phase and allow to sit for thirteen nights. To invoke or worship the Goddess.

Goddess Oil II

⅓ part Lemon
⅓ part Jasmine
⅓ part Camphor
A few grains of Sea Salt

To invoke or worship the Goddess.

Goddess Within Oil

½ part Sandalwood
¼ part Camphor
¼ part Lemon

To help you get in touch with your inner goddess.

Golden Lion Oil

⅓ part Frankincense
⅓ part Petitgrain
⅓ part Lime
Sweet Orange, a few drops

Good to use at Lammas, or in August, since it combines Leo and Sun energies.

High Altar Oil

½ part Frankincense
½ part Rose

A good-all purpose oil to use in anointing your altar or holy objects.

High Altar Oil II

½ part Van Van Oil
½ part Almond Fragrance Oil

Dress the altar and the candles with this potent oil. Burn only on an altar that has been blessed, and good spirits will come. Use oil to anoint heads during voudoun baptismal services. It attracts only good spirits.

High Altar Oil III

¼ part Frankincense
¼ part Vanilla
¼ part Heliotrope
¼ part Ylang-Ylang
Myrrh, a few drops

This oil is used to invite good spirits and angelic guides into your sacred space.

High Priestess Oil

½ part Wisteria
½ part Rose
Lavender, a few drops

For initiations and use within the sacred Circle during magical work.

High Priestess Initiation Oil

¼ part Gardenia
¼ part Lotus
¼ part Narcissus
¼ part Ylang-Ylang

A drop of Camphor may be added, if desired, to strengthen the lunar properties. This oil is specifically for the very special initiation of a third-degree priestess in the Wiccan tradition.

Holy Oil

Olive Oil carrier oil
½ part Lily of the Valley
½ part Rose
Cross in bottle

Special oil used only for blessing candles before they are used in a voudoun ritual. Very attracting.

Holy Oil II

½ part Rose
¼ part Frankincense
¼ part Neroli
Olive Oil, a few drops

A sacred oil for blessing of altars, candles, talismans, and persons.

Hoodoo Oil

⅓ part Honey
3 dried Pumpkin seeds
⅓ part Rose Oil
½ part Patchouli Oil
Honeysuckle, a few drops

When the Moon is full, crush the pumpkin seeds, using a mortar and pestle. Mix all of the ingredients together by the light of a new white candle. Bottle and keep in a dark place. Used for rituals.

Imbolc Oil

⅓ part Lavender
⅓ part Dill
⅓ part Rosemary

Use essential oils, blended with the carrier oil of our choice, in this recipe. Use this oil in Circle and to anoint candles for ritual. Use during the time of blessing and charging the seeds (February 2).

Imbolc Oil II

Equal amounts of all:
Jasmine
Rose
Chamomile
Lemon
Lavender

To wear on the grand Sabbat of Imbolc/Candlemas (February 2).

Initiation Oil

½ part Frankincense

½ part Myrrh

Sandalwood, a few drops

For works of initiation and consecration, ceremonies and Esbats. Use for mystic initiation ceremonies and also to increase your awareness of the spiritual realm.

Lammas Oil

⅓ part Lime

⅓ part Cinnamon

⅓ part Sandalwood

Clove, a few drops

Frankincense, a few drops

Mix well and bottle. Use in Lughnasadh/Lammas rituals.

Lammas Oil II

½ part Frankincense

¼ part Basil

¼ part Sunflower carrier oil

Patchouli, few drops

To wear on the Grand Sabbat of Lammas (Harvest Home).

Litha Oil

½ part Angelica

½ part Vervain

Sesame, a few drops

Helps with divination pursuits and for seeing beyond the veil on Midsummer's Eve.

Litha Oil II

¼ part Hazelnut

¼ part Elder

¼ part Lavender

¼ part Rosemary

Mix in bottle. Use to anoint altar and candles. Use at Midsummer's Eve.

Loban Oil

½ part Frankincense
¼ part Bergamot
⅛ part Lemon
⅛ part Lilac

A powerful purifier to use before and after a ritual.

Lugh Oil

½ part Heliotrope
½ part Sunflower Oil
1 citrine stone
1 piece gold, such as gold chain or piece of jewelry or shaved gold (get from a jeweler)

Use in Lughnasadh/Lammas rituals or when invoking Lugh.

Lugh Oil II

Equal parts of all:
9 drops Lime
9 drops Rose
9 drops Rose Geranium
9 drops Lavender
6 drops Sandalwood
6 drops Dragons Blood

Mix well and bottle. Use in Lughnasadh/Lammas rituals or when invoking Lugh.

Lughnasadh Oil

½ part Peppermint
½ part Elder
Fir, a few drops
Hazelnut, a few drops

Mix well and bottle. Use in Lughnasadh/Lammas rituals.

Lunar Oil

½ part Sandalwood
¼ part Camphor
¼ part Lemon

A general-purpose oil to celebrate Luna in all of her phases throughout the year.

Lupercalia Oil

¼ part Rose
¼ part Vanilla
¼ part Peach
¼ part Jasmine
Tonka, a few drops

Lupercalia is a Roman fertility festival. This oil is about bringing fertility and abundance, frivolity and happiness to your life.

Mabon Oil

⅓ part Rosemary
⅓ part Frankincense
⅓ part Apple Blossom
Chamomile, a few drops

Wear during the celebration of the Feast of Autumn.

Mabon Oil II

⅓ part Pine
⅓ part Sandalwood
⅓ part Ginger
Lemon, a few drops

A tree-inspired scent that harks upon the majestic qualities of an autumn harvest.

Mabon/Autumn Equinox Oil

¼ part Sandalwood
¼ part Pine
¼ part Allspice
¼ part Nutmeg
Musk, a few drops
Cinnamon, a few drops

Used to celebrate Mabon, the autumn season, and harvest celebrations. It brings love, beauty, bounty, and many blessings of the harvest season to your home.

Macha Oil (Lughnasadh)

½ part Grape Seed
½ part Corn
1 small piece of Obsidian
1 small crow feather

Use in Lughnasadh/Lammas rituals or when invoking Macha.

Magic Circle Oil
⅓ part Juniper Berry
⅓ part Frankincense
⅓ part Sandalwood
Rosemary, a few drops
Nutmeg, a few drops

For general magic work, especially in casting Circles.

Magical Power Oil
¼ part Dragon's Blood
¼ part Ginger
¼ part Tangerine
¼ part Allspice
Frankincense, a few drops
Vanilla, a few drops

Anoint your body prior to religious rituals to stimulate spirituality. Also, anoint others during mystical group rites.

Mermaids Oil
⅓ part Lotus
⅓ part Ambergris
⅓ part Carnation
Rain fragrance oil, a few drops (optional)

Mermaids can be both friends and foes of humankind. When they are your friend, they can be fierce and powerful protectresses. This oil can be used to anoint the watchtower in ritual to conjure the mermaids to guard and guide your Circle.

Midsummer Oil
¼ part Lavender
¼ part Rosemary
¼ part Rose
¼ part Sunflower
A pinch of gold glitter

A blend to assist in celebrating the longest day of the year, the Summer Solstice.

Midsummer Oil II
⅓ part Frankincense

⅓ part Orange
⅓ part Patchouli
Cinnamon, 2–3 drops

To wear during the celebration of the feast of the Summer Solstice.

Midsummer Oil III

½ part Neroli
¼ part Cedar
¼ part Sandalwood
Cinnamon, a few drops
Palmarosa, a few drops
Clove, 3 drops

The time for enjoying the first fruits of the season's bounty. A time for asking for abundance; also for fertility magic.

Midsummer Faerie Oil

½ part Rose
¼ part Chamomile
¼ part Lavender
3 Daisy Petals
3 pinches Vervain
3 pinches Elder Flower

For the magic that summer nights bring. Great for divination.

Moon Priest Cologne

¼ part Lemon Verbena or Lime
½ part Coriander
¼ part Camphor or Myrrh

Increasing the Myrrh gives a darker perfume; increasing the Camphor, a lighter and more spicy one. This oil is designed to assist males with any Moon magic.

Moon Priestess Perfume

¼ part Queen of the Night fragrance oil
½ part Rose

¼ part Lemon Verbena

This oil is designed to assist females with any Moon magic.

Mystic Rites Oil

¼ part High John
¼ part Galangal
¼ part Cinnamon
¼ part Squill

General oil for Sabbat and ritual. Vibrates on a powerful spiritual/magical level.

New Moon Oil

⅓ part Jasmine
⅓ part Chamomile
⅓ part Patchouli
Sandalwood, 2–3 drops

To work with the energies of the Dark Moon.

Oil for the Dark of the Moon

½ part Myrrh
⅛ part Cinnamon
¼ part Queen of the Night fragrance oil
⅛ part Rose

Blend, bottle, and shake well. Use in spellwork at the New Moon for contacting ancestors and the dead.

Ostara Oil

⅓ part Jasmine
⅓ part Geranium
⅓ part Patchouli
Juniper, a few drops

Worn to celebrate the Vernal Equinox, where light and day are balanced.

Ostara Oil II

Equal parts of all:
Almond
Patchouli

Elder
Lavender
Violet

This oil is great to have in a diffuser to celebrate the festival of rebirth of the Earth after the winter's death.

Ostara Oil III
½ part Vetiver
⅛ part Geranium
⅛ part Ylang-Ylang
¼ part Rose

Worn to celebrate the Vernal Equinox where light and day are balanced.

Ostara Oil IV
½ part Rosewood
¼ part Geranium
⅛ part Chamomile
⅛ part Myrrh
Cedarwood, a few drops
Bay, a few drops

Another oil to wear on the Grand Sabbat of the Vernal Equinox.

Power Oil
¾ part Orange
⅛ part Ginger
⅛ part Pine

To infuse yourself with additional power during potent rituals, anoint with power oil.

Power of Old Oil
¼ part Frankincense
¼ part Myrrh
⅛ part Sandalwood
⅛ part Vervain

⅛ part Mistletoe fragrance oil
⅛ part Mandrake fragrance oil (optional)
Piece of mandrake in the master bottle

Authentic old Druidic blend to increase power in any work.

Priestess Oil
⅛ part Violet
⅛ part Lemon
¼ part Honeysuckle
½ part Lavender
Lilac, a few drops

Enchanting oil that brings down the energies of the goddess and increases self-confidence and self-esteem.

Purification Oil
½ part Frankincense
½ part Myrrh
Sandalwood, a few drops

This oil can be placed in a diffuser or worn to help negativity and bad influences stay away. Very nice blend for Circle work.

Rosy Cross Oil
½ part Rose
½ part Lotus

A general-purpose ritual oil.

Sabbat Oil
½ part Frankincense
¼ part Myrrh
¼ part Sandalwood
Orange, a few drops
Lemon, a few drops

Add to an Olive Oil base and wear to Sabbat celebrations.

Sabbat Oil II
½ part Frankincense
¼ part Myrrh
¼ part Allspice

Clove, a few drops

This oil can help "set the stage" on the ritual area as the participants enter.

Sabbat Oil III

1 teaspoon Frankincense, powdered

1 teaspoon Myrrh, powdered

1 teaspoon Benzoin, powdered

Add to ¼ cup Olive Oil. Heat slowly over a live flame until the powders have melted into the oil. Cool and apply sparingly for the Sabbats.

Sacred Circle Oil

¾ part Frankincense

¼ part Sandalwood

Cinnamon, 2–3 drops

Anoint your body prior to religious rituals to stimulate spirituality. Also anoint others during mystical and religious group rites.

Sacred Oil

Same as above.

Samhain Oil

½ part Pine

¼ part Frankincense

¼ part Patchouli

Lavender, a few drops

To wear on the Grand Sabbat of Samhain (Halloween).

Self-Love Oil

¼ part Tuberose

¼ part White Rose

¼ part Geranium

¼ part Rose

Palmarosa, a few drops

Prepare and empower the oil before the ritual; used to enhance self-esteem.

Spirituality Oil

½ part Sandalwood

¼ part Cedarwood

¼ part Frankincense

¼ cup carrier oil

Blend oils and add a small piece of Sandalwood, Cedarwood and/or a Frankincense Tear, and any of the following: Calcite, Diamond, Lepidolite, or Sugilite. Wear before all spiritual works and rituals. Be sure to visualize your goal while using the oil.

Spring Goddess Oil

⅓ part Tuberose

⅓ part Sandalwood

⅓ part Myrrh

A very young and fragrant-smelling oil for working with the maiden aspect of the Goddess.

Spring Time Oil

¾ part Lemon

¼ part Bergamot

Bayberry, a few drops

A bright, cheerful, uplifting blend, excellent for working with the festival of rebirth of the Mother Earth after winter's death.

Stone Circle Power Oil

¼ part Rosemary

½ part Frankincense

¼ part Vetiver

Use this blend for banishing and for protection from physical and spiritual danger.

Summer Oil

¼ part Verbena

⅛ part Balm of Gilead

½ part Ylang-Ylang

⅛ part Magnolia

A blend for use in summer rites, spellwork, and rituals.

Summer Breeze Oil

⅛ part Neroli

¾ part Sweet Orange

⅛ part Chamomile
Rose, a few drops
Lavender, a few drops

Use essential oils only in this blend. Helps to bring a higher vibration of energy in yourself or your environment. Excellent in room diffuser, or place a drop on cotton balls and place around the room.

Summer Solstice Oil
½ part Lavender
½ part Rosemary
Pine, 2–3 drops

This oil is to be used on the longest day of the year, the time when the Sun is strongest. It is a time for asking for abundance, and for making fertility magic so the harvest will be a fine one.

Sun Goddess Perfume
⅓ part Cinnamon
⅓ part Lemon Verbena
⅓ part Ylang-Ylang

Use this blend as an offering to honor the goddess and to release the energy of the Sun God in order to ensure a plentiful harvest.

Sun King Anointing Oil
½ part Frankincense
½ part Sandalwood
3 pinches Saffron or Sunflower Oil

Concentrating on the Sun, rub the oil on the person or token representing the Sun. This blend invokes beneficial energy on the recipient.

Talisman Consecration Oil
2 parts Frankincense
1 part Cypress
1 part Ash leaves

1 part Valerian
1 pinch Alum
1 part Tobacco
1 pinch Asafetida
2 ounces Olive Oil

Let herbs and oils sit in the Olive Oil for two weeks, shaking every other day. Strain into bottle and use. Recommended, although it does not smell pretty!

Taper Perfume Oil

⅓ part Jasmine
⅓ part Cinnamon
⅓ part Patchouli
Olive Oil

Used to float wicks. Usually no more than perfumed Olive Oil, More for decoration than for ritual purposes, but the oils tend to attract love, healing, and positive forces.

Temple Oil

½ part Frankincense
¼ part Rosemary
⅛ part Bay
⅛ part Sandalwood

Wear during religious rites, those designed to promote spirituality, and temple workings.

Tetragrammaton Oil

⅓ part Myrtle
⅓ part Cedar
⅓ part Frankincense

For any ceremonial work or undertaking of Goetic Magic.

Tool Cleansing Oil

⅛ part Lemongrass
⅛ part Almond fragrance oil
¼ part Benzoin
½ part Peppermint

Blend and use during tool cleansing rituals.

Voudoun Oil

¼ part Myrrh

¼ part Patchouli

¼ part Galangal

¼ part Jasmine

Lemon, a few drops

This is a standard oil blend for any voudoun ritual or work.

Wicca Oil

½ part Frankincense

⅛ part Myrrh

⅛ part Sandalwood

$\frac{1}{16}$ part Orange

$\frac{1}{16}$ part Lemon

Blend designed for Wiccan rituals and initiations.

Winter Solstice Oil

½ part Pine

¼ part Frankincense

¼ part Myrrh

Wear this blend during the celebration and feast of the Winter Solstice.

Witch Oil

3 tablespoons Honey

6 drops Honeysuckle

13 drops Dragon's Blood

3 drops Patchouli

¼ cup Sunflower Oil

Mix all ingredients on a night of a Full Moon, and use it to anoint candles for all types of magic, divination, spirit communication, and invocations.

Witch Blood Anointing Oil

¼ ounce Artemesia (Wormwood powder)

¼ ounce Valerian Root (whole if possible)

¼ ounce Vervain Herb

¼ ounce Madder Root Powder

½ ounce Mandrake Root (White Bryony)

1 pint Olive Oil

9 drops Oak Moss

7 drops Elder

10 drops Pine Essence

5 drops Chamomile

2 drops of Honey or Sweet Sap

A pinch of White Sea Salt

When used solely by a high priest, leave out the Vervain; when used solely by a high priestess, leave out the Oak Moss.

It is difficult to make this recipe in small quantities. Most people will find the complete recipe perfectly satisfactory for general use, for example, in a ritual aspect of goddess or god to influence your spellcasting. This makes a wonderful gift for initiation.

Yule Oil

½ part Sunflower Oil

Musk, A few drops

Sesame Oil, a few drops

½ part Rosemary

Mix in bottle. Anoint on altar and candles.

Yule Oil II

¼ part Pine

¼ part Fir

¼ part Almond fragrance oil

1 Cinnamon Stick

¼ part Musk

4 Cloves

Peace, harmony, love, divination, a healthier planet, and increased happiness.

Yule Oil III

¼ part Cinnamon

¼ part Clove

⅛ part Mandarin

⅛ part Pine
¼ part Frankincense
¼ part Myrrh

Another oil to wear during the celebration of the feast of Winter Solstice.

Yule Oil IV

¼ part Allspice
⅛ part Cedar
⅛ part Orange
¼ part Vanilla
⅛ part Frankincense Tears
⅛ part Sandalwood
Bay, a few drops

Add Bay Leaf, Frankincense Tears, and gold glitter to individual bottles (optional) before adding the oil. This oil is for celebrating this glorious season of the Sun's birth.

Planetary Oils

The seven sacred planets (the five visible planets plus the Sun and Moon) relate to the days of the week and also planetary hours within days. The seven sacred planets were also associated with ancient gods and goddesses. The use of these planets and their hours has an ancient history in witchcraft and Paganism. These oils help invoke the powers and characteristics of the individual planetary power. You can use these oils to anoint candles, or wear them as personal scent to help convey the power of the deities represented by the planets. They may also be combined with zodiacal oils when you work an astrologically based spell.

Sun Oil—Sun, Sol, Apollo; Sunday; ruler of Leo

Mercury Oil—Mercury, Hermes, Wotan; Wednesday; ruler of Gemini and Virgo

Venus Oil—Venus, Freya; Friday; ruler of Taurus and Libra

Earth Oil—Terra, Gaia, Earth; our Mother

Moon Oil (located in Sabbat section)—Moon, Luna, Artemis; Monday; ruler of Cancer

Mars Oil—Mars, Twi; ruler of Aries; co-ruler of Scorpio

Jupiter Oil—Jupiter, Zeus, Thor; Thursday; ruler of Sagittarius; co-ruler of Pisces

Saturn Oil—Saturn, Kronos; Saturday; ruler of Capricorn; co-ruler of Aquarius

Uranus Oil—Urania; co-ruler of Aquarius

Neptune Oil—Neptune, Poseidon; co-ruler of Pisces

Pluto Oil—Pluto, Hades; co-ruler of Scorpio

Sun Oil

½ part Frankincense

¼ part Cinnamon

⅛ part Petitgrain

⅛ part Rosemary

This oil brings general prosperity and well-being, and positions of rank and title such as executive positions and civilian government positions. A wonderful blend to assist in new ventures, publicity and notoriety, honors and self-esteem, finances, and healing.

Sun Oil II

1 teaspoon Cinnamon, ground
1 teaspoon Juniper berries, mashed
1 Bay Leaf, crumpled
A scant pinch of genuine Saffron

Place ingredients in a double boiler and gently heat over low flame in ¼ cup of base oil. Strain and use for healing, vitality, strength, promotions, and all solar influences.

Sun Oil (Planetary)

½ part Frankincense
¼ part Myrrh
¼ part Amber

To attract the qualities of the planet, or to worship/invoke the god; enhances enjoyment, increases understanding of art and music, and brings solutions to problems and escape from bad situations.

Sun Self Oil

¼ part Sandalwood
¼ part Frankincense
½ part Orange

Use when you want to find the confidence to know and follow your own path, drawing strength from within and power from the universe.

Mercury Oil (Planetary)

½ part Lavender
½ part Eucalyptus
Peppermint, a drop or two

Wear to draw Mercurial influences, such as communication, intelligence, and travel.

Venus Oil (Planetary)

⅓ part Ylang-Ylang
⅓ part Geranium
⅓ part Cardamom
Chamomile, a few drops

Wear to attract love and friendships, to promote beauty, and for other Venusian influences.

Venus Oil

⅓ part Rose

⅓ part Gardenia

¼ part Frangipani

¼ part Wisteria

⅛ White Diamonds fragrance oil (optional)

To attract the qualities of the planet, or to worship or invoke the goddess; to create harmony and bring love, to ignite passion in a lover or calm an argument.

Earth Oil

½ part Patchouli

½ part Cypress

Wear to invoke the powers of the Earth to bring money, prosperity, abundance, stability, and foundation.

Earth Oil II (Elemental)

1 drop Patchouli

¼ part Pine

½ part Magnolia

¼ part honeysuckle

Earth is the realm of fertility, wealth, abundance, and stability.

Earth Oil III

⅓ part Sandalwood

2 drops Vetiver

⅓ part Myrrh

⅓ part Patchouli

2 drops Honeysuckle

Create this oil by adding the ingredients in the order they are listed.

Earth Dawn Oil

½ part Vetiver

½ part Rose

¼ part Vanilla

¼ part Cypress

To help bring in the elementals and energies of the Earth.

Earth Mother Perfume

⅓ part Musk
⅓ part Patchouli
⅓ part Rose

Blend in equal parts, bottle, and shake well. A delicious blend to assist you in working with the Mother Earth.

Mars Oil (Planetary)

½ part Ginger
½ part Basil
Black Pepper, a drop or two

Wear for physical power, lust, magical energy, and all Martian influences.

Mars Oil

⅓ part Ginger
⅓ part Cinnamon
⅓ part Civet
Add Iron Filings and Dragon's Blood to each bottle (optional)

Men particularly like this oil, as it adds to their energy, virility, and passion. Both men and women apply it liberally on the wrists and hands when facing any foe. Soldiers who believe it leads to military honors favor it. To cause ruin, discord, and hostility among one's enemies, sprinkle it in their home or rub it on their clothes.

Jupiter Oil (Planetary)

¾ part Oak Moss Bouquet
¼ part Clove
Tonka Bouquet, a few drops

Wear for wealth, prosperity, help in legal matters, and all other Jupiterian influences.

Jupiter Oil II

¼ part Hyssop
⅛ part Clove
⅛ part Nutmeg
⅛ part Sandalwood
⅛ part Rosewood
Bitter Almond, a few drops

Same as planetary, to attract the qualities of that planet. It can bring good fortune and cause people to become generous toward you. Increases joviality.

Jupiter Oil III

¾ part Sandalwood

¼ part Anise

Almond, a few drops

Among the Greek-Roman gods, Jupiter represents the supreme virtues of the judgment and the will. This oil is made for use by those who wish to acquire riches, protected from all earthly dangers, win honors and glory, and gain tranquility of mind.

Saturn Oil

⅓ part Pine

⅓ part Patchouli

⅓ part Myrrh

To attract the qualities of the planet, or to worship or invoke the god. Ease of learning and passing exams, brings tranquility to the home.

Uranus Oil

½ part Musk

½ part Sandalwood

Rose, 2 to 3 drops

To attract the qualities of the planet, or to worship or invoke the god. Use it in magical pursuits and especially when the magician wishes to hide his or her intentions for influencing popular opinion.

Uranus Oil II

½ part Labdanum

¼ part Musk

¼ part Frankincense

Uranus, the son of Gaea, the Greek goddess of the Earth, used to hide his children from the light in the hollows of the Earth. If you wish to hide anything, particularly secret information, write the secret on parchment that you have soaked in this oil and then dried. Burn the paper in the flame of a green candle. The secret will never be discovered unless you reveal it.

Neptune Oil (Planetary)

⅓ part Ambergris
⅓ part Lotus
⅓ part Cucumber
Hyacinth, a few drops

To attract the qualities of the planet, or to worship/invoke the god; to change fortune, to aid in politics, to command elementals.

Neptune Oil

⅓ part Lily of the Valley
⅓ part Magnolia
⅓ part Lavender

In primitive thought, Neptune was the god of Heaven (that is, the god of clouds and rain). Later he became the god of fresh water, and finally, he was seen as the god of the sea. It is he who unleashes storms, representing the passions of the soul, particularly in his most extreme role as destroyer. This oil, when used daily and applied in a circle around the waistline of the body, should serve to calm the turbulence of these upheavals in life, particularly when upheavals are caused by unleashed passion or rage.

Pluto Oil

¾ part Musk
⅛ part Frankincense
⅛ part Hyacinth

This oil brings about transformation and metamorphosis.

Pluto Oil II

½ part Cypress
¼ part Peppermint
⅛ part Eucalyptus
⅛ part Mimosa

To attract the qualities of the planet, or to worship or invoke the god. Designed for pursuits of war and politics, for broad-term financial endeavors and speculation.

Zodiacal Oils

Zodiacal Oils relate to the various signs of the zodiac and help symbolize and invoke the kind of activities and characteristics with which the various signs of the zodiac are associated. You can use these oils to anoint candles, or wear them with Planetary Oils as a personal scent to help strengthen weak astrological characteristics or to help heighten strong astrological characteristics. These formulas are used to attract the qualities of a particular astrological sign and to influence people born under that sign.

Aries Oil—The Ram; March 21–April 21; ruled by Mars; element Fire.

Taurus Oil—The Bull; April 21–May 21; ruled by Venus; element Earth.

Gemini Oil—The Twins; May 21–June 21; ruled by Mercury; element Air.

Cancer Oil—The Crab; June 21–July 21; ruled by the Moon; element Water.

Leo Oil—The Lion; July 21–August 21; ruled by the Sun; element Fire.

Virgo Oil—The Virgin; August 21–September 21; ruled by Mercury; element Earth.

Libra Oil—The Balance; September 21–October 21; ruled by Venus; element Air.

Scorpio Oil—The Scorpion; October 21–November 21; ruled by Pluto and Mars; element Water.

Sagittarius Oil—The Archer; November 21–December 21; ruled by Jupiter; element Fire.

Capricorn Oil—The Sea goat; December 21–January 21; ruled by Saturn; element Earth.

Aquarius Oil—The Water Bearer; January 21–February 21; ruled by Uranus and Saturn; element Air.

Pisces Oil—The Fishes; February 21–March 21; ruled by Neptune and Jupiter; element Water.

Archer Oil

¾ part Rosemary

¼ part Oak Moss

Clove, a few drops

Designed for one of my Sagittarius friends. I think it smells a little weird, but the Sagittarians who have sampled it seemed to enjoy it.

Aries Oil

¾ part Frankincense

⅛ part Ginger

⅛ part Black Pepper

Petitgrain, 2 to 4 drops

Aids in beginnings, in athletics, and in contests of skill and luck.

Ethereal Oil

⅓ part Sandalwood

⅓ part Clary Sage

⅓ part Lavender

Cypress, a few drops

I created this one with Aquarius and Air energies.

Taurus Oil

½ part Oak Moss Bouquet

¼ part Cardamom

¼ part Ylang-Ylang

Wear as a personal oil to increase your own powers.

Gemini Oil

¾ part Lavender

⅛ part Peppermint

⅛ part Lemongrass

Sweet Pea Bouquet, a few drops

Aids quickness of thought, wit, and energy; improves facility with ideas and learning; aids in dealings with family members, especially siblings.

Cancer Oil (Moonchildren)

¾ part Palmarosa

⅛ part Chamomile

⅛ part Yarrow

Aids domestic arts, humor, entrepreneurial skills and success in business, etc.

Leo Oil (Planetary)

½ part Petitgrain

¼ part Orange

¼ part Lime

This blend will help you keep active and clear thinking, as well as have enthusiasm working in your behalf.

Leo Oil

¼ part Frankincense

⅛ part Musk

⅛ part Rose

⅛ part Lemon

⅛ part Patchouli

Balm of Gilead, a few drops

Enhances drama, personal magnetism, individuality, hedonism.

Virgo Oil

½ part Oak Moss Bouquet

¼ part Patchouli

Cypress, a few drops

For pursuits involving work or food, powers of analyzing.

Libra Oil

½ part Rose Geranium

¼ part Ylang-Ylang

¼ part Palmarosa

Use to bring or strengthen a desired partnership, to influence a court case, to bring understanding and enjoyment of music.

Libra Oil II

½ part Rose Geranium
¼ part Ylang-Ylang
¼ part Palmarosa
Rose, 2 to 3 drops
Cardamom, 2 to 3 drops

Wear as a personal oil to increase your own powers and assist in loving the arts.

Scorpio Oil

½ part Pine
½ part Cardamom
Black Pepper, a few drops

Use in pursuits of sex, financial security, and in workings of deep spirituality/occultism.

Sagittarius Oil

¾ part Rosemary
¼ part Oak Moss Bouquet
Clove, 2 to 3 drops

To bring generosity, to increase understanding of broad concepts, to help in travel, especially long journeys.

Capricorn Oil

¼ part Valerian
¼ part Pine
¼ part Ylang-Ylang
¼ part Galangal
Wisteria, a few drops

Improve political skill, ability to manipulate people/events. Luck with money; regard from others.

Aquarius Oil

¾ part Lavender
⅛ part Cypress
⅛ part Patchouli

Enhances social skills, feeling of community, friendship, originality, spontaneity, and psychic ability in groups.

Aquarius Oil II

½ part Jasmine

¼ part Lavender

⅛ part Patchouli

⅛ part Vetiver

Wear as a personal oil to increase your own powers.

Pisces Oil

½ part Ylang-Ylang

½ part Sandalwood

Jasmine, a drop or two

Wear as a personal oil increase your own powers.

PART THREE

All About Oils

Magical Properties of Carrier Oils for Use in Spells, Rituals & Potions

Carrier oils are used in magic for making anointing oils, as well as potions for many spells and rituals.

Carrier oils, or oil bases or vegetable base oils, have an existence of their own, and this gets "behind" the additional ingredients to bring them all together and empower them further. It is also possible to "program" carrier oils simply with intention; for example, by writing the additional ingredients or the purpose for the oil on a piece of paper and placing it underneath the oil bottle for a period of 24 hours.

Although carrier oils are generally safe to be used on skin, the potion might or might not be safe depending on what other ingredients have been added. If they are to be used on the skin, conduct a small allergy test first. For example, Wheat Germ Oil is particularly dangerous to people with wheat or gluten allergies.

When anointing anything, you should test a small area in an inconspicuous place. The carrier oils themselves, whether they have been mixed with other ingredients or not, may have an adverse effect on certain types of cloth or material.

Carrier oils should always be purchased and stored in dark glass bottles to extend their shelf life.

Apricot Kernel Oil (*Prunus Armeniaca*)

Apricot Kernel Oil is very rich and nourishing, warm, and supportive.

Apricots have been traditionally associated with Venus, goddess of women, power, and love. Apricot Kernel Oil, as a carrier, gives protection to women as well as supports women's endeavors, from menopause to childbirth.

A love potion based on Apricot Kernel Oil will have a strong and powerful protective aspect about it. This is recommended for love potions for a virgin looking for a first love, for example.

Just because Apricot Kernel Oil has a Venus essence doesn't mean that men can't use it for self-protection as well. Use this oil for creating more of a resonance to the female cosmos in general, or needing a female base vibration in a potion or anointing oil.

Apricot Kernel Oil lasts for six to twelve months.

Avocado Oil (*Persea Americana* or *Persea Gratissima*)

Avocado trees come from the rain forest in South America and were an important item in Inca worship, where they were strongly related to all matters of procreation on account of their similarity to a female pregnant belly.

Avocado Oil is the oil of passion, and one of the passions, of course, is sex. The oil is very thick and dense, very earthy rather than ethereal. Used for love potions or love anointing oils, it will have a strong push toward physical sexuality, but also toward procreation. So unless these are desired, be a little careful with this oil.

The fruitfulness/passion/procreation aspects can be very helpful in business endeavors and money matters. In general, Avocado Oil can help bring an idea into absolutely reality.

Use within three months.

Starflower Oil (Borage Oil or *Borago Officinalis*)

The Starflower is an interesting plant that looks the part for the witch doctor—hairy and spiky, but with an amazing five-petal double flower in pale blue to violet.

Use this oil as a carrier when higher guidance needs to be applied to find out the truth about a situation, or to overcome a problem at hand, including legal and relationship problems. Starflower Oil will bring with it a resonance of courage, honesty, and aligning a situation.

A love potion using Starflower Oil as the carrier might be used in circumstances where there is confusion other people involved, or where matters such as previous marriages or current relationships are confusing the issue. Using Starflower Oil as the carrier will push any issue strongly towards resolution, so be careful what you ask for. The Starflower power doesn't give up easily.

Starflower Oil doesn't last much beyond three months, even in the refrigerator.

Evening Primrose Oil (*Oenothera Fiennis*)

The Evening Primrose plant came from America, where it was eaten and used in many different ways by the indigenous people. For example, the leaves were used in making poultices for wounds. People would rub the plant all over the body and the feet to mask one's scent prior to hunting. The fact that this plant has flowers which "glow in the dark" and that all parts of it are edible, from the roots to the seeds, would account for its popularity and high standing as a magical plant.

In modern days, Evening Primrose Oil is sold as a treatment for many things including the blocked kitchen sink. This has diluted its power field somewhat, so be careful when you use this oil as a carrier.

Evening Primrose's true magical properties lie in protection, shielding, and also sustaining. It is a "friend in need," with a line to the higher levels of existence. It opens its flowers to the night and thus can be used safely in potions designed to enhance vision, paranormal abilities, and clairvoyance whilst remaining safe.

Evening Primrose Oil lasts for three to six months.

Grape Seed Oil (*Vitis Vinifera*)

Grapes were once thought to be the food of the gods. As wine is made from grapes, there are many alive today who would agree! This "spirit" of the grape is especially strong in its seeds, where all the life of the plant is stored for future purposes.

Grape Seed Oil makes a good base for spiritual anointing oils for oneself, a statue of a deity or ritual objects with a spiritual bent, or to make potions that are designed to enhance or bring about spiritual development.

In love potions, using Grape Seed for the carrier oil gives a spiritual dimension to the entire potion. Grape Seed is very neutral, awaiting an imprint that will then be amplified and the message broadcast on a spiritual dimension. This, together with its low price, makes Grape Seed Oil the perfect oil for every day and all purposes.

Use within three to four months.

Jojoba Oil (*Simmondsia Chinensis*)

Jojoba Oil is waxy in structure and is the least "oily" of all the carriers. It penetrates deep into the skin and takes with it anything it carries. Its non-greasy consistency makes it a good choice for an anointing oil!

The Jojoba plant comes from the Sonora desert where it provides much-needed food in a difficult environment.

Jojoba Oil is a carrier used for times you need extra perseverance, are trying to overcome hardship, don't want to give up, and are flourishing even when you're not exactly in the Garden of Eden.

A powerful protector against doubt, depression, and giving up too soon, this is a carrier to use when you need some extra "oomph" in your anointing oil or potion, to keep the vision clear and focused, and keep on keeping on until it's been done.

Jojoba carrier oil has a shelf life of nine months to a year due to its waxy nature.

Olive Oil (*Olea Europaea*)

Called "Liquid Gold" by Homer, Olive Oil has a history of at least 6,000 years of service to the human race.

It is linked with vibrant health, well-being, and joy of life, as well as with success and enormous prosperity. Olive trees make the most of what other trees might find to be quite a difficult environment. They are strong and bestow practical prosperity and good health on their owners.

Olive Oil is a very good choice for hard-core money and success potions. It is also a very powerful base carrier oil for things that are designed to make a real change on the earthly plane.

In love spells, Olive Oil is used if a rich husband or wife is sought, or a partnership based on prosperity and earthly success is desired.

Use within nine months to a year.

Peach Kernel Oil (*Prunus Persica*)

The peach tree comes from China, where it is one of the oldest domesticated fruit trees. There are records of peach trees growing at least 6,000 years.

The peach tree is not long lived, but its fruit is said to bestow longevity, which the tree gave up in favor of transmitting longevity through its fruit to those who eat it. The peach tree is also very beautiful, with white or pink flowers when in bloom. Unlike many more mundane plants, the peach tree is special—exotic, experienced with people, and always welcome as a real treat and a lift to those who experience it.

Peach Kernel Oil is refined and retains the memory of its long ancestry in the service of humankind and all the other creatures that it nourishes.

Peach Kernel Oil is used in energy magic for special purposes. It has proven to be a reliable and powerfully active carrier. Its connection with longevity and immortality make it useful for angelic anointing oils, and for Faerie magic.

When used as a carrier for a love potion or anointing oil, Peach Kernel Oil will bring in the essence of a long-lived and spiritual relationship.

Use within three months.

Sweet Almond Oil (*Prunus Amygdalus*)

The Sweet Almond tree, with its multitude of white flowers, was held to be a place where friendly spirits of the land would gather. Planting one was held to be very fortuitous, leading to prosperity and a blessed existence.

The carrier energy of Sweet Almond Oil is one of gentle support and unconditional blessing.

It can be used for any purpose because it will simply pick up on any added ingredients and broadcast their energies without getting in the way. It is a very good oil for beginners because it is safe and positive, both physically and magically.

For this reason it is often used in protection potions and oils, and in spells to protect children and their innocence.

A love spell based on Sweet Almond Oil as a carrier would be suitable for a virgin, a young person, or someone who wants a flowing, protective relationship rather than something massively passionate. Practically, Sweet Almond Oil is the first choice among aromatherapists. It is rich in vitamins and many other elements, all of which are nourishing and supporting.

Use within nine months.

Sunflower Oil (*Helianthus Annuus*)

The wonderful Sunflower is one of the fastest-growing plants around. It is incredibly abundant, and in its season, it is the king of the flower world.

In order to achieve that growth, the Sunflower sucks in the Sun and makes it a part of its own structure. The oil from its seeds is thus imbued with sunlight, power, and life giving qualities.

Most people cook with Sunflower Oil and think it too "common" for use as anointing oil for ritual purposes, but that's a big mistake.

If you want superior results, fast growth, and the power of the Sun behind your potion, giving it extra, extra power, then Sunflower Oil is the carrier oil for you.

I don't even have to say it—how can you have a prosperity oil without Sunflower Oil involved in some way? This sunlight-golden oil is perfect for positive prosperity spells and works quickly, too.

If you use Sunflower Oil as the base for a love potion, better put on the seat belt and the shades! This is not always suitable for everyone. For many people, and for various reasons, it is probably safer to go with one of the gentler, more protective carrier oils.

Sunflower Oil lasts for a year if treated well.

Wheat Germ Oil (*Triticum Vulgare*)

A Safety Note: Wheat Germ Oil must be avoided by those who have wheat or gluten allergies. It can cause allergic reactions even if you are not allergic to gluten.

Wheat Germ Oil, being made from what was originally an abundant grass growing wild, is a powerful natural healer and restorer of life and vibrancy at a very basic and primal level.

Of course, wheat has such a long history—especially with the Celtic peoples—as being that which nourishes and feeds them, gives them daily bread, and keeps a family alive.

This is a good oil to use in potions for healing and protecting anything that is fear- and stress-related, also trauma, abuse, and accidental injury.

It can therefore also be used for love potions where extra help is needed, for example, if someone is still suffering from a broken heart, or was traumatized by earlier love relationships.

If you are unsure, always test in a small area of skin first. If you are sensitive to it, you can still use this oil for anointing with a brush while wearing gloves.

Use within three months.

Common Essential Oil Measurements:

1 drop = 0.05 ml
1 ml = 20 drops
1 teaspoon = 5 ml
1 teaspoon = 100 drops
1 tablespoon = 15 ml
1 tablespoon = 300 drops
1 ounce = 30 ml
1 ounce = 600 drops

Tincture of Benzoin Recipe:

Soak 1 tablespoon of powdered benzoin in ¼ cup of good-quality vodka or apple cider vinegar for three weeks. Strain and keep in a tightly capped dark bottle. Add tincture of benzoin to preserve your oils.

Essential Oil Profiles

Using Essential Oils

Many plants contain essential oils that can be extracted from flowers, leaves, roots, bark, seeds, and peels. Each of these essential oils is highly concentrated and has specific healing properties. They can be soothing, antispasmodic, antiseptic, calming, warming, or stimulating, for example. The quality of the essential oil depends on a number of factors: plant species, region, soil condition, and the climate in which the plant was grown; time of day the plant material was harvested; the extraction method used; and storage. It is believed that plants grown organically, or collected in the wild, yield the highest-quality essential oils.

Extracting the essential oils is done through various methods, but the best ones are steam distillation and cold-pressing. Avoid synthetic oils whenever possible and those extracted with chemical solvents. In all cases, very large quantities of plant materials are needed to extract even the smallest quantities of oil. This means that extraction methods are labor-intensive and expensive. Consequently, it's best to purchase essential oils from reputable sources.

Quality Oils

Be sure your essential oils are of high quality and pure. Read labels: Make sure an oil comes from the specific plant the product name indicates. Knowing Latin plant names may be helpful. Avoid blended and reconstituted oils and oils with synthetic or chemical additives. Anything labeled "fragrance oil" is not pure.

Therapeutic Effect: Research shows that the aromatic benefits of essential oils have a range of health-promoting qualities. They can also reduce anxieties and stress and generally enhance well-being. Essential oils are used with aromatherapy lamps, steam inhalations, baths, and massages.

Diluting for Use: Essential oils are very highly concentrated and should be diluted with water, plant extracts, or carrier oils before being applied to the skin.

Carrier Oils: Carrier oils do exactly what they say. They "carry" the potent essential oil for use on the skin. They are fatty, plant-based oils—usually vegetable, nut, or seed oils, such as Sweet Almond, Apricot Kernel, Olive, and Wheat Germ Oils. Each has its own therapeutic value to add to the essential oil's value. Use up to 15 drops of essential oil per ounce of carrier oil. Prepare small quantities as needed.

Other Bases: There are several extracts that work well as bases for diluting essential oils which may be used in the same way as carrier oils. For example, Witch Hazel is astringent and combats inflammation; Aloe Vera is a moisturizing healer for burns, cuts, and irritated skin; and Rose Water imparts its scent and is antiseptic.

Controversial Beliefs: In Europe, the ingestion of essential oils is generally accepted, primarily because it's done under a physician's care. But American herbalists are more conservative: Because the active ingredients in essential oils are highly concentrated, they can be dangerous if used improperly or in excess. You should only ingest essential oils upon the advice and recommendation of a qualified herbalist.

Extra Tip: Store essential oils in clearly labeled, opaque glass bottles in a cool, dark place. Refrigerate citrus oils. Properly stored, most essential oils will keep over a year.

Popular Oils

Allspice-Leaf Oil

The allspice, or pimento, tree is indigenous to Mexico and the West Indies. A relative of the Clove tree, it reaches a height of about 40 feet and bears tiny white flowers that produce small berries, which are dried and used as a spice. The name allspice refers to the fact that the berries' warm flavor is reminiscent of cloves, nutmeg, and cinnamon. Like the berries, the essential oil extracted from the leaves of the allspice tree smells mildly spicy. It has a powerful and stimulating effect on both the body and the mind. Allspice-Leaf Oil warms the body and promotes circulation when it is added to massage oils and baths, helping to relieve pain from muscle cramps and strains. Inhaling the oil has a beneficial effect on respiratory-tract infections, as it can alleviate coughing and thin mucus. In addition, using it as a massage oil can ease cramps. The warm, spicy scent of Allspice-Leaf Oil can lift the spirits and help in overcoming fatigue and listlessness.

For Mild Depression

The stimulating, harmonizing effect of Allspice-Leaf Oil can help to ease mild depression, especially when it is blended with soothing Lavender and Bergamot Oils. Try this blend in an aromatherapy lamp:

    3 drops Allspice-Leaf Oil
    2 drops Bergamot Oil
    2 drops Rosewood Oil
    1 drop Lavender Oil

Therapeutic Effect: The caryophyllene, eugenol-methyl ether, eugenol, and phellandrene in Allspice-Leaf Oil stimulate circulation and have a warming, relaxing effect in cases of physical and mental fatigue. The oil also helps to relieve stomachaches and intestinal colic. In addition, the strengthening effect of Allspice-Leaf Oil may support recovery from contagious illnesses.

For a Good Night's Sleep: A bath containing Allspice-Leaf Oil can have a relaxing, balancing effect and can help promote a restful sleep. Mix 2 drops each of Allspice-Leaf and Clary Sage Oils and 3 drops Lavender Oil with 2 ounces of Jojoba Oil. Blend well; add to your bathwater.

For Firmer Skin: Lotion containing Allspice-Leaf Oil can help nourish the skin and protect it from dryness. It also has a firming effect. Mix 3 drops of Allspice-Leaf Oil in 2 ounces of lotion. *Caution: Do not use as a facial lotion.*

For Coughing: An inhalation of Allspice-Leaf Oil can suppress coughing and speed recovery from colds. Mix 2 drops each of Allspice-Leaf, Frankincense, and Roman Chamomile Oils. Add them to a big bowl of steaming water. Cover your head with a towel and inhale the vapors.

To Relax Muscle Tension: Mix 2 drops each of Allspice-Leaf and Juniper Oils, 3 drops of Rosemary Oil, and 1 drop of Cinnamon Oil in 4 ounces of Sweet Almond Oil. Gently rub it into sore muscles.

Extra Tip: A compress with Allspice-Leaf Oil can ease headaches. Mix 2 drops in ½ gallon of cool water. Dip a cloth in it and put the cloth on your forehead.

! **Take Care!** Be sure to dilute Allspice-Leaf Oil thoroughly and use it only in very small amounts, because large doses of the oil can lead to irritation of both your skin and your mucous membranes. Avoid using Allspice-Leaf Oil around your eyes, mouth, and nose.

Applications

- Allspice-Leaf Oil can be effective for alleviating mild toothache pain. Mix 1 drop of the oil in 1 teaspoon of cider vinegar and blend it into a glass of warm water. Use it to rinse your mouth, but do not swallow any of the liquid. *Note: Always consult your dentist immediately about any kind of tooth pain.*

- A bath with Allspice-Leaf Oil can help to improve your circulation when you have a bad cold. Mix 2 tablespoons of milk and 3 drops each of Allspice-Leaf Oil, Thyme, Lemon, and Rosemary Oils. Fill your tub with warm water and add the mixture to the bathwater. Bathe for 20 minutes, and then rinse off under a lukewarm shower. This bath can help you feel stronger and hasten your recovery while preventing further infection.

- To help relieve cramps and gas pains, mix 2 drops of Allspice-Leaf Oil and 3 drops of Lavender Oil in 2 ounces of Sweet Almond Oil. Blend the mixture thoroughly and rub on your abdomen.

- Allspice-Leaf Oil possesses mild disinfectant properties and can be used to help clean the home and your clothes. Blend 3 drops each of Allspice-Leaf, Lemon, and Pine Oils in 1 gallon of water and mix thoroughly. Use it to mop your floors or clean the kitchen. You can also add it to the water in your washing machine.

Angelica Oil

The elegant plant known as *Angelica archangelica* was named for its famed habit of blooming on the feast day of Saint Michael the Archangel. A tall, stately, and expansive plant, Angelica is considered one of the most potent herbs in the botanical world—a panacea for all ills. Similarly, the herb's essential oil seems to impart rejuvenation and strength to everyone who uses it. Extracted from either the fresh roots or the seeds, Angelica Oil is obtained from one of two different methods: steam distillation or solvent extraction. Both are available, but it's best to use the distilled oil for medicinal purposes. In addition, the root oil is more readily available and stronger than the seed oil. However, regardless of which type you use, Angelica Oil boosts blood circulation and eases respiratory ailments, including coughs, congestion, and colds; soothes digestive complaints, such as stomachaches, poor appetite, cramps, and indigestion; and promotes sweating to relieve fevers. On an emotional level, its balsamic musky aroma lifts the spirits, eases anxiety, and promotes relaxation.

For Renewed Vitality

Angelica Oil's fragrance has a stimulating effect that can promote emotional stamina and inspire new strength for daily living. Scent any room in the house by evaporating the following mixture in your aromatherapy lamp:

    3 drops Angelica

    2 drops Basil

    1 drop Ginger

Therapeutic Effect: Angelica Oil contains lactones, acids, borneol, coumarins, and terpens, such as pinene. These components give the oil its strengthening effect on the body and mind. The oil can also stimulate the immune system and protect the body against infection. In addition, it relieves menstrual and intestinal cramps and alleviates indigestion, bloating, and gas. Because it loosens mucus and quiets coughs, the oil helps relieve symptoms commonly associated with colds, flu, and bronchitis.

For Headaches: The relaxing, soothing effect of Angelica Oil gently relieves headaches caused by mental overextension. Blend 1 drop of Angelica Oil with 20 drops of Sweet Almond or Olive Oil. Massage the mixture onto your forehead and temples.

For Colds: Inhalations with Angelica Oil relieve respiratory ailments, such as bronchitis, colds, flu, and congestion. The oil also loosens mucus and promotes expectoration, which helps to alleviate stubborn coughs.

For Insomnia: Angelica Oil's aromatic scent has a very beneficial effect on sleep. Place 1–2 drops on the pillow to ease insomnia and promote a restorative sleep.

For Fevers: Added to a bath, Angelica Oil can promote sweating, which helps reduce fevers as well as speeds the removal of toxins and wastes from the body.

For Flu Prevention: Angelica Oil boosts immunity and can help prevent viruses, including flu. Blend a few drops of the oil in a bowl of hot water. Place a towel over your head and bend over the bowl, inhaling the vapors.

For Motion Sickness: For anxiety and nausea while traveling, dab a drop of oil onto a handkerchief or carry it in a vial to inhale the scent.

Extra Tip: Add a few drops of the oil to a humidifier or an aromatherapy lamp. It helps restore vitality and stamina after an illness.

Applications

- For intestinal cramps, bloating, and gas, take a sitz bath with Angelica Oil to soothe and relax the digestive tract. Add 1 drop of Angelica Oil and 2 drops of Fennel Oil to a half-full bath and soak for 20 minutes. Rest for at least 30 minutes afterward with a hot-water bottle on your abdomen.

- Massages with Angelica Oil can alleviate joint and muscle pain from arthritis and rheumatism. Combine 2 drops of Angelica Oil, 5 drops of Rosemary Oil, and 2 drops of Juniper Oil with 1 ounce of Sweet Almond Oil. Massage the blend into affected areas using a gentle circular motion.

- Angelica Oil loosens mucus and calms coughs due to respiratory ailments, including bronchitis. Add 2 drops of the oil to a pot of boiling water, drape a towel over your head, and inhale the vapors.

- To alleviate menstrual cramps, mix 3 drops of Angelica Oil in 1 ounce of Olive Oil. Massage the blend into your lower abdomen using gentle circular motions. You can also rub the mixture on your chest to ease coughs, or on the upper abdomen for intestinal cramps.

Take Care! The components of Angelica Oil can increase the skin's sensitivity to light. Don't use the oil before going out in the sunlight because pigment spots can form. Angelica Oil may also irritate the skin, so only its diluted form is suitable for use. In addition, because excessive amounts of Angelica Oil may overstimulate the nervous system, use the oil only in very small amounts.

Anise Oil

The Anise plant, native to the Near East, is now grown in warm regions throughout the world. The grayish, brown seeds of *Pimpinella anisum* were highly prized in Ancient Greece as a natural digestive aid. Known for their ability to reduce bloating and flatulence, the seeds effectively address nervous-stomach ailments that are accompanied by nausea or vomiting. Also of note is the plant's ability to sweeten bad breath. Anise Oil, obtained from the seeds, can be used to settle the stomach as well. In addition, the oil can have a regulating effect on the entire digestive tract—especially in cases of colic and diarrhea. The oil is also appreciated for its ability to relieve headaches and menstrual cramps, but it may irritate the skin unless it is first diluted. An inhalation prepared form Anise Oil can provide relief from colds and bronchitis. With its pungent scent—which is similar to that of licorice—Anise Oil is useful in reducing mental fatigue and improving concentration.

For Brightening Your Mood

The scent of Anise Oil has an uplifting effect and can lend a pleasant atmosphere to any room. Try this blend in your aromatherapy lamp:

3 drops Anise

2 drops Mandarin Orange

2 drops Petitgrain

Therapeutic Effect: Anisic acid, anisic ketone, anethole, and acetaldehyde, the key components of Anise Oil, are responsible for its antispasmodic, expectorant, and digestive properties. The oil is effective in countering menstrual cramps and migraine headaches, and it can be effective in alleviating colic, nervous-stomach ailments, and bad breath. In addition, Anise Oil is beneficial for addressing coughs and other respiratory illness.

For Menstrual Cramps: A soothing bath with Anise Oil can alleviate pain in the back and lower abdomen during menstruation. Add 2 drops of Anise Oil and 3 drops of Clary Sage Oil to your bathwater. Soak for about 20 minutes.

For Migraines: The antispasmodic and pain-relieving properties of Anise Oil can help relieve migraines. Mix 2 drops of Anise Oil with 1 teaspoon of base oil. Rub the blend into your forehead and the nape of your neck; then rest for a while. If you prefer, you can apply 2 drops of undiluted Anise Oil to your hair. Be sure to wash your hands thoroughly after use.

For Fresher Breath: Anise Oil inhibits the growth of bacteria, thereby helping to prevent bad breath and gum inflammation. To freshen your breath, add 1 drop of Anise Oil to ½ cup of warm water. Mix well. Swish the wash in your mouth, spit it out, and then rinse with plain water. ***Caution***: *Anise oil may cause oral irritation. If this happens, discontinue use.*

For Detoxifying: Anise Oil can gently detoxify your body. Mix 2 drops each of Anise, Juniper, and Cypress Oils with 1 cup of fine-ground sea salt; then scrub your damp body with the mixture before taking a bath or shower.

Extra Tip: Inhaling Anise Oil can provide gentle relief from cold symptoms and allow you to breathe more freely. Add 2 drops each of Anise, Eucalyptus, and Peppermint Oils to a pan of simmering water.

Applications

- The fresh, mildly pungent scent of Anise Oil is helpful in cases of nausea and vomiting. To make a compress, add 2 drops of Anise Oil to a bowl of hot water, Dip a small towel or washcloth in the water, wring it out gently, and apply to the stomach. If desired, you may add 1 drop of Ginger or Peppermint Oil to the water.

- For colicky pain that occurs suddenly, a massage-oil blend can bring relief. Mix 2 tablespoons of Sweet Almond Oil and 2 drops each of Anise Oil and Fennel Oil. Rub the oil onto your abdomen, using gentle circular motions. This will help relieve the cramps. Afterward, apply a hot-water bottle to enhance the effect. Regular inhalations with Anise Oil can be effective in relieving chronic bronchitis as well as other respiratory conditions. Add 2 drops of Anise Oil and 1 drop of Roman Chamomile Oil to 1 quart of water in a bowl. Put a towel over your head, lean over the bowl, and deeply inhale the vapors for 5 to 10 minutes. Do this every day until all of your symptoms have been relieved.

Take Care! It is not recommended to apply undiluted Anise Oil directly to the skin, since it may cause irritation or other allergic reactions. Be sure to mix the oil well with other ingredients before using, and wash your hands thoroughly after use. Anise Oil should also not be used for an extended period of time or if you are pregnant.

Basil Oil

Basil (*Ocimum basilicum*) is a native herb of Africa and Asia that is cultivated in North and South America, Europe, and the Mediterranean. The name comes from the Greek word *basilokos*, meaning "royal," and indeed, Basil was once a very important ingredient in the oil used to anoint kings. Basil was also a sacred plant to the Hindu gods Krishna and Vishnu, and was widely applied in India's traditional

Ayurvedic medicine. Through steam distillation, the herb's oil is extracted, then used in many medicinal preparations. When inhaled, the oil relieves coughs, emphysema, asthma attacks, bronchitis, congestion, and colds. The oil is effective in treating nausea, indigestion, constipation, and gas, as well. Basil Oil is also valued as a tonic to reduce stress, tension, and mental fatigue. Further, the stimulating effects and spicy aroma of this oil help to clear the head, alleviate a headache, sharpen the senses, enhance concentration, and even revive someone from a fainting spell. Since Basil Oil also aids circulation, it can stimulate menstrual flow and ease discomfort, too.

To Reduce Lethargy

Possessing both sedating and stimulating medicinal effects, Basil Oil blends very well with Bergamot Oil and Lemon Oil. When the mixture is heated in an aromatherapy lamp, it is an ideal way to lighten the mood, fight mental fatigue, ward off nervous tension, and build self-confidence. Try this blend for an extra lift at the end of a stressful day.

    4 drops Basil

    2 drops Bergamot

    2 drops Lemon

Therapeutic Effect: The main chemical components of Basil Oil are phenol methylchavicol, estragole, linalool, cineol, caryphyllene, ocimene, pinene, eugenol, and camphor. Basil Oil is an antiseptic for hard-to-heal wounds and inflammations. Its antispasmodic properties help ease indigestion, tension, and muscle pain. When inhaled, the spicy freshness brings relief to respiratory ailments.

For Relaxation: A soothing blend of 4 drops each of Basil Oil and Lemon Balm Oil in your aromatherapy lamp calms and relaxes the entire body and may even lower your blood pressure. It also helps to relieve nervous tension and to ensure a deep, restorative sleep.

For Menstrual Pain: A nice warm bath with 2 drops each of Basil and Juniper Oils stimulates menstrual flow to ease pain at the start of your period.

For Cold Feet: The properties of Basil Oil help stimulate the circulatory system. To make an effective remedy for cold extremities, combine 3 drops each of Basil and Ginger Oils in 2 gallons of warm water. By regularly soaking your feet in this mixture, you can help prevent unpleasant foot perspiration and odor.

For Colds: To protect your immune system by reducing bacterial growth in the body, place 3 drops each of Basil and Peppermint Oils and 5 drops of Eucalyptus Oil in an aromatherapy lamp.

As an Insect Repellent: When it's placed in an aromatherapy lamp, Basil Oil can be quite effective in warding off insects. Combine 3 drops each of Basil, Cinnamon, and Clove Oils.

Extra Tip: Used regularly, a hair tonic of 2 ounces of Witch Hazel and 3 drops each of Basil and Rosemary Oils promotes circulation of the scalp, adds luster to hair, and reduces hair loss.

Applications

- Compresses with Basil Oil help treat slow-healing wounds: Mix 1 cup of luke-warm water, 1 tablespoon of cider vinegar, 1 drop of Basil Oil, and 2 drops of Lavender Oil. Soak gauze in the mixture, and place it on the wound. Cover the gauze with a bandage for the night. Change the compress as needed.

- For a headache, the spicy aroma of Basil Oil both refreshes and eases tension. Place 2 drops of Basil Oil in a handkerchief and deeply inhale the aroma. Be sure to avoid direct contact with the mouth and nose.

- A bad cold diminishes the sense of smell. The invigorating and strengthening properties of Basil Oil help to rebuild irritated mucous membranes. Vaporize 2 to 3 drops on an aromatherapy lamp. Do not use more than 2 hours a day since overstimulation dulls the nerves that transmit the sense of smell.

- For gastrointestinal cramps caused by indigestion: Mix 1 drop of Basil Oil into 1 tablespoon of Sweet Almond Oil. Then massage your upper abdomen with this soothing mixture, using a gentle circular motion in a clockwise direction.

- An abdominal massage with 3 drops Basil Oil, 3 drops of Lavender Oil, and 2 ounces of either Evening Primrose Oil or Sweet Almond Oil eases menstrual discomfort and cramps.

Take Care! It's best not to use Basil Oil during pregnancy, as it induces menstruation. People who have seizure disorders should avoid the oil as well. Because Basil Oil can irritate skin, be careful not to use it undiluted. To test your skin's sensitivity to the oil, place a drop on the inside of your forearm. While aromatherapists have used the oil for centuries, a component of Basil, estragole, has been investigated for carcinogenic effects. Consult your health provider before using.

Bay Laurel Oil

The bay laurel, a tree native to the Mediterranean, can reach a height of thirty feet. Its fragrant, smooth, leathery dark-green leaves have been treasured for many centuries, both as a culinary seasoning and as a medicinal herb. The leaves also symbolized honor and wisdom to the ancient Greeks and Romans. Now, the leaves are valued as a seasoning in marinades, sauces, stews, and fish. In addition, Bay Laurel leaves are treasured for their ability to alleviate a variety of health problems. The leaves' medicinal properties are due to the essential oil, which is extracted through a process of steam distillation. When applied externally, the oil's pain-relieving effects make it wonderful for treating muscle cramps, rheumatism, arthritis, and sprains. It also promotes sweating and urination, which can help eliminate wastes. Use this oil in moderation, however, since it has a mild narcotic effect and is very strong, even in the tiniest amounts; be sure to dilute first.

For a Sense of Peace
The warm scent of Bay Laurel Oil, which resembles that of Cinnamon, helps to relax the mind and body. The fragrance clears your mind, eliminating stress and anxiety. To create a sense of peace, warmth, and security, add this oil blend to an aroma-therapy lamp:

    3 drops Bay Laurel
    2 drops Cedarwood
    2 drops Sweet-Orange

Therapeutic Effect: The components phellandrene, pinene, terpineol, and cineole account for Bay Laurel Oil's soothing and relaxing properties. The oil alleviates pain and is very effective for treating bruises sprains and arthritic and rheumatic pain, when added to massage oils, baths, and compresses. Bay Laurel Oil also has an antispasmodic effect on colicky diarrhea.

For a Warming, Calming Bath: Bay Laurel's warm, slightly sweet scent helps to impart a sense of calmness and stability to your mind and body. Add 2 drops of the essential oil to a tub full of warm bathwater.

For Bronchitis: The scent of Bay Laurel Oil can help to thin the mucus in the bronchial tubes, while also easing coughs. A steam inhalation is the best way to do this. Fill a bowl with hot water and add a few drops of Bay Laurel Oil to it. Inhale the vapors.

To Ease Headaches: Since Bay Laurel Oil possesses gentle anesthetic and pain-relieving properties, it can alleviate headaches and migraines. Add 3 drops of Bay Laurel Oil to a bowl of cool water. Dip a small towel or cloth in it. Wring out the excess liquid and place the cloth on your forehead. If necessary, repeat after about 5 minutes.

To Promote Hair Growth: A shampoo containing a few drops of Bay Laurel Oil helps to stimulate circulation in the scalp. When used regularly, it promotes healthy, strong hair growth and adds shine. Add 2 drops of Bay Laurel Oil to 8 ounces of a mild and neutral-scented shampoo and shake it thoroughly. Be sure to keep it away from your eyes.

Extra Tip: To customize a Bay Laurel Oil blend, try experimenting with Rose, Lavender, Lemon, Orange, Rosemary and Eucalyptus Oils. All of these oils mix easily and effectively with Bay Laurel Oil.

Applications

- Massage oil with some Bay Laurel Oil added to it can help to alleviate pain from bruises, muscle cramps, and sprains. Mix 6 drops of Bay Laurel Oil and 4 drops each of Juniper and Rosemary Oils with 3 tablespoons of Sweet Almond or Avocado Oil. Mix it thoroughly and rub the blend into the affected areas several times each day.

- Compresses and wraps with Bay Laurel Oil help heal bruises and swelling. Mix 4 cups of cold water, 1 teaspoon of cider vinegar, and 4 drops of Bay Laurel Oil. Dip a clean towel in the liquid, wring out the excess, and apply the towel to the affected area. If you wish, apply a bandage over it to hold it in place.

- Bay Laurel Oil can help alleviate rheumatic and menstrual pain when added to your bathwater. Blend 3 tablespoons of milk, 4 drops of Bay Laurel Oil, 3 drops of Clary Sage Oil, and 2 drops of Roman Chamomile Oil. Add the mixture to a tub of warm bathwater.

- To relieve abdominal cramps, blend 2 drops of Bay Laurel Oil and 2 drops of Peppermint Oil in 2 tablespoons of Sweet Almond Oil. Use it to massage your abdomen.

Take Care! Bay Laurel Oil is one of the strongest oils used in aromatherapy. It should never be used by women who are pregnant, since it may cause spotting. The oil should also not be taken internally. In addition, Bay Laurel Oil can irritate the skin and mucous membranes. Be sure to always dilute the oil well and use it in very small amounts.

Black Pepper Oil

Native to Asia, Black Pepper (*Piper nigrum*) thrives best in shady, forested locations. Its dried berries, known as peppercorns, have multiple uses. In the past, they were of notable value as a trading commodity. Black Pepper Oil is obtained from the berries and features a mildly pungent scent. Up to half a ton of peppercorns must be processed by steam distillation to produce 1 quart of Black Pepper Oil. The oil is useful for warming the body and promoting circulation, as well as for alleviating muscle pain and tension. When used as a bath or massage oil, it provides relief from chronic rheumatic ailments. Black Pepper Oil also strengthens the entire digestive tract and alleviates bloating and colic by regulating activity in the large intestine while inducing a mild laxative effect. The oil's intense aroma invigorates the whole body and is effective for people who feel listless.

For Renewed Energy

The scent of Black Pepper Oil can have stimulating effects on people who experience mental and physical fatigue. Combining the following oils in an aromatherapy lamp will activate your body and mind, promote concentration, and enhance your performance.

> 3 drops Black Pepper
>
> 2 drops Cypress
>
> 2 drops Juniper
>
> 2 drops Lemon

Therapeutic Effect: The components of black pepper oil, including piperine, phellandrene, pinene, citral, and caryophyllene, have potent stimulating properties. Baths and massages with the oil warm the muscles and alleviate tension. The oil helps intestinal colic and stomach pain as well. It supports digestion and increases intestinal muscle activity.

For Aiding Digestion: To aid digestion after a meal, mix 2 drops each of Black Pepper Oil with 4 tablespoons of Sweet Almond Oil. Gently rub the mixture onto your abdomen.

For Detoxifying: Adding Black Pepper Oil to a warm bath helps stimulate sweat production and thereby increases the effectiveness of a detoxifying effect. The bath also increases kidney activity, promoting the excretion of additional toxins. Add 3 drops each of Black Pepper and Juniper Oils to your bath.

For Bruises: To decrease the swelling from a bruise, mix 2 tablespoons of Avocado Oil with 2 drops each of Black Pepper and Helichrysum Oils. Dip a clean cloth in the mixture and apply it to the bruise twice daily.

For Nausea: With its pungent scent, Black Pepper Oil can help to relieve queasiness and nausea quickly with no side effects. Apply a few drops of oil, as needed, to a handkerchief, and then inhale the scent deeply.

For a Fever: Black Pepper Oil can reduce a fever when mixed with cool water. It is also used to prepare a calf wrap. Dissolve 2 drops of Black Pepper Oil in about ½ teaspoon vodka. Add the mixture to a bowl of cool water, soak two bandages in it, and then loosely wrap each calf. Keep the wraps in place for about 20 minutes.

Extra Tip: White Pepper Oil is similar in scent to Black Pepper Oil, though it's less pungent. Their effects are similar, too, but the latter is more readily available.

! **Take Care!** Always exercise caution when using Black Pepper Oil, because over-use may result in kidney damage. The oil is toxic when taken internally. It should always be thoroughly diluted prior to external use, since it can be irritating to the skin. In general, it is best to use Black Pepper Oil sparingly.

Applications

- For muscle pain: A massage with highly diluted Black Pepper Oil can improve circulation and warm tissues, thus alleviating muscle pain and tension. To make massage oil, mix 3 tablespoons of Sweet Almond Oil, 5 drops of Lavender Oil, and 3 drops of Black Pepper Oil. Gently apply the blend to the affected areas and massage it into your skin.

- For rheumatic ailments: Warm baths with Black Pepper Oil can be beneficial in alleviating pain and joint stiffness associated with rheumatism. Blend 2 table-spoons of an unscented cream, 2 drops of Black Pepper Oil and 3 drops each of Rosemary and Hyssop Oil. (You can substitute Frankincense Oil for the Hyssop Oil.) Add the mix to your bathwater and then soak for 20 minutes. After drying off, cover up warmly and rest for at least two hours. *Caution: If you are suffering from acute inflammation, with symptoms such as redness, soreness and very pain-ful areas, you should not use this remedy, as it can exacerbate your symptoms.*

- Before exercise: Black Pepper Oil's stimulating effect can help prevent muscle pain as well as cramps. Massage your entire body with 3 tablespoons of Sun-flower Oil, 5 drops each of Black Pepper Oil and Rosemary Oil, and 4 drops of Orange Oil.

Cajuput Oil

A member of the family Myrtaceae, the Cajuput tree is native to Australia, Malay-sia, India, and the Spice Islands. The aromatic tree can grow to a height of 130 feet and bears pale green oval leaves and clusters of small white flowers on long spikes. It is cultivated for its lumber and essential oil. Cajuput Oil, extracted by a process of steam distillation from the tree's leaves and twigs, has long been valued for its anti-inflammatory and analgesic properties. It can help to treat upper-respiratory ailments, such as bronchitis, asthma, laryngitis, colds, and flu. The oil also eases ar-thritis, rheumatism, and such nervous-stomach complaints as cramps and gas. In ad-dition, Cajuput Oil can alleviate neuralgia, neuritis, toothaches, bleeding gums, and symptoms caused by urinary-tract infections. Furthermore, the oil possesses many antiseptic qualities and may relieve skin blemishes, acne, psoriasis, and dermatitis. On an emotional level, Cajuput Oil's fresh and eucalyptus-like fragrance can invigo-rate the senses, helping to clear the mind and banish fatigue and poor concentration.

To Clear the Air

Cajuput Oil's slightly pungent, woodsy, herbal scent quickly purifies and freshens stale air. Try the following blend in your aromatherapy lamp to help deodorize musty rooms:

> 4 drops Cajuput
> 2 drops Lime
> 2 drops Bergamot

Therapeutic Effect: Cineol, pinene, valeric acid, limonene, and terpenes give the oil its antiseptic, analgesic, antimicrobial, and antispasmodic effects. Cajuput Oil strengthens the body and mind in cases of physical and mental exhaustion. It also eases intestinal complaints, promotes expectoration, and relieves joint and nerve pain.

For Skin Conditions: Cajuput Oil helps clarify and cleanse the skin in cases of psoriasis and neurodermatitis. It soothes itching and speeds the healing of scaly patches. Add 2 drops each of Cajuput and Frankincense Oils to 2 tablespoons of Sweet Almond Oil. Stir into warm bathwater.

For Nausea: To help alleviate nausea, put 1 drop of Cajeput Oil onto a handkerchief. Hold the cloth away from your nose in order to avoid skin contact. Deeply inhale the aroma and repeat as needed.

For Laryngitis: To soothe a sore throat and relieve laryngitis, mix 1 drop each of Cajuput and Tea Tree Oils, and 1 teaspoon vodka in 4 ounces of water. Gargle with the solution 3 to 4 times a day until the symptoms have completely subsided.

For Bladder Inflammations: Sitz baths with Cajuput Oil can relieve bladder inflammations and urinary-tract infections. Mix 2 drops each of Cajuput, Myrtle, and Thyme Oils and 1 drop of Lemon Oil with ½ cup heavy cream. Blend well and add it to a half-full bath. Soak for about 20 minutes, then rest in bed for an hour.

For Bleeding Gums: For toothaches and bleeding gums, mix 2 drops of Cajuput Oil with 1 cup of warm water. Use the solution to rinse your mouth several times a day. Spit out this rinse completely, as with all mouth washes.

Extra Tip: For an invigorating pick-me-up, add 3 drops of Cajuput Oil to a bowl of hot water. Drape a towel over your head and the bowl; inhale the vapors.

Take Care! As with all essential oils, Cajuput Oil should not be used internally. It is also unsuitable for pregnant women. When applying Cajuput Oil externally, do a test patch first to check skin for sensitivity. It is important to dilute the oil before using it too.

Applications

- Make a chest rub with Cajuput Oil to help alleviate respiratory ailments, such as bronchitis and asthma. Mix 5 drops of Cajuput Oil, 3 drops each of Thyme and Frankincense Oils, and 2 drops of Lemon Oil with 3 tablespoons of Sweet Almond Oil, petroleum jelly, or lotion. Apply to your chest and upper back several times daily.

- Cajuput Oil can help relieve pain due to arthritis. Blend 4 drops of the oil with 2 tablespoons of Sunflower Oil. Gently massage the oil into the painful joints. However, if the area is inflamed, you may want to try a compress (below).

- Cajuput Oil has a soothing and antispasmodic effect that can help alleviate nervous-stomach complaints, including diarrhea, gas, and abdominal cramps. Mix 2 drops of Cajeput Oil and 1 drop of Peppermint Oil with 1 ounce of Sweet Almond Oil. Use the blend to massage your stomach in a clockwise motion.

- For joint inflammation, make a cool compress with Cajuput Oil instead of massage oil. Blend 3 drops of the oil in a large bowl of cool water. Dip a cloth in the mix and apply to the affected areas, as needed.

Calamus Oil

The Calamus plant, which belongs to the family Araceae, is native to the areas of Southeast Asia. Also called sweet flag, it was introduced to Europe and North America hundreds of years ago; now it grows wild along bodies of standing water. Essential oil of Calamus, obtained from the root via steam distillation, stimulates the appetite and helps relieve gastrointestinal ailments. Due to its antibacterial properties, the oil is also used in gargles. (Similarly, people in India chew pieces of Calamus Root as a remedy for toothaches and to cleanse the mucous membranes of the mouth.) The oil also promotes blood flow through the tissues and stabilizes circulation. Thus, it can provide the body with lasting warmth, prevent muscle tension and cramps, and alleviate rheumatic aches and joint pain. Finally, the oil's fresh, mildly pungent aroma can be beneficial in relieving exhaustion. *Caution: Calamus Oil can irritate the skin, so be careful when using it.*

Aromatic Strengthening

The fresh aroma of Calamus Oil has a revitalizing effect on the body and the mood. Try this blend in an aromatherapy lamp to help get you on your feet again in times of stress and emotional strain.

2 drops Calamus

2 drops Basil

2 drops Clary Sage

Therapeutic Effect: The active ingredient in Calamus Oil is asarone, which has a stimulating effect. The oil also contains asaryl aldehyde, camphene, and limonene. It strengthens the body, stimulates the appetite and has an antispasmodic effect in cases of colic and stomach pain. The oil also relieves gas and acts as a mild laxative. Its sweat-inducing and diuretic effects help remove wastes from the body.

For Exhaustion: Blend 2 drops each of Calamus, Lemon, and Rosemary Oils in a bowl of steaming water and use as a steam facial. This combination can help to relieve fatigue and poor concentration.

For Self-Care: A bath with Calamus Oil warms and strengthens your entire body. It also increases your immunity to infectious illnesses and protects against hypothermia during wet, cold weather. Add 2 drops each of Calamus, Eucalyptus, and Lavender Oils to your bath.

Massage for Varicose Veins: A daily massage with diluted Calamus Oil relieves pressure in the legs and can help prevent varicose and spider veins. Mix 2 drops each of Calamus, Rose, and Cypress Oils with 2 ounces of Sweet Almond Oil.

For Low Blood Pressure: A shower gel with Calamus Oil can stimulate blood flow in your skin. Alternating with warm and cool showers will further stimulate your blood pressure. Add 2 drops each of Calamus, Juniper, and Rosemary Oils to 4 ounces of unscented gel and then mix them well.

For Dental Care: Toothpaste containing Calamus Oil invigorates the gums and protects against bleeding and periodontal disease. Such toothpaste can be found in stores that carry natural cosmetics.

Extra Tip: Obtain Calamus Oil from a reliable source that can guarantee its authenticity.

Applications

- Massages with Calamus Oil can relieve cramps and pain in the lower abdomen. Mix 1 drop of Calamus Oil with 2 tablespoons of Sweet Almond Oil and massage the blend into your abdomen, using circular motions. Hold a hot water bottle wrapped in a towel against your abdomen and rest in bed for 30 minutes.

- A bath additive consisting of 2 tablespoons of Wheat Germ Oil, 1 drop of Calamus, and 2 drops of Ginger Oil promotes circulation and provides relief from chronic rheumatic pain. After bathing, it's best to rest for at least one hour.

- Calamus Oil promotes sweating and acts as a diuretic, helping to cleanse the body. To support a fasting regimen, take a hot shower, and while still damp, rub your skin well with a blend of 3 tablespoons Olive Oil and 2 drops of Calamus Oil. Wrap yourself in a large linen towel and rest in bed for two hours, covered up warmly. Then take another shower, this time in lukewarm water, to wash away the waste products you've excreted through sweating.

- To help keep moths and other insects out of your clothes, blend 2 drops each of Calamus and Patchouli Oils, 10 drops of Lavender Oil, and 1 ounce of dried Lavender flowers. Place the blend in a sock, knot the end, and hang it in a closet.

Take Care! Because of its potentially carcinogenic effects if used in large quantities over an extended period of time, Calamus Oil is banned in some countries. It is also banned in fragrances which is one of its traditional uses. Like the majority of essential oils, Calamus should not be taken internally or applied undiluted to the skin. It is also not suitable for use during pregnancy.

Caraway Oil

Caraway (*Carum carvi*) has been used as a medicine and a spice for millennia. An aromatic member of the Umbelliferae family, it is closely related to Anise and Fennel and thus bears similar medicinal qualities. Caraway seeds have been prized as a natural digestive aid since the ancient Romans baked them into their cakes and pastries to promote proper digestion after sumptuous banquets. In fact, the therapeutic value of the seeds is derived from the presence of essential oil. The oil, extracted from the seeds by steam distillation, can help relieve digestive complaints. Caraway Oil has carminative properties that help regulate intestinal function, dispel gas, alleviate abdominal cramps, ease bloating, and boost the appetite. When used in steam inhalations, the oil promotes expectoration and alleviates congestion due to bronchitis, colds, and sinus infections. It can also be applied topically to soothe joint pain caused by rheumatism and arthritis. Cosmetically, the oil helps regulate sebum production and reduces acne, oily skin, and unsightly blemishes.

Banish Fatigue and Listlessness

The peppery, pungent scent of Caraway Oil stimulates the body's senses and awakens new energy. To help relieve physical exhaustion, mental fatigue, and listlessness, burn the following blend in your aromatherapy lamp:

3 drops Caraway

3 drops Lime

1 drop Petitgrain

Therapeutic Effect: Caraway Oil contains carvone, dihydropinol, carvol, and limonene, which have an invigorating effect on the entire body. The oil strengthens and regulates digestion, boosts the appetite, and relieves intestinal cramps, diarrhea, gas, and bloating. Inhaling the oil loosens mucus and eases congestion. Applied topically, the oil helps treat acne and oily skin.

For Oily Skin: When used regularly, a cleansing lotion with a few drops of Caraway Oil can combat acne and regulate the oil production of the sebaceous glands.

For Rheumatism: Caraway Oil's ability to warm the body and stimulate blood flow helps ease joint pain due to rheumatism, arthritis, and gout. Mix a few drops with Sweet Almond Oil and rub into joints.

For Abdominal Cramps: Caraway Oil is beneficial for a variety of intestinal complaints. Add about 3 to 4 drops to a base oil, such as Sweet Almond Oil, and massage onto your abdomen with gentle, circular motions.

For Milk Production: Caraway Oil prompts milk flow and has been used as a natural nursing aid. Place 3 drops in your aromatherapy lamp; inhale before nursing.

For Respiratory Congestion: For sinus inflammations, head colds, respiratory congestion, and flu, Caraway Oil loosens mucus and fights the germs that can cause infection. Mix 3 drops of the oil in a bowl of steaming water. Drape a towel over your head, bend over the bowl and inhale the vapors with your eyes closed.

! Take Care! Because Caraway Oil can irritate the skin, it should always be diluted and used only externally in very small doses. Young children and pregnant women may instead want to consider using Fennel and Anise Oils, which offer similar medicinal effects.

Applications

- For a sore throat, dilute 3 drops of Caraway Oil in ½ cup of water and gargle with it several times each day. Spit out the mixture. The oil's antiseptic action helps fight germs, and its astringent property helps heal inflamed mucous membranes.

- Caraway Oil has an antispasmodic effect on the lower abdomen that helps ease menstrual pain. Mix 4 drops of Caraway Oil with 2 tablespoons of cream and add the mixture to a half-full bath. Soak for 20 minutes and then rest for one hour.

- For coughs and congestion, mix 1 drop each of Caraway, Lavender, and Frankincense Oils in 2 ounces of Sweet Almond Oil. Massage the blend onto your chest and back to help promote expectoration.

- Try sweetening bad breath with Caraway Oil. Add 1 drop of oil to 2 tablespoons baking soda and blend well. Dip your toothbrush in the mixture and brush your teeth as usual. Spit out the mixture and rinse your mouth thoroughly.

- For nausea, put a few drops of Caraway Oil onto a clean cloth. Inhale, keeping the folded cloth from touching your skin.

- Prepare a household cleaning solution with 2 to 3 drops of the oil mixed in 1 gallon of water and some liquid Castile soap. The oil has disinfectant, antibacterial properties and helps get rid of bathroom and kitchen germs.

Cedarwood Oil

Atlas cedar (*Cedrus atlantica*) is an evergreen native to Africa that is cultivated in Asia and can grow up to 130 feet. It has needle-like leaves and, if left undisturbed, can live as long as 2,000 years. Cedarwood was one of the first fragrant plants used by the Egyptians as an ingredient for cosmetics, perfumes, and the mummification process. In addition, Native Americans burn Cedar for purification. Today, Cedarwood Oil is used in cosmetics, fragrances, and household products. The oil is extracted from the sawdust and wood of cedar trees and has a scent that is deep, sweet, and camphor-like. Cedarwood Oil is known for its calming quality and numerous healing properties. An antiseptic and astringent, it relieves skin conditions, such as eczema, dermatitis, psoriasis, oily skin, and acne, as well as upper-respiratory infections. Its aroma helps to promote spirituality, balance, and a sense of tranquility.

For Sensuality

Cedarwood Oil is believed to heighten the senses and relax the body. People have long relied on the oil to create an atmosphere of romance and sensuality and to enhance sexual desire: in fact, the oil is a renowned aphrodisiac. To use, place 5 to 10 drops in an aromatherapy lamp in your bedroom, add it to a warm candlelit bath or apply it to clothing. You can add one or more of these aphrodisiac oils as well: Jasmine, Sandalwood, Clary Sage, Patchouli, Rose, Neroli, and Ylang-Ylang.

Therapeutic Effect: Cedarwood contains alantone, caryophyllene, cedrol, and cadinene. It has astringent, antifungal, and antiseptic properties, which make it useful in treating infections and skin conditions. As a diuretic, it helps to relieve urinary-tract infections. As a sedative, it can also relieve anxiety and nervous tension.

For Emotional Balance: Cedarwood helps to alleviate anxiety, stress, and tension. It also improves mental clarity and concentration and assists meditation. Blend 6 drops of Cedarwood and 2 drops each of Geranium and Lemon Oils in 1 ounce of Sweet Almond Oil. Use the blend to massage the neck and shoulders.

For Body Care: Cedarwood, an astringent and antiseptic, is a common ingredient in many body-care lotions and creams. Add 2–4 drops of Cedarwood Oil to 1 tablespoon of your favorite lotion and massage it into the skin. It will help tighten your pores and even out your skin tone.

For Muscle Pain: Cedarwood Oil has a cooling effect that can help to relax your sore, tight muscles and lessen pain. Fill a bath with warm water, add 4–6 drops of Cedarwood Oil, and soak for 20–30 minutes.

For Congestion: For coughs, upper-respiratory congestion, bronchitis, colds, and sinusitis, Cedarwood Oil's expectorant effect opens the sinuses, thins mucus, relieves congestion, combats infection, and eases difficult breathing. Add 7 drops of Cedarwood Oil, 3 drops of Lavender Oil, and 2 drops of Juniper Oil to 1 ounce of Sweet Almond or Olive Oil and blend well. Gently massage this mixture into your chest and upper body.

Extra Tip: Cedarwood Oil is a moth deterrent. Add a few drops to a cloth, and store it in your linen closet.

Take Care! High doses of Cedarwood Oil added to body oils, bath oils, or facial treatments may irritate the skin. Stop using the oil immediately if your skin shows signs of irritation. **Note:** Since this oil can stimulate menses, don't use it if you are pregnant.

Applications

- Cedarwood Oil's calming effect eases tension and anxiety that may cause insomnia and helps to promote a deep, restorative sleep. Before bed, fill a bath with warm water, and add 3 drops of Cedarwood Oil and 3 drops of Ylang-Ylang and Rosemary Oils. Soak for 15–20 minutes.

- Cedarwood Oil relieves many skin conditions. Add 3 drops of Cedarwood Oil and 2 drops of Lavender Oil to ¼ cup of warm water. Soak a soft washcloth in the water, wring it out, and then apply it to the affected areas. Be careful to avoid the eyes. When the cloth cools, soak it again in warm water, and reapply.

- To help relieve dandruff, control oily hair, improve hair condition, and stimulate the scalp and hair follicles, combine 2 drops of Cedarwood, 1 drop of Cypress, and 2 drops of Rosemary Oils in 1 tablespoon of Olive Oil. Massage the mixture into the scalp for three minutes. Leave it on the hair for 20 minutes; then shampoo. Repeat weekly.

- To keep insects out of the home, use 3–5 drops of Cedarwood Oil in an aromatherapy lamp or in a spray bottle for misting.

- Make a traditional fragrance to enhance meditation. Mix 2–3 drops each of Cypress, Juniper, Frankincense, Sandalwood, and Cedar Oils, and add to your aromatherapy lamp.

Cinnamon Oil

Cinnamon, one of the most commonly used spices in the world today, has been an essential ingredient in both Indian and Arabic cooking for centuries. Cinnamon's familiar aroma continues to warm kitchens throughout the world. The spice was first used medicinally in ancient Egypt; we now know it has antiviral properties due to its volatile oil, which is extracted from both the bark and leaves of the cinnamon plant. These oils emit a sweet scent that aromatherapists believe can provide warmth and a sense of security. The bark oil is quite potent and can irritate the skin; oil from the leaves is more delicate, but it, too, may irritate. Each has its own set of uses. Oil from the bark is appropriate for a diffuser; its aroma is thought to arouse the senses. Used topically as a beauty aid, Cinnamon Leaf Oil is astringent, antiseptic, and soothingly warm. The warmth also soothes aching muscles due to cold symptoms. Avoid skin irritation by diluting either oil before use.

Gentle Strength for When You Feel Fragile

The aroma of Cinnamon Oil can calm your anxieties and strengthen self-confidence. A few drops of the following blend in an aromatherapy lamp has a soothing effect on the spirit, strengthens the heart, and may bring comfort in times of painful loss.

Therapeutic Effect: The primary components of Cinnamon Oil are eugenic acid and cinnamic aldehyde. These constituents are highly antiseptic and have a warming, stimulating effect on both the body and the mind. They may help alleviate pain from muscular, bone, and joint problems, including arthritis.

For Head Lice: To repel head lice, add a few drops of Cinnamon Oil to 1 tablespoon of Jojoba Oil. Rub the mixture into your scalp daily until the parasites are gone. Be extremely careful to avoid your eyes.

For Strengthening Nerves: When you're feeling tense or overexcited from the stresses of life, the sweet, spicy aroma of Cinnamon Oil offers peace and composure. The scent of cinnamon in a simmer pot or diffuser acts as a gentle tonic without side effects.

As a Custom Perfume: For an antiseptic perfume, a single drop of Cinnamon Leaf Oil may be added to 2 ounces of vodka for a warm, spicy base. Other essential oils like Lavender, Bergamot, or Ylang-Ylang could be added—up to 10 drops total—to create your own personal scent. Spray your hair (using caution to avoid your eyes) or on your clothes. If you add Bergamot Oil, do not spritz your skin, as it's phototoxic. Add Jasmine Oil for a rich scent; Vanilla Oil will lend an exotic edge.

To Combat Chills: A warm bath with Cinnamon Leaf, Ginger, and Juniper Oils may dispel the chills that can accompany colds. The bath stimulates circulation and warms the entire body. Add 1 drop of each of the oils to your bathwater, and be sure to mix them well.

Extra Tip: If you decide to use Cinnamon Oil topically, choose oil from the leaf and dilute it first with a fatty carrier oil, such as Olive Oil. Discontinue use if any skin irritations occur.

Applications

- Daily massages with 3 tablespoons of Sweet Almond Oil mixed with 8 drops of Cinnamon Leaf Oil, 5 drops of Orange Oil, and 4 drops of Juniper Oil stimulate blood flow and help to firm up and tone the skin. The mixture can also help you battle cellulite: Massage the oil into the skin with firm upward strokes toward the heart. In addition, this oil works well as a foot massage.

- Cinnamon Oil strengthens and firms up gums and helps prevent gum disease. Add 1 drop of Cinnamon Leaf Oil to 1 teaspoon of vodka and 2 tablespoons of water. Shake the mixture well, and swish your toothbrush in it. Brush your teeth as usual.

- In a room spray, Cinnamon Oil will refresh damp, mildewy areas. Mix 2 ounces of vodka, 3 drops of Cinnamon Oil (bark or leaf), 5 drops of Bergamot Oil, and 2 ounces of water in a spritzer; shake the bottle well, and then spray the room. You can add this mixture to a simmer pot or diffuser for the same effect.

- For a warming footbath, fill a deep tub with 2 gallons of warm water. Add 1 drop of Cinnamon Leaf Oil, 2 drops of Rosemary Oil, 1 teaspoon of vodka, and 2 drops of Juniper Oil. Mix well, and submerge your feet in the mixture for a relaxing soak.

Take Care! Cinnamon Oil should only be used sparingly for topical applications. Even when diluted, it can irritate the skin if the amount is too high. As with most volatile oils, Cinnamon Oil is always diluted first with a carrier oil. Oil extracted from the bark of the cinnamon plant is suitable only for use in a diffuser or simmer pot. Don't use more than 3 drops, since its high potency may cause headaches. Wash your hands well after each use.

Clary Sage Oil

As an esteemed member of the Labiatae family—which also includes Lavender, Lemon Balm, and Thyme—Clary Sage is a well-loved perennial that is native to France, Italy, and Syria and is now cultivated worldwide for medicinal use. Its heart-shaped, fuzzy leaves and pale purple flowers yield a highly aromatic essential oil with both antispasmodic and anti-inflammatory properties. As such, it has been a widely prescribed natural treatment for eczema and psoriasis, as well as for minor cuts and wounds. Clary Sage Oil is also estrogen stimulating; the oil's ability to balance fluctuating hormones makes it a highly beneficial remedy for PMS, painful menstrual cramps, and the hot flashes associated with menopause. The oil has even been used during childbirth to minimize labor pains. In addition, Clary Sage Oil's sweet, nutty scent is said to revitalize those who are suffering from depression, tension, stress, and fear. Herbalists also recommend the oil for inspiring creativity and awakening intuition.

To Awaken the Imagination

To spark the creative impulse or create a stimulating and inspiring atmosphere, blend Clary Sage Oil with Sandalwood and Bergamot Oils. Place the oils, along with Lemon Oil for a refreshing scent, in a diffuser or in an aromatherapy lamp:

> 3 drops Clary Sage
>
> 3 drops Bergamot
>
> 3 drops Sandalwood
>
> 3 drops Lemon

Therapeutic Effect: Composed of such therapeutic components as linalool, sclareol, monoterpenes, and tannins, Clary Sage Oil is antispasmodic, antiseptic, and calming. When used as a massage oil—or in a bath or aromatherapy lamp—the oil can help soothe menstrual cramps, treat acne, alleviate headaches and muscle strain, promote calm and lift the lowest of spirits.

For Peace and Tranquility: A warm and aromatic bath enhanced with Clary Sage Oil will help to ease tension and encourage calm, paving the way for a good night's rest. Mix 3–5 drops of the oil in your bathwater just before you enter the tub. Remember, too, that less is best when it comes to using essential oils; as pure concentrates, they should be used sparingly.

Facial Bath for Acne: Clary Sage Oil's antiseptic and anti-infectious effects are said to work together to effectively treat acne. Add 2 drops each of Clary Sage, Geranium and Roman Chamomile Oils to a bowl of steaming water; then cover your head with a towel and breathe deeply for 2–5 minutes. Do not use if you have broken facial capillaries.

For Dry Hair and Dandruff: Clary Sage will not only help prevent dandruff but also condition dry hair, giving it a silky shine. When used as a scalp massage, it is said to encourage hair growth. Mix 4–5 drops of Clary Sage Oil with 5 drips of Lavender Oil in 2 tablespoons of shampoo.

For Labor Pains: Mix 3 drops of Clary Sage Oil and 2–3 drops each of Jasmine and Rose Otto Oils, as well as 2 tablespoons of a carrier oil, for a blend to help ease labor pains. Using gentle strokes, massage your entire lower abdomen and lower back. This blend can also help to reduce the fear and stress that often accompany childbirth.

A Little Lore: Derived from the Latin *clarus*, for "clear," Clary Sage was a medieval remedy for blurred vision and eyestrain.

! **Take Care!** Clary Sage Oil has been known to create a state of euphoria in certain cases. Refrain from using Clary Sage Oil with drugs or alcohol. It can cause their effects to become exaggerated, while also intensifying intoxication and hangovers. The oil can cause drowsiness as well and severely impair the ability to drive. In addition, Clary Sage Oil should not be used if you are pregnant or are trying to conceive.

Applications

- Clary Sage Oil's warming and relaxing effects make it an excellent massage oil for stiff, sore muscles. Mix 15 drops of the essential oil with 3 tablespoons of Sweet Almond Oil, and then massage into affected muscles.

- For colds and coughs, try the following mixture: In a diffuser or aromatherapy lamp, place 6 drops of Clary Sage Oil, 3 drops of Thyme Oil and 1 drop of Eucalyptus Oil. *Caution: Avoid using red-or-white Thyme Oil. Use Thyme-linalool Oil instead.*

- Clary Sage Oil can lower blood pressure and is said to have a calming effect during times of stress. Place 2 drops of Clary Sage Oil and 1 drop of Ylang-Ylang Oil on a tissue and inhale to settle the mind and restore emotional equilibrium.

- For menstrual cramps, fill a bowl with steaming water and add 2 drops each of Geranium Oil, Roman Chamomile Oil, and Clary Sage Oil. Dip half of a large cloth into the water; fold the cloth and apply the warm compress to the abdomen, with the oil-soaked side away from the skin.

- Clary Sage Oil can help heal minor cuts, wounds, and burns. Make a compress (above), using 3 drops of Clary Sage Oil, 3 drops of Lavender Oil, and 2 drops of Tea Tree Oil. Apply to the skin.

Clove Oil

Cloves are the dried flower buds of the Clove tree, native to the Molucca Islands of Indonesia. The trees grow up to fifty feet tall and bear aromatic leaves and buds. They rarely flower, however, because buds are harvested as soon as they turn pink.

When the buds are completely dried, these Cloves resemble small, dark brown nails; indeed, the word *Clove* is derived from the Latin word *clavus*, or nail. Cloves have been treasured for more than 2,000 years in Asian countries, as both a spice and a remedy. During China's Han dynasty, courtiers chewed on them to help freshen their breath when speaking to the emperor. In medieval Europe, Cloves were valued for medicinal and culinary uses. Today, they are mainly used for cooking. The oil made from Cloves retains their spicy, warm, sweet scent and possesses antispasmodic, antiviral, and antiseptic effects. It is used to relieve flatulence, diarrhea, stomachaches, and toothaches. In addition, Clove Oil is very effective for killing germs and bacteria, making it useful as an ingredient in mouthwashes, toothpastes, and wound disinfectants.

A Natural Insect Repellent

Aromatic Clove Oil can ward off mosquitoes. Use this blend in an aromatherapy lamp, placing it outside to help prevent bugs from disturbing a peaceful evening:

   4 drops Clove

   3 drops Lavender

   3 drops Lemon

   3 drops Orange

Therapeutic Effect: The components eugenol, acetyleugenol, and oleanolic acid are responsible for Clove Oil's mildly anesthetic properties, which can alleviate pain from toothaches and gum inflammations. It is also effective for disinfecting canker sores and wounds and can help treat intestinal ailments that result in diarrhea, flatulence, and stomach pain.

For a Relaxing Scent: Clove Oil can lend a warm and pleasant note to natural perfumes. It harmonizes with Citronella, Orange, Grapefruit, Nutmeg, and Cinnamon Oils.

Following Childbirth: The strengthening effect of Clove Oil may help to tone the uterus following delivery. Mix 1 drop each of Clove and Cinnamon Oils and 3 drops of Orange Oil into your bathwater. Soak for about 15 minutes, once a week.

For Muscle Cramps: A massage oil that contains Clove Oil can ease muscle pain and cramps, as it stimulates circulation. Mix 3 drops each of Clove, Juniper, and Rosemary Oils with 2 ounces of Sweet Almond Oil. Massage it into sore muscles as needed.

For Toothache Pain: Clove Oil is very effective for alleviating toothache pain. Mix 1 drop each of Clove and Myrrh Oils and 1 teaspoon vodka. Put the mixture on a cotton ball and use it to gently swab the gums that surround the painful tooth.

For Disinfecting Wounds: Clove Oil is anti-inflammatory and antiseptic. To make a
   Clove tincture for wounds, mix 2 drops of Clove Oil and 2 ounces of vodka in a
   glass bottle. Shake and apply as needed. *Caution: Never put undiluted Clove Oil on
   your skin, as it may cause irritation.*

Extra Tip: To ward off bugs and insects while you are outside, thoroughly mix 3
   drops of Clove Oil in a bottle of suntan lotion and apply it to exposed skin several
   times a day.

Applications

- A mouthwash with Clove Oil in it can help to disinfect your gums and mouth.
  Mix 2 drops of Clove Oil in 4 ounces of vodka. You can also add a pinch of Cinnamon if you wish. Dilute 1 teaspoon of the blend in ½ cup warm water and
  use it to rinse out your mouth.

- Clove Oil's strengthening effect and its ability to relieve coughs can help soothe
  inflamed and irritated bronchial tubes. People with asthma can also benefit from it. An inhalation of Clove Oil is easy to make: Mix 2 drops each of
  Clove and Eucalyptus Oils and 1 drop of Peppermint Oil in a bowl of hot water.
  Lean over the bowl and drape a towel over your head and the bowl. Take deep
  breaths of the vapors for a few minutes.

- The relaxing, mildly anesthetic effect of Clove Oil can alleviate tension headaches. Add 2 drops of Clove Oil to a bowl of warm water. Soak a clean cloth in
  the liquid, wring out the excess, and place the cloth on your neck for 5 minutes
  to ease the headache.

- Clove Oil helps ease abdominal discomfort from cramps and diarrhea. Mix 1
  drop each of Clove, Cypress, and Peppermint Oils in 2 ounces of Jojoba Oil.
  Use this blend to massage your abdomen whenever you have pain or cramping.

Take Care! There are three different types of Clove Oil: Clove-Bud Oil, Clove-
Stem Oil, and Clove-Leaf Oil. But only use Clove-Bud Oil, which has the lowest
eugenol content and is the safest. Clove-Stem and Clove-Leaf Oils are too strong.
Use Clove Oil sparingly and only when diluted because it may irritate skin. Also,
avoid Clove Oil if you are pregnant, since it can trigger contractions.

Cypress Oil

A prominent feature of the Mediterranean landscape, the slender evergreen cypress
tree (*Cupressus sempervirens*) can live up to 2,000 years. As a medicinal plant, cypress
is of particular significance due to its ability to constrict blood vessels. Medicinal
salves with Cypress Oil have been in use since ancient times as a way of staunching

wounds. The oil's astringent properties facilitate the flow of lymph in cases of tissue edemas, particularly in the legs. This helps prevent waste products from being deposited in the connective tissue and can protect against cellulite as well as varicose veins. As an aromatherapy inhalation, Cypress Oil has a dilating effect on the bronchial tubes and can be quite useful in alleviating ailments of the respiratory tract, including asthma, bronchitis, spasmodic coughing, and symptoms that are associated with hay fever. Its aromatic scent clears the mind, strengthens the nerves, and has a comforting effect during times of stress. Cypress Oil can be diluted and applied to the body in a variety of ways, including massage oils, shower gels, and sitz baths.

For Promoting Concentration

The fresh scent of Cypress Oil soothes and strengthens the nerves, thereby helping you keep a cool head in stressful situations. When added to an aromatherapy lamp, this blend has a balancing effect that can improve your ability to focus your attention.

3 drops Cypress

2 drops Bergamot

2 drops Rosemary

Therapeutic Effect: The main component of Cypress Oil includes sabinol, cymene, sylvestrene, camphene, and pinene. Due to its astringent properties, the oil can be beneficial in rubs and baths, which help remove waste products, eliminate blockages in the tissues, strengthen the veins, and clear up oily, large-pored skin.

To Refresh and Invigorate: A shower gel with Cypress Oil can be both deodorizing and refreshing. The oil stimulates blood flow in the tissues and stabilizes circulation. Combine 5 drops of Cypress Oil, 3 drops of Rosemary Oil, and 2 drops of Juniper Oil, and add the mixture to 4 ounces of an unscented shower gel or liquid castile soap.

For Wounds: An ointment made with Cypress Oil can help heal wounds, due to its antibacterial effect. Combine 5 drops of Cypress Oil, 2 drops of Tea Tree Oil, and 2 drops of Lavender Oil with 1 ounce of ointment base or aloe vera gel.

For Repelling Insects: Cypress Oil acts as an insect repellent and protects clothing from moths. Many stores carry untreated wooden balls that you can scent with a few drops of oil. Or add a couple of drops of Cypress Oil to a cotton ball, put it into a sock, and place in a storage trunk or a drawer.

For Relieving "Heavy" Legs: If your legs are tired, carefully rub them with highly diluted Cypress Oil (mix 5 drops into 2 ounces of Avocado Oil). The rub eases the reabsorption of lymphatic fluid into the tissues. It will also help the venous blood to flow back out of the overtaxed vessels.

Extra Tip: Cypress Oil can be useful in treating people who experience extreme mood swings and tend to have an excessive flood of thoughts. The oil helps restore equilibrium to their emotions.

Applications

- A sitz bath with Cypress Oil can help alleviate the symptoms of hemorrhoids, including itching. Mix 4 drops of Cypress Oil with 1 drop of Tea Tree Oil and 1 tablespoon of milk; add the mixture to a half-filled bathtub. Sit in the tub for about 20 minutes; then cover up warmly and rest in bed.

- Since Cypress Oil has the ability to remove waste products, it can help firm the connective tissue and may prevent cellulite from forming. After you take a warm shower, massage your body—especially the cellulite prone areas—with a mixture of 3 tablespoons each of Sweet Almond Oil and aloe vera gel, 10 drops of Cypress Oil, 5 drops of Grapefruit Oil, and 3 drops of Juniper Oil. Blend well before applying.

- To stop bleeding gums and help inhibit inflammation, combine 2 drops of Cypress Oil and 1 teaspoon of cider vinegar in warm water. Gargle with the solution; spit it out. Repeat several times daily.

- Cypress Oil dilates the bronchial tubes, making expectoration easier, and relieving the urge to cough. Add 2 drops of Cypress Oil and 2 drops of Frankincense Oil to a bowl of steaming water. Drape a towel over your head, and then hold your face over the bowl. Inhale the vapors deeply.

! **Take Care!** Cypress Oil should not be used during pregnancy, because it can stimulate uterine contractions. When buying Cypress Oil, be sure the label reads *Cupressus sempervirens*. The essential oils of some other types of cypress are less effective medicinally.

Dill Oil

Dill belongs to the carrot family and is a close relative of fennel. The aromatic plant, a native of the Mediterranean region, southern Russia, and central and southern Asia, is widely cultivated in England, Germany and North America. Its name is derived from the Norse *dilla*, which means "to soothe." In fact, Dill has been valued for thousands of years not only for its culinary uses, as is common today, but also for its healing properties. It was an essential ingredient in a common Egyptian remedy to ease pain and promote healing. The ancient Greeks used Dill, too. They believed it caused drowsiness, so they covered their eyes with the herb's fronds before going to sleep. The plant's therapeutic properties are also present in Dill Oil extracted by steam distillation of the seeds and the plant. This oil can help strengthen the stomach and relieve intestinal spasms and cramps. It is also a mild antiseptic and antispasmodic. In addition, Dill Oil may help to suppress severe coughs, promote milk in nursing mothers, ease flatulence and hiccups, and relieve anxiety.

For Stress and Panic

Dill Oil's balancing, relaxing effects help to soothe feelings of panic, stress, and nervous exhaustion. Also, the oil's aroma, which is sweet, spicy, and minty at the same time, can promote sleep and help relieve cramps. Try this blend in an aromatherapy lamp:

  3 drops Dill
  2 drops Lavender
  2 drops Lemon Balm

Therapeutic Effect: The major component of Dill is carvone, but the oil also contains terpinine, phellandrene, and limonene. The combination of these substances gives the oil its antispasmodic, pain-relieving, and soothing effects. It can ease the cramping that accompanies diarrhea and menstrual periods. When it's used to treat colic, Dill Oil may help regulate intestinal activity. It is also an effective remedy for bloating and nervous tension.

For Fidgety Children: Children who are hyperactive and unable to concentrate can benefit from Dill Oil. Mix 3 drops of Dill Oil and 3 drops of Roman Chamomile Oil with 5 drops of Lavender Oil in an aromatherapy lamp. This blend helps promote concentration and a sense of calm.

To Refresh the Senses: Use Dill Oil in the shower to get a mildly refreshing and relaxing feeling after an illness. The oil can strengthen circulation and stimulate your entire body. Add 3 drops to some of your favorite shower gel.

For Menstrual Pain: Massage oil containing Dill Oil simultaneously relieves pain from menstrual cramps and stimulates circulation in the areas being massaged. It may also help to facilitate menstrual flow. Thoroughly blend 2 drops each of Dill, Clary Sage, and Lavender Oils with 2 tablespoons of Jojoba Oil; rub it onto your abdomen.

To Stimulate Milk Flow: Nursing mothers who have a problem with milk flow may find that diluted Dill Oil can help trigger milk production. Blend 1 drop of Dill Oil and 1 tablespoon of Jojoba Oil and rub it into your breasts. Then wash it off before you nurse, as babies do not like its taste.

A Little Lore: Gladiators in ancient Rome believed that Dill Oil made them invincible, strong, and quick; they rubbed it all over their bodies prior to each and every fight.

Applications

- The relaxing effect of Dill Oil can relieve spasmodic abdominal pain. Mix 6 drops of Dill Oil and 2 drops each of Lavender and Roman-Chamomile Oils with 3 tablespoons of Olive Oil. You can rub this blend into your abdomen several times each day.

- To treat hiccups, add 3 drops of Dill Oil to some boiling water in a bowl. Cover your head with a towel, lean over the bowl, and inhale the vapors for 2 minutes.

- For whooping cough and croup, blend 5 drops each of Dill and Frankincense Oils with 1 teaspoon of Sweet Almond Oil. When gently massaged onto your upper chest, this oil blend can help ease severe coughing fits.

- Dill Oil helps promote a deep, restful sleep.

- It is very useful after a long, stressful day. Add 2 to 3 drops of Dill Oil to your pillow before going to bed to relax your senses. Or add a few drops to your sleeve or handkerchief and deeply inhale the vapors occasionally throughout the day to keep you feeling relaxed and calm.

- To soothe tense, sore muscles, blend 1 drop of Dill, 2 drops of Roman-Chamomile, and 3 drops of Lavender Oil in 1 tablespoon of Sweet Almond Oil. Massage into the affected areas.

Take Care! Pregnant women should not use Dill Oil because it may have a stimulant effect that can trigger premature labor. The substance carvone, which is present in the oil, can be toxic in large doses and is dangerous to certain parts of the nervous system. For this reason, Dill Oil should be used only in the amounts specified. If you have an allergic reaction, discontinue its use immediately.

Eucalyptus Oil

The essential oil of eucalyptus is obtained from the leaves and branches of the eucalyptus tree, *Eucalyptus globulus*. A steam distillation process is used to extract the oil from the tree parts, and some 110 pounds of plant material is required to produce about 2 pounds of Eucalyptus Oil. The medicinal properties of Eucalyptus Oil were most likely first discovered by the Aborigines, the native inhabitants of Australia (where the tree originated). They used the oil as a remedy for skin problems and fever; not surprisingly, the eucalyptus tree has long been called the "fever tree." Modern herbalists rely on Eucalyptus Oil to treat these conditions, as well as colds and other bothersome respiratory ailments. The oil is a fine decongestant and has strong germicidal and antibacterial effects.

For Mental Fatigue

Eucalyptus Oil stimulates the nervous system and promotes concentration. Combined with Lemon Oil in a diffuser, it is ideal to use when the psyche is affected by mental exhaustion and listlessness.

> 4 drops Eucalyptus
> 2 drops Lemon

Therapeutic Effect: The principal active ingredient in Eucalyptus Oil is eucalyptol, which has strong germicidal and disinfectant properties. It also functions as a diuretic, lowers blood sugar, and helps to relieve cough and fever. Eucalyptus Oil is an effective analgesic and is often used in preparation designed to relive muscle, nerve, and joint pain. On a psychological level, it helps to combat exhaustion and dispels mental sluggishness.

For a Sense of Well-Being: A few drops of a blend of Eucalyptus and massage oils have a cooling and stimulating effect on both mind and body. Apply to pulse points.

To Purify the Sickroom: Eucalyptus Oil is the ideal essence to use in a sickbed environment. Five drops of the oil in a diffuser will kill germs in the air and reduce the number of bacteria. This will help keep germs from spreading.

For Wounds and Abscesses: The strong germicidal effect of Eucalyptus Oil can help heal wounds, burns, ulcers, and insect bites or stings. Place a few drops of the essential oil in a dressing or bandage before covering the area with it.

To Suppress Coughs: Make a chest compress with Eucalyptus and massage oils to loosen phlegm and improve lung function.

For Scarlet Fever: A few drops of Eucalyptus Oil added to a diffuser can help relieve the flu-like symptoms of scarlet fever.

To Improve the Sauna: To get the best detoxifying effects of a sauna, place 3 drops of Eucalyptus Oil in a ladleful of water and pour it over the hot stones.

! Take Care! Too much Eucalyptus Oil can potentially irritate the skin, so be sure to use the exact amount specified in the preparations listed here. Combining Eucalyptus Oil with massage oil reduces the chance of irritation. Keep Eucalyptus Oil away from children under age six.

Extra Tip: Insects dislike the odor of Eucalyptus Oil. To make an insect repellent, add a few drops of the oil to massage oil. Or place a few drops in a diffuser to keep the room pest free.

Applications: External use

- Lower a fever with a Eucalyptus Oil calf wrap. Add 5 drops of Eucalyptus Oil to 1 quart lukewarm water. Soak linen or cotton cloths in the mixture. Then, wrap the cloths around your calves and secure with dry cloths. Calf wraps should be used only when the feet are warm.

- To rid dandruff, mix 10 drops of Eucalyptus Oil with your shampoo. Massage well into your scalp. Wait a few minutes before rinsing.

- To alleviate cold symptoms, place a few drops of Eucalyptus Oil on a handkerchief and deeply inhale the aroma.

- To relieve sinus and chest congestion, combine 5 drops of Eucalyptus Oil with 1 drop of Peppermint Oil. Add crushed Eucalyptus, Peppermint, Coltsfoot, and Comfrey herbs. Place ½ ounce of mixture in a clean sock, knot the end, and place inside your pillowcase overnight.

- For relief from muscular aches and pains, mix 10–15 drops of Eucalyptus Oil and 2 ounces of Sweet Almond or Grape Seed Oil. Massage into your muscles.

Frankincense Oil

Frankincense—the very word conjures up images of ancient, smoke-filled temples and aromatic offerings to the gods. This legendary substance actually comes from an unspectacular scrubby tree that's native to Africa, India, and Saudi Arabia. When the bark of the tree is peeled away, resin oozes out and forms "tears." Those tears are scraped off and distilled to yield an oil that's both fragrant and medicinal. When used as a massage oil, or in a warm bath or diffuser, Frankincense is a fine remedy for colds, bronchitis, asthma, and skin wounds. Once an ingredient in ancient Egyptian cosmetics, Frankincense is still prescribed to rejuvenate and restore wrinkled skin and promote the healing of scars. The oil is said to notably affect emotion and mood, as well. Used for many centuries as an incense to create a spirit of peace and contemplation, Frankincense has a uniquely warm and rich fragrance. Aromatherapists today recommend the oil for times of stress and anxiety. Frankincense Oil is also said to calm and focus a restless soul, alleviate mental fatigue, and mend a broken heart.

For Deep Relaxation

Frankincense Oil is believed to have a sedating effect on the central nervous system. Its soothing scent also slows and deepens breathing. To foster a sense of peace and serenity, combine these oils in an aromatherapy lamp:

2 drops Frankincense

2 drops Lavender

1 drop Sandalwood

Therapeutic Effect: The primary healing components of Frankincense Oil are pinene, dipentene and phellandrene; all are responsible for the oil's anti-inflammatory, antiseptic, and antidepressant properties. In addition, Frankincense Oil is *cytophylactic*; in other words, it can stimulate new cell growth and help prevent wrinkles. This may account for its long-standing use to heal wounds and scars and to counter the effects of aging.

To Ward Off a Cold: Essential oils can often help fight off viral infection. Add 3–4 drops of Frankincense, 3 drops of Eucalyptus Oil, and 2–3 drops of Lemon Oil to a steaming bath. This anti-infectious blend is soothing and immune boosting to boot.

For Aging Skin and Wrinkles: While aging is inevitable—and at times accelerated by smoking, poor diet, too much sun, and stress—Frankincense Oil can help counter the telltale signs by strengthening connective tissue. Combine 3 drops of Frankincense Oil with 1 teaspoon Wheat Germ Oil. Apply to your face, especially to the area around your eyes, and leave on overnight. Or, make a facial steam bath: mix 4 drops each of Frankincense and Lavender Oils, 3 drops of Rose-Otto Oil, and 5 teaspoons of a base oil. Add to a bowl of steaming water and drape a towel over your head. Lean over the bowl and steam for about 10–15 minutes.

To Minimize Scarring: Frankincense Oil encourages skin to heal and reduces the possibility of both infection and scarring. In those cases where a wound is slow to heal, mix 2 drops of Frankincense Oil, 1 drop of Neroli or Lavender Oil, and 1 teaspoon of Wheat Germ Oil. Massage the ointment into wounds and scars on a daily basis until the skin is healthy again.

Extra Tip: For an essential oil bath blend that's aromatic and uplifting, mix 2 drops each of Frankincense, Clary Sage, Bergamot, Rosewood, and Sandalwood Oils in a tub filled with warm water.

Applications: External Use

- To alleviate sinus congestion or other symptoms of a head cold, add 3 drops of Frankincense Oil to 1 quart of steaming water. Place a towel over your head and the bowl, creating a tent. Inhale the steam deeply through your nose and exhale through your mouth. If your symptoms are acute, use the steam bath twice daily until there's a marked improvement. Reduce the treatment to once daily until all of your symptoms have subsided completely.

- Frankincense is antiseptic, and is effective in combating urinary-tract infections. Add 3 drops each of Frankincense Oil, Lavender Oil, and Roman-Chamomile Oil to a sitz bath. Soak for 15 minutes and repeat during the day as needed.

- As an anti-inflammatory, the Frankincense Oil can help ease an asthma attack. Place 3 drops each of Frankincense Oil and Tea Tree Oil in an aromatherapy lamp to promote deep breathing and reduce inflammation of airways.

- The use of aromatic essential oils can help relieve anxiety and bring about a welcome change in your outlook. Frankincense Oil is often used for calming frayed nerves, and has been useful during times of stress. Place a few drops of the oil on a tissue or handkerchief and inhale the scent as needed during the day.

Take Care! Like all essential oils, Frankincense Oil should only be used externally. If taken internally, it can lead to intoxication and may cause damage to the delicate membranes of the digestive tract. In addition, always dilute it with a base oil or a cream first.

Geranium Oil

Geranium Oil is extracted from the green leaves of the Geranium (*Pelatgonium graveolens*), which grows primarily in Madagascar, Egypt, and Morocco. Even though there are approximately 700 varieties of Geranium, only about 10 supply the valuable essential oil, which is obtained by distilling the leaves and shoots with steam. The oil, with its fresh, rosy, citrusy scent, stimulates the senses. It can renew your energy when you feel exhausted and calm, when you feel angry or irritable. Geranium Oil also helps balance the hormones, making it a good option for women who are troubled by menopausal symptoms. Because of its cleansing and antiseptic properties, the oil has proved valuable in healing wounds and fighting infections. Many cosmetic lotions contain Geranium Oil, as it soothes irritated skin and helps control acne. Geranium Oil blends well with other oils, including Lemon, Grapefruit, Lavender, Rosemary, Jasmine, Bergamot, and Ginger essential oils.

Insect Repellent

Geranium Oil is especially suited to warding off insects, particularly mosquitoes. The following mixture used in an aromatic diffuser provides the perfect insect-free evenings.

5 drops Geranium

3 drops Clove

Therapeutic Effect: The main constituents of Geranium Oil, geraniol, linalool, and citronellol have strong cleansing and antiviral effects. They also help maintain healthy skin. It is used in bath preparations as well as for facials, hair rinses, and compresses. The tannins found in Geraniums have a strongly constrictive effect, making it anti-inflammatory and antispasmodic; it also serves as a decongestant.

For Insect Bites: Geranium Oil can help with the aggravation of swollen, itching mosquito bites. Simply dilute 2 drops of Geranium Oil in 1 ounce of Witch Hazel. Dab on the affected area with a cotton ball to help the swelling go down.

To Feel Good: If plants could speak, the message from the Geranium would be, "Don't do a thing, let yourself be pampered." The pleasant scent of Geranium, Oil when mixed with Rose Oil is ideal for making a body oil combination to pamper yourself in a bath, with a facial, or in a hair rinse. The oil relaxes the body and softens the skin.

For Concentration Problems: You can begin to feel more in control of your hectic life and decrease absentmindedness by inhaling the scent of Geranium Oil. The clear, light scent will aid you in organizing your thoughts and improving your memory. You can also mix 2 drops of Geranium Oil with 2 drops of Rosemary Oil to enliven your senses. Add some to a tissue and keep it in your purse when you travel.

For Beauty: Geranium Oil can help most skin types because its stimulating action helps boost the regeneration of skin cells and aids the healing of acne and blemishes. Diluted, it also helps control excessive oiliness of the skin and soothe dry, sensitive skin. Geranium Oil will give your skin a healthy glow, making it appear more youthful and radiant.

Extra Tip: Geranium Oil eases premenstrual syndrome (PMS) symptoms. With its diuretic action, it combats fluid retention; it may also reduce breast tenderness.

Applications

- To reduce swelling in the legs, rub them with a mixture of 3 tablespoons of Sweet Almond Oil, 8 drops of Geranium Oil, and 5 drops of Lemon Oil, After applying the mixture, elevate your legs slightly and rest for 30 minutes. The oils unblock the lymph nodes and prevent edema.

- To help fade scars, use Geranium Oil mixed with Neroli Oil: Mix 5 drops of Geranium Oil, and 3 drops of Neroli Oil into 3 tablespoons of odorless, enriched skin cream. Massage thin cream daily into scar tissue to keep it supple.

- A bath with Geranium Oil provides relief from menstrual pain and cramps. Add 6 drops of Geranium Oil, 3 drops of Jasmine Oil, and 2 drops of Clary Sage Oil to 1½ cups of whole milk and pour it into your bathwater; soak in the tub for at least 30 minutes or more.

- Geranium Oil can give you new optimism when you're feeling worn out and apathetic. Evaporate 3 drops each of Geranium and Bergamot Oil, using an aromatic diffuser.

German Chamomile Oil

Three different species of chamomile—German, Roman, and wild—are cultivated for their essential oils. All are members of the Asteraceae family, and all share similar properties, although research has shown that the German type, *Matricaria chamomilia* (also known as blue or true chamomile), may be more potent in its effects. It owes its dark blue color as well as its greater anti-inflammatory action to a compound known as *chamazylene*. This action makes German Chamomile Oil an especially good choice for treating infections, wounds, headaches, skin irritations, and menstrual pain. However, all the Chamomile Oils have a prominent place in botanical medicine and have long been used to cool fevers, alleviate aches and pains and relieve muscle soreness and spasms. We still profit from these centuries-old remedies, especially from German Chamomile Oil's ability to calm jittery nerves. Indeed, some believe that the oil can relieve almost any ailment.

For Tranquility

German Chamomile Oil is a wonderful relaxation agent when your nerves are tense and frazzled. Put this mixture in an aromatherapy lamp to help create a sense of peace.

   3 drops German Chamomile
   2 drops Lemon Balm
   2 drops Orange

Therapeutic Effects: German Chamomile Oil contains chamazulene, which has strong antispasmiodic qualities that relax tense, aching muscles. The volatile oil is also anti-inflammatory and is particularly effective in healing burns and preventing infection.

For Menstrual Cramps: German Chamomile Oil is a recommended treatment for menstrual pains. Take a five-minute sitz bath in 1 gallon of warm water to which you've added 2 drops each of German Chamomile and Lavender Oils.

To Help Heal Burns: For minor burns and wounds, blend 2 drops of German Chamomile oil with 2 drops of Lavender Oil. Add 2 cups of warm water. Used in a compress, this will prevent scarring and inflammation.

For Candida Infections: A warm sitz bath will relieve the itching and inflammation associated with yeast fungus in the vaginal area. Add 1 drop German Chamomile oil and 2 drops of Tea Tree Oil to 1 gallon of warm water, and mix well before using.

For Joint and Muscle Pain: For painful joints and tense, stiff, or cramping muscles, blend 2 tablespoons of Sweet Almond Oil and 2 drops each of German Chamomile Oil and Rosemary Oil. Massage this blend into the affected areas to relax muscles, reduce inflammation, and increase circulation.

Extra Tip: Don't waste time being grumpy. Add this oil to an aromatherapy lamp to lift your mood.

Take Care! Of the different varieties of chamomile—German, Roman, and wild— the most readily available are German and Roman. While they share similar properties, German Chamomile Oil has a higher volatile-oil content, making it preferable for healing treatments. If you are pregnant, use only in the later stages of your pregnancy, and mix it with Rose Oil to relieve the restlessness and fear associated with childbirth.

Applications

- Following a day in the sun, mist your skin with this moisturizing after-sun spray: Blend 2 drops of German Chamomile Oil, 2 drops of Lavender Oil, 1 drop of Rose-Otto Oil, and 4 ounces of purified water in a spray bottle.

- A compress made with German Chamomile Oil may be applied to wounds to help form healthy scar tissue. Moisten a cloth with a few drops of the pure oil, and place it on the wound with the essential oil facing away from the skin. The oil's properties penetrate the cloth, but the skin is spared any irritation. Replace the compress once a day until the wound is healed.

- An oil treatment will leave your hair soft and easy to comb and your scalp conditioned. Blend 2 drops each of German Chamomile Oil, Rosemary Oil, and Lavender Oil with 4 tablespoons of Sweet Almond Oil, and massage your head and hair with the mixture once a week. Add a dab of shampoo before rinsing, or for best results, leave on overnight. *Note: Use caution around your eyes.*

- German Chamomile Oil relieves pain and reduces tension during migraine attacks. For very severe cases, moisten a towel with cool water and add a few drops of German Chamomile Oil. Place the cloth on your forehead, close your eyes, and breathe normally.

Helichrysum Oil

Also called Everlasting, Strawflower, and Immortelle, Helichrysum is best known as a flower that keeps its shape and color when dried. It is, therefore, often included in dried flower arrangements and wreaths. Originally from the Mediterranean region, the hardy evergreen bears long stems with velvety needles and clusters of ball-shaped, golden flower heads. Used by the ancient Romans to repel moths. Helichrysum gained a following for its honey-like fragrance. In fact, the flower is often strewn on floors in Europe, crushing it underfoot releases a sweet aroma. The plant's essential oil is distilled from several species, such as *Helichrysum italicum* and *Helichrysum angustifolium*, and has a soothing, pleasant scent. Helichrysum essential oil can help alleviate skin irritation, aching muscles and joints, and upper-respiratory congestion. On an emotional level, the essential oil assists creativity and intuition. It blends well with many other oils, including Cypress, Clary Sage, Juniper, Lavender, Pine, Bergamot, Lemon, Rosemary, Tea Tree, and Geranium.

For Inner Peace

The unique aromatic scent of Helichrysum Oil helps to clear the mind, awaken the senses, and promote inner peace and serenity. Allow the following blend to evaporate in your aromatherapy lamp.

3 drops Helichrysum

2 drops Clary Sage

1 drop Lavender

Therapeutic Effect: Helichrysum's primary components of pinene, nerol, uvaol, and amyrin give the oil its anti-inflammatory and antiseptic properties, which are useful when applied to inflamed, blemished skin, acne, and burns. The oil's powerful expectorant effect makes it a good addition to steam inhalations, relieving respiratory congestion, bronchitis, and coughs.

For Soft Skin: A body oil with 2 ounces of Sweet Almond Oil, 10 drops of Helichrysum Oil, and 5 drops of Rose Geranium Oil leaves the skin soft and smooth. The oil protects skin from drying and helps to relieve psoriasis. Massage the oil into the skin immediately after a shower or bath to enhance absorption.

For Congestion: Mix 5–7 drops of Helichrysum Oil in a bowl of boiling water. Place a towel over your head and inhale the vapors to ease congestion, hacking coughs, bronchitis, and sinusitis.

For Menstrual Cramps: A hot bath with Helichrysum and Clary Sage Oils can help ease painful cramping during menstruation. Helichrysum Oil's relaxing and analgesic effect can also relieve menstrual tension.

For Gum Inflammation: Helichrysum Oil has a powerful anti-inflammatory action that alleviates gum inflammation. Mix 1 drop of Helichrysum Oil in ½ teaspoon of Witch Hazel extract. Dip your toothbrush into the blend and gently rub over the inflamed areas.

For Sore Muscles: Make a massage oil for sprains, strains, aching muscles, and arthritic joints. Mix 2 drops of Helichrysum, Lavender, and Clary Sage Oils in 2 tablespoons of Sweet Almond Oil. Massage it into affected areas.

Extra Tip: Since Helichrysum Oil stimulates the flow of lymph and firms the skin, it relieves varicose veins and edema. Massage the oil into the affected areas.

! **Take Care!** Helichrysum Oil should not be used by children younger than 12 or by pregnant women. In addition, Helichrysum Oil can evoke powerful emotions in some individuals and should therefore be used in moderation.

Applications

- For psoriasis: Make a skin oil to ease inflammation and painful itching. Blend 5 drops of Helichrysum Oil and 2 drops of Lavender Oil in 2 tablespoons of Sweet Almond Oil. Massage as needed into affected areas.

- For varicose veins: Make a daily massage oil by mixing 10 drops of Helichrysum Oil and 5 drops each of Lemon and Cypress Oils in 3 tablespoons of Grapeseed Oil. This oil blend helps alleviate swelling and congestion in the veins. It also works to relieve the typical feeling of heaviness in the legs that sometimes results from varicose veins.

- For coughs: The antispasmodic and expectorant properties of Helichrysum Oil help to relieve congestion, loosen mucus, and soothe coughs. Blend 3 drops each of Helichrysum, Eucalyptus, and Frankincense Oils in 2 tablespoons of Sweet Almond Oil. Massage the blend onto the entire chest area.

- For rheumatic complaints: Mix 3 drops of Helichrysum Oil, 5 drops of Lavender Oil, and 2 drops of Roman-Chamomile Oil in 2 tablespoons of Sweet Almond Oil. Massage the mixture into your rheumatic joints to relieve pain and inflammation.

- For skin care: Add 2–3 drops of Helichrysum Oil to your favorite lotion and use it to moisturize daily.

Hyssop Oil

The bushy perennial *Hyssopus officinalis* is native to the Mediterranean region and has been used for healing purposes for more than 2,000 years. Indeed, the plant's ability to detoxify the blood was recognized by the ancient Hebrews and Greeks, who used it as part of ritual cleansings. Hyssop Oil, which is extracted from the plant by a process of steam distillation, retains this healing property. Aromatic, fresh, and spicy, Hyssop Oil is most often used to alleviate respiratory ailments, such as coughs, colds, bronchitis, and asthma. It boosts circulation and invigorates the body and mind, making it very useful in cases of recuperation, fatigue, and listlessness. In addition, Hyssop Oil has antiseptic and antibacterial qualities; when applied topically, it can help heal acne and eczema. Gum inflammation also responds well to mouth rinses with the oil. On an emotional level, it enhances mental focus and stimulates creative thinking. However, Hyssop Oil is not in common use and can be hard to find; mail-order suppliers may be able to help locate it.

For Mental Clarity

The stimulating fragrance of Hyssop Oil increases mental clarity, boosts concentration, and enhances creativity. Try the following blend in your aromatherapy lamp when you need to focus your mind:

3 drops Hyssop
2 drops Fennel
2 drops Rosemary
1 drop Lemon

Therapeutic Effect: Hyssop Oil contains pinocamphone, thujone, pinene, and sesquiterpene, all of which have expectorant, antiseptic, and invigorating effects. The oil helps ease respiratory ailments, such as coughs, asthma, and bronchitis. Applied topically, it can speed the healing of bruises and blemishes. Hyssop Oil also helps restore vigor and cleanse the blood, which boosts overall health.

For Skin Care: To condition dry skin and to alleviate itchy eczema, blend 2 drops of Hyssop Oil, 3 drops of Lavender Oil, and 2 drops of Rose-Geranium Oil with 2 tablespoons of Sweet Almond Oil. Add to warm bathwater and soak for 20 minutes.

For a Fever: Hyssop Oil can help promote sweating, thereby reducing a fever. Mix 2 drops of the oil in a bowl of cool water. Dip a cloth in it, wring it out, and wrap it around your calves.

For Oral Hygiene: Mouthwash containing highly diluted Hyssop Oil promotes blood circulation in the gums, which may help prevent gum disease. Blend 2 drops of oil and 2 tablespoons of vodka with 4 ounces of spring water. Use the mixture to rinse your mouth, and then spit it out.

For Vaginal Infections: For vaginal inflammation and discharge, add 2 drops each of Hyssop and Lavender Oils to a half-full bath. Bathe daily until your symptoms subside.

For Convalescence: Following an illness, try this blend in an aromatherapy lamp: 3 drops each of Hyssop, Bergamot, and Cinnamon Oils and 2 drops of Basil Oil. This can restore energy and get you back on your feet.

Extra Tip: To help speed the healing of bruises, blend 2 drops of Hyssop Oil and 1 drop Helichrysum Oil in a bowl of very cold water. Soak a cloth in the mixture and apply to the affected area for 20 minutes.

Applications

- Hyssop Oil stimulates sweating, which helps cleanse the body of toxins and waste products. To make a body-cleansing oil, mix 9 drops of Hyssop Oil with 1 cup of pure Olive Oil. Apply the mixture to your entire body and wrap yourself in a linen cloth. Rest, covered, for one hour and then rinse off.

- To combat colds and flu and to help expectorate mucus, add 4 drops of Hyssop Oil to 1 quart of hot water. Put a towel over your head and the bowl, bend over, and deeply inhale the vapors.

- For swollen, painful acne, blend 1 drop of Hyssop Oil in 2 tablespoons of Witch Hazel. Dip a cotton swab in the mixture and dab onto the affected areas to speed healing.

- To relieve a state of exhaustion and invigorate a sluggish body, add 2 drops of Hyssop Oil to 1 quart of water and simmer uncovered on low heat. Check the pot often to make sure the water hasn't evaporated and replenish the mixture as needed.

- Hyssop's powerful antibacterial properties make it an excellent household cleaner to eliminate germs. Add 6 to 10 drops of the oil to 2 gallons of warm water and use the solution to wipe down any surfaces or object in the home prone to infectious microbes.

Iris-Root Oil

Iris, a member of the Iridaceae family and native to North America, Asia, and Europe, is probably best known for its beautiful and dramatic flowers. Ranging in color from white to blue to purple, the blossoms have been prized for centuries by many cultures. However, it is the root—not the flowers—of the iris that produces its oil. This essential oil is very rare and expensive, as more than 1,500 pounds of iris roots are needed to make 1 quart of the oil through a process of steam distillation. Iris-Root Oil has a violet-like, sweet, soft, warm, and highly comforting fragrance. The oil not only possesses an appealing scent, but it also has health and beauty benefits. It can loosen mucus and quiet dry coughs, making it good for treating bronchitis and whooping cough. Iris-Root Oil also has a regulating effect on nervous disorders. Cosmetically, the oil helps to maintain healthy skin and nourishes sensitive skin. It is frequently used in exclusive skin-care products. Iris-Root Oil can also gently deep-clean oily, blemished skin, and may even help regulate overactive sebaceous glands.

To Create a Festive and Relaxing Mood

Iris-Root Oil is often too expensive for regular use. It can also be difficult to find. However, if you are fortunate enough to have a little extra oil on hand, you can create a fun and festive mood for a special event or party. Use a blend of the following essential oils in your aromatherapy lamp to help set an exhilarating moods.

   1 drop Iris-Root
   2 drops Rose
   1 drop Ylang-Ylang

Therapeutic Effect: Iris-Root Oil's relaxing and calming effect on the body is due to the action of its primary components, naphthalene, and iridin. Because of its mucus-thinning properties, Iris-Root Oil is frequently used to soothe coughs that occur with flu, colds, and bronchitis. It can help clear up blemished skin and also possesses laxative and diuretic effects that can help cleanse the blood.

For Soothing Skin Care: A skin oil containing Iris-Root Oil can help soften and tone dry, sensitive skin. Blend 1 drop each of Iris-Root and Frankincense Oils in 1 teaspoon of Wheat Germ Oil and 2 teaspoons of Sweet Almond Oil. Apply as needed.

For Fatigue: Place a few drops of Iris-Root Oil in a room diffuser to help minimize fatigue and poor concentration.

A Delicate Note in Perfume: Iris-Root Oil's delicate, flowery fragrance makes it popular for use as a fixative in violet-scented perfumes. Dissolved in a base oil, it is like an elegant, floral bouquet. Make a custom scent by mixing 2 drops each of Iris-Root and an essential oil of your choice in 2 teaspoons of Jojoba Oil.

To Comfort the Soul: To relieve tension and create a calming, harmonious mood, mix 1 drop each of Iris-Root, Lemon Balm, and Rose Oils in 2 teaspoons of Jojoba Oil. Add the blend to a handkerchief and tuck it into your pocket.

For Blemishes and Oily Skin: A skin toner that contains Iris-Root Oil can be useful in clearing up blemished skin. It regulates oil production and gently deep-cleans the skin. Blend 1 drop each of Iris-Root and Lavender Oils into 5 teaspoons of Witch Hazel.

Extra Tip: Pure Iris-Root Oil is very concentrated; its true scent manifests only when it is extremely diluted. For this reason, as well as the expense of the oil. Use pure, undiluted essence as sparingly as possible.

Applications

- Using Iris-Root Oil in a warm bath helps to ease sore muscles and rheumatic pain. Add 2 drops each of Iris-Root, Lavender, and Juniper Oils and 3 tablespoons of honey to very warm bathwater. Bathe for 20 minutes, and then rest while warmly covered for one hour.

- Itchy skin that results from psoriasis can be treated with a blend of 3 drops of Iris-Root Oil and 2 tablespoons of Olive Oil. Dab the oil onto your skin 3–4 times a day. This oil blend will also help itchy affected skin to heal more quickly.

- Sinus inflammations can benefit from an inhalation of Iris-Root Oil, as it has a mucolytic and soothing effect on the mucous membranes. Add 1–2 drops of Iris-Root Oil to 1 quart of boiling water in a bowl. Cover your head and inhale the vapors.

- For blemished skin, thoroughly mix 1 drop of Iris-Root Oil, 1 teaspoon of kaolin clay, and 2 tablespoons of water. Apply the clay blend to your face and allow it to dry; then rinse it off.

- To help freshen the air in a sickroom, mix 2 drops each of Iris-Root, Frankincense, and Ravensara Oils. Add the blend to an aromatherapy lamp.

Take Care! Because Iris-Root Oil is so scarce and expensive, it is often adulterated. If you decide to buy some, be sure to check that it is guaranteed to be pure, 100 percent Iris-Root Oil. The color should be a golden amber, while the scent is reminiscent of violets, with a slightly sharp, aromatic, fruity, and flowery fragrance. *Caution: Never use Iris-Root Oil, or any essential oil, internally.*

Jasmine Oil

In India, Jasmine was called "Queen of the Night" because its earthy scent was thought to be an aphrodisiac. Native to Arabia, India, and China, the flowers of *Jasminum gradiflorum* are harvested before dawn so that the delicate aroma won't evaporate in the Sun. Perhaps this is why Jasmine has long possessed an air of mystery, sensuality, and romance. The absolute oil is extracted using a special solvent that is later evaporated. This yields a rich, heavy, and thick oil with a floral scent—one of the most popular ancient oils used in perfumes. This oil's healing properties are many: Familiar to midwives as a "woman's oil," it can be used during labor to induce contractions, ease cramps, stimulate milk production, and banish fear. In addition, Jasmine is known to encourage self-confidence, optimism, and intuition. The oil's antispasmodic, analgesic, and sedative properties help relieve pain, muscle spasms, and tension. Furthermore, its antiseptic and conditioning qualities make it an excellent remedy for acne or dry skin.

For Mild Depression
The potent aroma of Jasmine Oil dispels dark thoughts and worries, while instilling self-confidence and hope. It helps balance moodiness, alleviate anxiety, and ease tension. Let the following oils evaporate in an aromatherapy lamp.

   1 drop Jasmine-Absolute
   1 drop Rose-Absolute
   2 drops Bergamot Oil

Therapeutic Effect: Jasmine Oil contains benzyl acetate, geraniol, linalool, benzyl alcohol, and Jasmine, which calm and relax the body and mind. As a mild analgesic and antispasmodic, the oil is especially effective for easing menstrual cramps. Jasmine Oil also has a skin-softening action that treats dry skin and dermatitis; its astringent and antibacterial actions treat skin conditions as well.

For Coughs: For fits of coughing, Jasmine Oil helps relax the bronchial tubes and calms the urge to cough. It can be evaporated in an aromatherapy lamp or mixed with Sweet Almond Oil for a chest balm.

For Skin Tears and Stretching: During pregnancy and labor, massaging the skin of the abdomen and genital area with a blend of Frankincense, Jojoba, Jasmine, and Sandalwood Oils can help to protect connective tissue from tears caused from overstretching.

For Skin Conditioning: Blend Jasmine, Sweet Almond, Lavender, and Sandalwood Oils and use in a bath to nourish dry skin, dermatitis, and eczema. Jasmine Oil will also help to treat oily skin and acne by killing bacteria and regulating sebum production. As an astringent, it can help tighten wrinkled skin.

For Insomnia: The relaxing, warm aroma of Jasmine Oil helps soothe and release any physical tension caused by anxiety, stress, and depression. When mixed with Clary Sage and Ylang-Ylang Oils in an aromatherapy lamp, Jasmine Oil helps to assure a sound sleep.

Extra Tip: Jasmine-Absolute Oil is laborious to produce and thus quite expensive: To use less of it in your aromatherapy lamp, mix 3 drops of Jasmine Oil with 1 tablespoon of Jojoba Oil.

❗ Take Care! Jasmine Oil possesses a very intense aroma and should therefore not be used too much or for too long. When Jasmine Oil is administered in too high a concentration for a long period of time, the sweet, heavy aroma might lead to dizziness, headaches, and even nausea. It is therefore important not to let Jasmine-absolute oil evaporate in your aromatherapy lam for longer than 2 hours.

Applications

- The analgesic effect of Jasmine Oil relieves menstrual cramps: Mix 2 tablespoons of Sweet Almond Oil with 2 drops Roman-Chamomile and Clary Sage Oils. Massage the entire lower abdomen with the blend, using gentle circular motions; then cover with a heating pad.

- Jasmine Oil's skin conditioning and emollient properties make it an effective agent against scaly, reddened skin. Gently massage the affected areas several times daily with 2 tablespoons of Avocado Seed Oil and 2 drops each of Jasmine, Lavender, and Neroli Oils.

- During late pregnancy, weekly sitz baths with Jasmine Oil help prepare the uterus for birth and prevent perinatal tears. Mix 2 tablespoons of heavy cream and 2 drops each of Jasmine, Rose, and Lavender Oils. Add to a half-filled bathtub. Soak for 30 minutes.

- Make a nourishing treatment for dry hair: Mix 4 tablespoons of Jojoba Oil with 4 drops of Jasmine, 5 drops of Sandalwood, 3 drops of Rosemary, and 2 drops of Clary Sage. Add to hair and leave it on for at least one hour or leave it on overnight. Apply shampoo without water, blend in, and rinse.

- Jasmine bath salts soothe and relax. Mix 2 cups of fine sea salt with 2 drops each of Jasmine and Rose Oils, and add to bath.

Juniper Oil

The evergreen Juniper may grow as a shrub that sprawls on the ground or stand erect as a bush that grows up to twelve feet tall. It bears needles, yellow flowers, and blue berries that turn black upon maturity. These ripened berries are the source of the aromatic Juniper Oil. Its spicy, pine-like scent has earthy undertones, and it is most notably associated with the characteristic smell of gin, to which Juniper berries are added for flavoring. The oil, however, has been used for medicinal purposes for many years. Juniper essential oil fights infection, warms, and soothes painful arthritic joints, and minimizes the pain from muscle spasms. It can also speed the healing of cuts and bruises. Since it helps to rid the body of toxins and purify the skin, the oil may even relieve cellulitis. In addition, it can ease anxiety and calm irritable nerves during times of stress and overwork. And, the oil is cleansing to more than spirit; the antiseptic action of Juniper Oil makes an excellent addition to water used in housecleaning.

To Enhance Your Mood

The fresh scent of Juniper Oil can eliminate crankiness and irritability caused by tension. The following mixture in an aromatherapy lamp helps calm stress and anxiety.

4 drops Juniper

2 drops Lavender

2 drops Clary Sage

Therapeutic Effect: Juniper Oil's most important constituents are pinene, terpinine, and terpineol. These make the oil quite useful for increasing circulation, fighting skin inflammations such as acne, and easing joint pain. Juniper Oil also lifts the spirit and balances emotions.

For a Warming Bath: Combine 3 drops each of Juniper and Rosemary Oils, and mix the blend well into your bathwater. This uplifting mixture will stimulate blood flow, induce sweat, eliminate toxins, and clear your mind.

Sitz Baths for Hemorrhoids: Mix 1 drop each of Juniper and Roman-Chamomile Oils into a warm sitz bath. Sit for about five minutes to allow the oil's properties to help relieve painful hemorrhoids.

Toner for Oily Skin: To combat oily skin, combine 1 drip of Juniper Oil with ½ cup of Witch Hazel, and ½ cup cool water, and shake well. Cleanse your skin with cotton pads soaked in the rinse. This toner works to help protect against additional infection or inflammation.

For Joint Pain: Mix 4 drops of Juniper Oil, 4 drops of Lavender Oil, and 2 drops of Rosemary Oil with ¼ cup of either Sweet Almond Oil or another base oil of your choice. Gently massage your skin with this blend; it may alleviate and soothe any muscles and joints that are painful due to arthritis.

Extra Tip: Juniper cleanses the atmosphere of a room and supports meditation. Add a few drops of Juniper and Frankincense to self-igniting charcoal blocks to create a custom incense.

Overall Health: The scent of Juniper Oil has been associated with improved overall health. It is astringent and antiseptic and helps balance mood swings.

! Take Care! Like all essential oils, Juniper should never be taken internally. Avoid using the oil if you have kidney problems or are pregnant, since it may prove too stimulating. Remember to dilute it with a carrier oil, such as Sweet Almond, before applying to your skin.

Applications: External

- Juniper's stimulating effect on circulation counteracts cellulitis and firms the connective tissue. Blend 2 drops of Juniper Oil, 2 drops of Cypress Oil, and 2 drops of Orange Oil in approximately 3 tablespoons of Sweet Almond Oil. Before taking a shower, massage the affected areas with a skin brush. Shower, and apply the oil blend to the flushed areas; massage the area in a circular motion.

- To relax muscles: Add 4 drops of Juniper Oil, 3 drops of Rosemary Oil, and 4 drops of Lavender Oil to 1 cup of sea salt. Add the mix to your bathwater; bathe for about 20 minutes, and then rest for one hour, to avoid excess stimulation.

- Be kind to your hair by applying an aromatic hair oil. Combine 6 drops of Juniper Oil with ½ ounce of Jojoba Oil. Pour oil in your hands and run it throughout your hair. Leave it on for one hour and rinse.

- For improving a pet's skin while bathing, add 4 drops of Juniper Oil to the bathwater. Another effective pet formula is 5 drops of Juniper and 10 drops of Lavender blended in an 8-ounce spritz bottle of water; use it to spray a pet's sleeping quarters or the areas they frequent in the home. Add 2 drops of Eucalyptus Oil to the spray to help freshen your pet's sleeping quarters and deter unwanted fleas and ticks.

Labdanum Oil

Cistus ladanifer is a small, resinous bush that grows in dry, rocky regions of the Mediterranean, especially the Greek Islands. Also known as the Rock Rose, the shrub bears fragrant white blossoms and lance-shaped leaves that exude a viscous gum called Labdanum Oil. This resin was so highly valued; it was an ingredient in a holy ointment mentioned in the Bible. The plant's essential oil, extracted from the resin and the branches by a process of steam distillation, was used by the ancient Greeks and Romans to help freshen the air. Today, Labdanum Oil is most often used as a fixative for perfumes; it also lends a musky, balsamic fragrance to balance heavy floral scents. Medicinally, the oil promotes circulation, which may ease muscle and menstrual pain. Labdanum Oil has numerous benefits for the skin as well. Its antiseptic and stringent properties help heal wounds, strengthen connective tissue, speed skin regeneration, dry acne and oily skin, and treat eczema and itchy rashes. On an emotional level, Labdanum Oil boosts self-confidence and soothes restless anxiety.

Tenderly Fragrant

For a relaxing fragrance to banish restlessness and self-doubt, try this blend in your aromatherapy lamp.

> 2 drops Labdanum Oil
> 2 drops Rose-Otto
> 1 drop Ylang-Ylang

Therapeutic Effect: Labdanum Oil contains terpenes, phenol, eugenol, and acetic and formic acids, all of which contribute to its antiseptic, astringent, expectorant, sedative and anti-inflammatory qualities. In addition, the oil stimulates the flow of blood, which helps reduce swelling.

For Oily Skin and Acne: Try this toner if you have oily or acne skin. Blend 2 drops of Labdanum Oil and 1 drop of Rose-Otto Oil with 2 ounces of Witch Hazel. Apply to your face every day to stabilize the oil production and moisture content of your skin.

For Menstrual Pain: Added to a warm bath, this mixture eases menstrual pain and helps relax the abdomen. Blend 3 drops each of Clary Sage and Labdanum Oil and add to bathwater. Soak 20 minutes; then rest in bed.

To Warm Your Feet: Labdanum Oil helps promote blood circulation, which can warm cold feet and alleviate chills. Add 2 drops each of Labdanum Oil and Rosemary Oil to 2 gallons of water. Mix well and submerge your feet for a relaxing soak.

To Condition Your Skin: To strengthen and condition your skin's connective tissue, combine 2 drops each of Labdanum Oil and Rose-Geranium Oil, 3 drops of Lavender Oil, 2 ounces of Sweet Almond Oil. Regular massages with the oil mixture can help to prevent the development of unsightly spider veins.

As a Perfume Fixative: A great fixative for perfumes, Labdanum Oil helps round off fragrances that are either too heavy or too floral. The oil also blends very well with Citrus, Rose, and Mimosa Oils for a subtle, earthy aroma.

Extra Tip: Pure Labdanum Oil has a rather unusual and clingy aroma. However, when it's diluted in lotion, alcohol, or other suitable base oils, it emits a subtle and flowery fragrance.

Applications

- For poorly healing and infected wounds, Labdanum Oil will help stop the growth of bacteria and speed the regeneration of the tissue. Mix 2 drops of Labdanum Oil with 1 ounce of Witch Hazel. Dip a clean piece of gauze into the solution, apply to the affected areas, and secure it in place. Change the compress twice daily until the wound is completely healed.

- A sitz bath with Labdanum Oil relieves bladder inflammation and supports the body's natural resistance to infection. Combine 3 drops of the oil with 1 tablespoon of apple cider vinegar. Blend the mixture into a half-full bathtub. Bathe for about 10 minutes; then cover your body with a blanket and rest in bed for one hour.

- The cleansing action of Labdanum Oil helps to stimulate the flow of lymph and blood. This is particularly effective for preventing the development of cellulite. Dry-brush your skin, then mix 4 drops of Cypress Oil and 3 drops of Labdanum Oil in 4 tablespoons of sea salt. Add the blend to the bathwater. While soaking, gently massage your skin under the water.

Take Care! Since Labdanum Oil can promote menstruation, it should never be used during pregnancy. Also, as with all essential oils, do not use Labdanum Oil internally. Accidental ingestion could lead to feelings of dizziness and nausea or even a toxic overdose. Always check the label to make sure you buy pure oil.

Lavender Oil

Although now cultivated primarily in Provence, in the south of France, Lavender is native to the Mediterranean. It grows in open fields and on mountain slopes, giving off an intense, spicy aroma when it blooms. The most potent medicinal form of Lavender is the oil, which contains a high concentration of active ingredients. The finest oil distilled from *Lavandula officinallis*, a variety of Lavender that grows only at altitudes above 3,000 feet and is particularly resistant to heat and cold. The herb's flower buds are harvested by hand at midday, when the oil content is highest; the essential oil is then extracted using steam distillation. Lavender Oil has many uses. It is a powerful antiseptic containing more that 200 compounds that are active against fungi, viruses, and other microbes. The oil is also valued for its ability to balance the emotions. It restores vitality in people suffering from nervous exhaustion and also has a calming effect on people who have trouble sleeping.

Lavender Oil

- Is antibiotic
- Soothes headaches

- Helps heal wounds
- Repels insects

To Purify Indoor Air

Place this mixture of essential oils in a simmer pot to help freshen the air. The oils have a powerful cleansing action. The fresh scent also exerts an uplifting effect on the mind, body, and spirit. Lavender combines particularly well with citrus oils.

4 drops Lavender

2 drops Bergamot

2 drops Lemon

Therapeutic Effect: The best-known active components in Lavender Oil are geraniol, cineole, and coumarin. These ingredients have a strong cleansing and germicidal effect and are believed to be particularly valuable for the treatment of inflammatory conditions and pain. Lavender also brings swift relief from digestive problems and various skin irritations.

For the breasts: Lavender Oil can be rubbed onto the breasts to help tone and tighten the skin. Add 2 drops of the oil to 3 tablespoons of a base oil, such as Sweet Almond, and apply to breasts daily.

For skin irritations: Lavender water promotes good circulation in the skin and prevents infections of the sebaceous glands. For a facial lotion, add 3 drops of Lavender Oil to 1 quart of distilled water; dab on daily.

For insomnia: Lavender Oil has a calming effect and can be used to induce sleep when you're feeling stressed or anxious. Put a few drops of Lavender Oil on an aromatherapy stone (available at most herbal stores) and place it in your bedroom. Its soothing effects will help you sleep soundly through the night.

For nerve pain: Lavender Oil helps to relieve pain and inflammation due to neuralgia. Mix 10 drops of the oil with 2 tablespoons of St. John's Wort Oil and gently rub it into the affected areas for pain relief.

For sunburn relief: Add 10 drops of Lavender Oil to 4 ounces of water. Store the liquid in a plastic spray bottle and take it with you to the beach to spritz on sunburned skin as needed.

Take Care! Lavender Oil is one of the few essential oils that is safe to use "neat," or undiluted, on the skin. Keep a small bottle in your kitchen cabinet to treat first-degree burns. One to two drops directly on the burn will relieve pain and reduce the risk of blisters.

Extra Tip: For an aromatic Lavender bath, use a natural emulsifier to help the oil blend well with the bathwater. Mix 5 drops of Lavender Oil with 1 cup of heavy cream or 1 teaspoon of honey and add it to the tub.

Applications

Steam Inhalation: Try inhaling fragrant steam to treat colds, sinus problems, or coughs. Add 5 drops of essential oil to a bowl of steaming water. Drape a towel over your head and hold your face over the bowl. Breathe in deeply, keeping your eyes closed.

Dry Inhalation: Put 1 to 3 drops of essential oil on a handkerchief and hold it under your nose. Breathe deeply.

Healing Compress: A hot, damp compress can soothe abdominal cramps, and a cold one can relieve fevers, headaches, or sunburn. Add 5 drops of essential oil to ½ cup of cold or hot water. Dip a cloth in the water, wring it out, and apply it where necessary.

Humidifiers: To fight the symptoms of colds, bronchitis, and asthma, add a few drops of Lavender essential oil to a humidifier or vaporizer.

Herbal Sauna: Use essential oils in the sauna to aid the lungs and help strengthen the immune system. Add 5 drops of an essential oil, such as Tea Tree, to 1 cup of water and pour over the heated sauna stones.

Applications: External use

- For middle ear infections, saturate a cotton ball in Olive Oil, drip 5 drops of Lavender Oil onto it an place it on the outer part of the affected ear. The Lavender Oil will help relieve the pain and inhibit the inflammation that often accompanies ear infections.

- Lavender essential oil can also be used externally to alleviate stomach aches, cramping or colic. Combine 30 drops of Lavender Oil, 10 drops of Chamomile Oil, and 3½ ounces of cold pressed Olive Oil in a bottle and shake vigorously. Massage this essential oil mixture gently onto the abdomen for 10 minutes, using broad circular movements. Rest for a brief period, and then apply a hot-water bottle to the affected area for 30 minutes.

Applications: Around the house

- Add several drops of Lavender Oil to the washer's final rinse cycle, or scent a cloth with a few drops of Lavender Oil and throw it in the dryer to freshen a load of newly laundered clothes.

- Place a handful of Lavender buds in an old sock, knot it, and store it in a drawer with your linens.

Lemongrass Oil

Lemongrass is a type of tropical grass that's native to Nepal, Sri Lanka, and India. Used in the cuisines of India and Asia, Lemongrass has long been an important part of Ayurvedic, or traditional Indian medicine. The essential oil is extracted by steam distillation from the harvested leaves, which are left on the ground for a few days to further increase their oil content. While there are many species of Lemongrass, only *Cymbopogon citratus* originally from western India, and *Cymnopogon flexuosus*, from eastern India are used to make essential oil. The oil is cooling, stimulating, and refreshing to both the body and the mind. Its powerfully astringent, antibacterial, and analgesic properties make it a useful remedy for muscle pain, bruises, skin conditions, and respiratory infections. In addition, Lemongrass Oil is an effective insecticide that can repel mosquitoes. It may also relieve depression and fatigue and improve mental concentration.

As a Room Freshener

The fresh, citrus-like fragrance of Lemongrass Oil can dispel stale air, cigarette smoke, pet odors, and unpleasant kitchen scents. The following blend in an aromatherapy lamp helps to purify and improve the air quality in any room of your house that needs deodorizing. Use it to prepare the house for company or festive occasions.

4 drops Lemongrass

2 drops Lime

2 drops Lemon

Therapeutic Effect: The most important components of Lemongrass Oil are citral, geraniol, linalool, and limonene, which give the oil its refreshing and invigorating effect. These substances also have analgesic, antibacterial, antiseptic, insecticidal, and astringent properties, as well as a sedative action on the nervous system.

For Cellulite: Mix 2 drops of Lemongrass Oil in 2 ounces of Sweet Almond Oil. Massage the blend onto areas with cellulite deposits, such as the thighs, hips, and buttocks. The oil stimulates blood circulation to the area while it removes any excess toxins and lymph fluid.

For Fatigue and Depression: A warm bath with Lemongrass Oil refreshes the whole body and helps relieve fatigue and depression after a strenuous day or a poor night's sleep. It also helps revive those with jet lag after a long trip.

For Skin Blemishes and Acne: A toner that contains 1 drop of Lemongrass Oil in 2 ounces of Witch Hazel firms the skin. The oil's anti-inflammatory and antiseptic properties help reduce blemishes and acne. Shake well before each use.

As an Insect Repellent: A blend with 2 drops each of Lemongrass and Cedarwood Oils, as well as 3 drops each of Lavender and Geranium Oils, repels insects. Place a few drops of the blend on cotton balls and bring outdoors. Or burn it in an aroma-therapy lamp in the bedroom to repel pesky mosquitoes. Add the mix to 1 ounce of vodka and spray throughout the house.

For Better Concentration: To boost concentration, put 1 drop each of Lemongrass and Rosemary Oils on a handkerchief. Deeply inhale the scent, avoiding skin contact.

Extra Tip: A blend of 3 tablespoons of Apricot Oil and 10 drops of Lemongrass Oil makes a great furniture polish. It is effective and completely nontoxic to both people and animals.

! **Take Care!** Because of its high citral content, Lemongrass Oil may increase the skin's sensitivity to sunlight. Avoid being in the Sun for six hours after using Lemongrass Oil. Also, if you have sensitive skin, you could experience an irritation or allergic reaction. Always dilute Lemongrass Oil before applying it to the skin. If you have glaucoma, don't use this oil at all.

Applications

- Inhalations of Lemongrass, Tea Tree, and Frankincense Oils help alleviate respiratory congestion and swollen nasal membranes, allowing you to breathe easier. Add 2 drops of each oil to a bowl of boiling water. Drape a towel over your head and bend over the bowl. Close your eyes and inhale the rising vapors.

- Antiseptic Lemongrass Oil helps ease the symptoms of bladder infections. Combine 5 drops of Lemongrass and 3 drops of Tea Tree Oils in 3 tablespoons of cream. Add the mixture to a warm, half-filled bath. Soak for 30 minutes and then rest for one hour.

- Lemongrass Oil is safe to use on pets. To deter lice, scabies, fleas, and ticks, blend 2 drops each of Lemongrass, Lavender, Geranium, and Cedarwood Oils in 1 ounce of alcohol, such as vodka. Add it to the mister and spray on pets, being careful to avoid their eyes.

- For minor muscle aches and pains, blend 3 drops each of Lemongrass and Rosemary Oils in 1 ounce of Sweet Almond Oil. Use the blend to massage sore muscles and aching joints.

- Lemongrass Oil is renowned for its calming effect on the nervous system. It also helps people who react to stress with indigestion and abdominal cramps. Burn it in an aromatherapy lamp or put 2–3 drops on a cloth and inhale.

Longleaf Pine Oil

In Colonial times, magnificent, thick forests of longleaf pine grew throughout the southeastern United States. Thousands of the trees were appropriated by the King of England, who set them aside for the Royal Navy's exclusive use. Lumber from long-leaf pine trees was considered the best grade of southern yellow pine; it was in great demand for flooring and construction. Although these majestic trees are not as plentiful now as they were then, they are still found in temperate coastal climates, where they can reach a height of 100 feet. Longleaf pines are named for their aromatic, fresh-smelling needles, which are between 10 and 15 inches in length. Longleaf Pine Oil is similarly scented. Its strong, balsamic fragrance is often effective in clearing bronchial passages and treating respiratory-tract ailments. It can also alleviate pain from arthritis, muscle soreness, and rheumatism, as well as stimulate circulation and even inhibit swelling. In addition, Longleaf Pine Oil acts to invigorate the senses, providing relief from fatigue.

To Relieve Asthma

Anyone who has a breathing problem, such as asthma, can benefit from the fresh, clean scent of Longleaf Pine Oil. Use the following blend in an aromatherapy lamp to help make breathing easier:

2 drops Longleaf Pine

1 drop Eucalyptus

1 drop Hyssop

Therapeutic Effect: Longleaf Pine Oil has potent antiseptic, antiviral, expectorant, and stimulant properties. Massages, compresses, and baths with the oil can boost blood circulation and ease neuralgia and the discomfort associated with muscle and joint conditions. Inhalations of Longleaf Pine Oil help to clear congested bronchial passages. The oil can also counteract effects of fatigue and stress.

For a Fresh, Masculine Scent: The scent of Longleaf Pine Oil gives men's cologne a clean, masculine note. Add 2 drops of the oil to ¼ cup of Witch Hazel or a dollop of shaving cream for a refreshing scent.

To Protect Your Clothes: To help prevent moths from ruining your wool sweaters, drip about 10 drops of Longleaf Pine Oil onto a few small pieces of untreated wood. Place the wood in your closets and drawers.

To Freshen the Air: Longleaf Pine Oil can help eliminate cigarette smoke and stale air. Add 4 drops of the oil to 1 cup of water in a spray bottle. Shake it well and mist into the air, avoiding furniture.

For Fatigue: The fresh, balsamic scent of Longleaf Pine Oil can stimulate the circulation and help revive you when you're feeling tired and weak. Place a few drops of the oil on a handkerchief and inhale the scent deeply.

Before or After Exercise: A massage oil with Longleaf Pine Oil helps prevent pulled or strained muscles before or after a workout. Mix 3 drops each of Longleaf Pine, Juniper-Berry, and Rosemary Oils with 2 ounces of Jojoba Oil.

Extra Tip: Carry a tiny bottle of Longleaf Pine Oil and take a whiff of its fresh, clean scent whenever you feel stressed, depressed, or claustrophobic.

Take Care! Longleaf Pine Oil may cause skin irritation and sensitivity; it should be diluted before use. Be careful when using the oil in inhalations and saunas. Always keep your eyes closed, as the vapors can irritate your eyes and the surrounding mucous membranes. Keep all essential oils away from small children and pets; don't use them internally either.

Applications

- Cooling compresses containing Longleaf Pine Oil can ease pain from rheumatism, arthritis, and pulled muscles. Mix 3 drops of Longleaf Pine Oil, 1 teaspoon of apple cider vinegar, and 2 drops each of Roman-Chamomile and Lavender Oil, with 1 quart of cold water. Slip a clean, folded cloth into the solution; wring out the excess liquid. Place it on the affected area and cover with a towel. Repeat after 15 minutes.

- People with inflamed skin or a fever may find a skin wash with Longleaf Pine Oil to be helpful. Add 1 drop each of Longleaf Pine and Peppermint Oils and 1 teaspoon of apple cider vinegar to 2 cups cold water. Use this skin wash solution up to 3 times a day.

- This invigorating blend perks up your senses and dispels fatigue: In a pot, mix 6 drops of Longleaf Pine Oil with 3 drops of Cinnamon-Bark, Rosemary, and Fir Oils in 1 quart of water. Simmer the blend on the stove or add the oils to an aromatherapy lamp.

- An inhalation containing some Longleaf Pine Oil can loosen mucus and clear the respiratory passages. Pour 1 quart of water into a bowl and add 2 drops of Longleaf Pine Oil. Then cover your head with a towel. Bend over the bowl, draping the towel over you, and take several, slow deep breaths.

Mandarin Oil

A member of the orange family, the mandarin tree, *Citrus nobilis*, originated in China. It was named for the Mandarins, the high officials of the former Chinese empire. Today, the mandarin tree is most commonly found in southern Europe, South America, and Japan. Its fruit is known to some as the tangerine orange. Pressed from the peels, Mandarin Oil emits a flowery, sweet aroma, which is especially popular with children. To produce an oil free of contaminants. The fruit should come from certified organic groves. The oil is believed to improve mood and relieve anxiety. Its gentle action is safe for pregnant women, children, and aging adults. Add it to bathwater, massage oil, or household cleaning solutions.

For Mental Strain

Put this mixture in an aromatherapy lamp on your desk top help relieve exhaustion and stress in the workplace:

> 5 drops Mandarin
> 3 drops Bergamot

Therapeutic Effect: It is mandarin's tart, fresh aroma that makes the oil useful for combating depression and sadness. It is considered to be an antiseptic as well as an antispasmodic; it is also helpful for relieving gas. Its properties enable it to ease distress, and it can even act as a gentle sedative.

For Grooming and Well-Being: Not only is an aromatherapy bath relaxing, but it also can relieve muscle cramps. Dissolve 10 drops of pure Mandarin Oil and 5 drops of Geranium Oil in about 1 cup of milk, and add the mixture to a warm bath.

During Pregnancy: To prevent stretch marks during pregnancy, rub your breasts and abdomen everyday with a massage oil made of ½ cup Sweet Almond Oil and 50 drops of Mandarin Oil.

At the Hospital: Lighten the sober, sterile atmosphere of a hospital with a few drops of Mandarin Oil. The aroma of mandarin can improve the mood of patients and chase away the septic odor common in hospital rooms. Drizzle some oil on a handkerchief, tissue, or cotton pad, and place it under the patient's pillow.

Mandarin Massage oil: For a relaxing massage, mix 1 tablespoon of any base oil, such as Sweet Almond Oil, with 2 drops of Mandarin, 2 drops of Bergamot, and 1 drop Rose-Otto Oil. This light, tangy blend is fresh, fragrant, and delightful to the senses. Massage it into tense muscles. Both the person receiving the massage and the person giving it will enjoy mandarin's uplifting effects. Rest the muscles for about 30 minutes after the massage.

Home Hint: Mandarin Oil can be used as a natural cleaner around the house. Simply add a few drops of Mandarin Oil to water, moisten a clean cloth with the mixture, and wipe down children's rooms and school bags.

Mood Lifting: Mandarin Oil can help lift the oppressive feelings of anxiety and depression.

! **Take Care!** Mandarin Oil is slightly yellow and leaves a residue in the aromatherapy lamp. If you apply Mandarin Oil to your skin, be sure to avoid any exposure to the Sun—or even ultraviolet radiation—for six hours after application. Skin that has been treated with Mandarin Oil can develop stubborn brown spots when exposed to the rays of the sun.

Applications: External Use

- Some women suffering from PMS have found that Mandarin Oil eases their distress prior to and during menstruation. Place a few drops on a handkerchief or tissue and tuck into your pocket or purse. Pull it out when you're feeling tense or blue. Also consider using Mandarin Oil in household cleaning solutions for an added lift during stressful times.

- Combat rough skin on the legs and buttocks with a daily massage using the following formula: Add 10 drops each of Mandarin Oil, Geranium Oil, Juniper Oil, and Cypress Oil to about ½ cup of Sweet Almond Oil. Before the massage, stimulate blood flow to the skin by brushing legs and buttocks in a circular motion with a skin brush.

- To purify the skin, add 15 drops of Mandarin Oil to about ½ cup of face lotion. Apply the lotion twice daily, in the morning and in the evening after washing.

- For a room spray, put ½ cup spring water in a spray bottle with 10 drops of Mandarin Oil, 5 drops of Lavender Oil, and 2 drops of Clary Sage Oil. Spritz around a room or on drapes for a pleasing scent. Shake the bottle while spraying and be careful to not spray on woodwork.

Marjoram Oil

The bushy perennial herb marjoram, or *Origanum majorana*, grows in the dry and sunny regions of the eastern Mediterranean. The plant has long been used for its culinary and medicinal value. Marjoram essential oil, extracted from the leaves and flowering tops by a process of steam distillation, also has therapeutic benefits. A thick, pale-yellow liquid, Marjoram Oil has a warm, herbaceous, slightly spicy scent that many people find comforting. The oil is often used to treat muscle and joint pain due to overexertion, rheumatism, and arthritis. Inhalations with the oil help alleviate respiratory ailments, such as congestion, coughs, and sinusitis, as well. When Marjoram Oil is applied to the lower abdomen, it can relieve indigestion and soothe menstrual cramps. Marjoram Oil also has beneficial effects on the hair and scalp; it helps condition the hair, promotes blood circulation to the scalp and supports healthy growth. On an emotional level, the oil is especially valuable during the grieving process, as it can comfort and relax both the body and the mind.

For Exhaustion and Nervous Tension

Marjoram Oil's sweetly spicy aroma strengthens the whole body. The following blend in an aromatherapy lamp helps relieve physical and mental exhaustion, nervous tension, and poor concentration:

> 3 drops Marjoram
> 2 drops Lime
> 2 drops Peppermint
> 1 drop Basil

Therapeutic Effect: The primary components of Marjoram Oil are original, geraniol, linalool, and terpinine, which have relaxing and balancing effects on the body and the mind. The oil soothes muscle and joint pain and promotes circulation. Inhalations of Marjoram Oil relive respiratory ailments and asthma as well.

For Headaches: Cool compresses made with Marjoram Oil can help relieve headaches. Add 2 drops of oil to a large bowl of cool water. Mix well. Dip a cotton cloth in the mixture, wring out the excess, and apply it to your forehead. Place another cool compress on the back of your neck to enhance the effect.

For Peaceful Sleep: To promote restful sleep, add 5 drops each of Marjoram Oil, Lavender Oil, and Cedarwood Oil to an aromatherapy lamp and let it burn for one hour.

For Sinusitis: Place 2 drops of Marjoram Oil on a handkerchief and inhale the scent deeply to clear your sinuses and ease breathing.

For Menstrual Pain: To ease menstrual pain, add 3 drops of Marjoram Oil and 2 drops of Clary Sage Oil to a half-full bath. This promotes circulation, relieves cramps in the lower abdomen and helps facilitate menstrual flow. Soak for about 20 minutes. Then rest in bed with a hot-water bottle on your abdomen.

For Muscle Cramps: To prevent muscle soreness and cramps after a workout, make a massage oil. Combine 2 drops each of Marjoram Oil, Cajeput Oil, and Rosemary Oil with 1 ounce of Sweet Almond Oil. Massage the blend into your muscles as often as needed. It also helps reduce pain caused by strains and sprains.

Applications

- To relieve rheumatic pain and swelling in the joints, combine 6 drops of Marjoram Oil and 3 drops of Ginger Oil with 2 tablespoons of whole milk. Add to a warm bath. Soak for about 20 minutes; then rest for one hour. Cover up warmly to prevent stressing your circulatory system.

- Marjoram Oil helps promote expectoration and can calm stubborn coughs. Mix 5 drops of Marjoram Oil and 2 drops each of Cajeput and Roman-Chamomile Oils with 3 tablespoons of Sweet Almond Oil. Massage the blend onto your chest and back several times each day until the symptoms subside.

- Marjoram Oil has a comforting and relaxing property that is particularly helpful for people who are grieving. Blend 1 drop each of Marjoram, Lemon Balm, and Rose-Otto Oils and mix with bath salts. Add to a warm bath and soak for 20 minutes. Or put the oils on a handkerchief; inhale the aroma as needed.

- Hair treatments with Marjoram Oil condition the hair and boost healthy growth. Mix 6 drops of Rosemary and 3 drops each of Marjoram and Sandalwood Oils with 3 tablespoons of Jojoba Oil. Apply to dry hair; leave on overnight. Shampoo and style as usual.

Take Care! Since Marjoram Oil may stimulate contraction and promote blood flow, it should never be used during pregnancy. Also, the oil can sometimes dull the senses, so it should be used only for short periods of time. Always dilute the oil well before applying it to the skin, since it may cause irritation in susceptible individuals. As with all essential oils, don't take Marjoram Oil internally.

Myrrh Oil

Myrrh has a long and interesting history. It has been used since antiquity as an ingredient in perfumes, incense, cosmetics, and even embalming formulas. Valued as a scarce commodity along ancient trade routes, the herb was one of the costliest items in the world. As such, myrrh—along with frankincense and gold—was said to have been given to Jesus at his birth. The plant's aromatic essential oil has long been prized, as well. Extracted by steam distillation from the resin of the thorny shrub *Commiphora myrrha*, the oil has astringent, antiseptic, and anti-inflammatory effects. Myrrh Oil helps treat arthritis, gum inflammations, wounds, hemorrhoids, and infections. Its expectorant action loosens mucus and eases congestion due to bronchitis, colds, and coughs. Cosmetically, Myrrh Oil heals rough, chapped skin, and firms the tissue to lessen the appearance of wrinkles. It is particularly effective for alleviating eczema and fungal infections, including athlete's foot. On an emotional level, Myrrh Oil boosts motivation and promotes mental clarity.

For Inner Peace and Serenity

The sweet, smoky aroma of Myrrh Oil soothes the nerves and creates a deep feeling of serenity. Myrrh Oil also clears the mind and has a stimulating yet relaxing effect on the body. Burn the following essential-oil blend in an aromatherapy lamp to counteract overwrought nerves after a long and stressful day.

   3 drops Myrrh

   2 drops Benzoin

   1 drop Sandalwood

Therapeutic Effect: Myrrh Oil contains the terpenes, limonene, pinene, sesquiterpenes, cinnamon aldehyde, and coumarin aldehyde, all of which provide anti-inflammatory and astringent properties. The oil has antifungal and antiseptic qualities as well. As a result, Myrrh Oil helps relieve pain and swelling, tones tissues, heals wounds, prevents infection, and promotes expectoration.

For Rejuvenation: After a stressful event or an extended illness, spicy Myrrh Oil revitalizes both body and mind. Combine 3 drops each of Frankincense, Sandalwood, and Myrrh Oils and burn them in an aromatherapy lamp.

For Mature Skin: A steam facial with Myrrh Oil stimulates and firms the skin. Add 2 drops of Myrrh and Frankincense Oils and 1 drop of Lavender Oil to a bowl of warm water. Put a towel over your head and bend over the bowl for five minutes and then splash your face with cool water.

For a Disinfectant: The disinfectant components in Myrrh Oil combat germs in sickrooms. Combine 3 drops each of Myrrh, Ravensara, and Thyme Oils in an aromatherapy lamp to reduce the risk of spreading an infection.

For Menstrual Complaints: A bath with Myrrh Oil soothes menstrual pain and tension. Blend 3 drops of Myrrh and 2 drops of Jasmine Oils; add to a bath and soak for 20 minutes.

For Scars: Mix 2 drops of Myrrh Oil with 1 ounce of Sweet Almond Oil. Massage into scars to soften them and promote healing.

For Dry Skin: Blend 3 drops of Myrrh Oil in 2 ounces of facial cream and apply each night to help nourish and protect sensitive, dry skin.

! Take Care! Since Myrrh Oil promotes menstruation, it should never be used during pregnancy, as it can cause breakthrough bleeding and possibly miscarriage. While the oil shouldn't be used internally, myrrh tincture is readily available and safe for internal use.

Applications

- For wounds, add a few drops of Myrrh Oil to a sterile gauze pad. Put the compress on the wound and fasten in place to prevent infection and speed healing.
- Myrrh Oil treats athlete's foot. Blend 3 tablespoons of distilled water, 1 teaspoon of vinegar, and 8 drops of Myrrh Oil. Add the mixture to a spray bottle. Be sure to shake well before using. After showering, thoroughly spray your feet and between your toes.
- Mix a few drops of Myrrh Oil in a glass of warm water to freshen your breath and keep your teeth and gums healthy. Use it to rinse your mouth each morning after brushing your teeth; spit out. Or add a drop to your toothbrush.
- To ease congestion due to colds and bronchitis, add a few drops of the oil to a bowl of hot water. Put a towel over your head and bend over the bowl; inhale the vapors. Keep your eyes closed.
- Myrrh Oil is a helpful remedy for gum inflammations and mouth ulcers. Add 2 drops of Myrrh Oil to ½ cup of water and use it as a gargle. Spit out the mixture. You can also dab mouth ulcers with Myrrh Oil using a cotton pad.
- For whooping cough, combine 2 drops of Myrrh Oil with 2 tablespoons of Sweet Almond Oil. Massage your chest with the oils to loosen mucus, promote expectoration, and alleviate the urge to cough.

Myrtle Oil

In late spring, Myrtle's beautiful flowers, with their slender, delicate stamens bursting from the centers, start to bloom, sprinkling the bush with fragrant white clusters. A native of the Mediterranean, the attractive plant has been a symbol of innocence for many centuries. In fact, Aphrodite—the Greek goddess of beauty and love—apparently found refuge in a Myrtle bush after she was created as a beautiful nude woman. This association with purity and chaste beauty becomes more apparent when one smells the clean, uplifting fragrance of Myrtle and the oil extracted from its flowers. The scent of Myrtle Oil can have a clarifying, strengthening effect on the senses, helping to allay fear. The oil is also valuable for treating acute and chronic chest and lung ailments, such as bronchitis, sinus infections, colds, and coughs. In addition, Myrtle Oil acts an antiseptic, an astringent, and a deodorant and helps both ease and eliminate infections of the urinary tract and skin.

To Ease Breathing

Myrtle Oil's fresh, herbal scent facilitates breathing. It relaxes and strengthens the body and mind. Try this blend in an aromatherapy lamp to create a gentle, soothing mood when you are feeling tense or fearful.

3 drops Myrtle

2 drops Siberian-Fir

1 drop Lemongrass

Therapeutic Effect: The components myrtenol, geraniol, and pinene are responsible for Myrtle Oil's antibacterial, expectorant, and anti-inflammatory properties. It can help treat many respiratory problems when added to inhalations and rubs. Baths with a little Myrtle Oil may ease bladder inflammations and the pain from hemorrhoids. The fresh scent also banishes fatigue.

For Muscle Cramps: Massage oil containing Myrtle Oil can promote blood flow through the tissues, creating a warming effect, and helping prevent cramps that may occur after exercise. Mix 5 drops of Myrtle Oil and 3 drops of Rosemary Oil with 2 ounces of Sweet Almond Oil. Use to massage your muscles.

To Firm the Skin: Myrtle Oil can help stimulate connective tissue, firming and toning the skin. Add 5 drops to your bathwater.

To Ease Head Colds: Inhaling Myrtle Oil may alleviate the discomfort caused by a stuffy nose and even help prevent colds from getting worse. Several times a day, place a few drops of the oil on your sleeve or a handkerchief and inhale the scent deeply.

To Freshen the Air: Antibacterial Myrtle Oil helps to clear the air, especially in sickrooms. Add 3 drops each of Myrtle, Lemon, and Thyme Oils to an aromatherapy lamp.

To Heal Pimples: A toner with Myrtle Oil may help heal acne. Mix 2 drops of Myrtle Oil and 1 drop of Lavender Oil with 1 ounce of Witch Hazel. Apply as needed.

Extra Tip: The next time you go to a sauna, add about 4–6 drops of Myrtle Oil to a wet towel and take it with you. The fresh scent will help to enhance the relaxing effect and make breathing easier.

Applications

- Inhalations with Myrtle Oil are anti-inflammatory and relieve symptoms caused by infections. For frontal or paranasal sinus inflammations accompanied by pus, add 4 drops of Myrtle Oil to 4 cups of hot water and inhale the vapors for a few minutes. Repeat several times daily.

- To treat painful ear inflammations, mix 3 drops of Myrtle Oil and 2 tablespoons of Olive Oil. Place 3–4 drops in each ear canals, and then put a cap or headband to keep them in place. Leave the cotton in your ears overnight.

- For relief from the itching and swelling of hemorrhoids, blend 3 drops of Myrtle Oil and 2 drops of Cypress Oil with 1 ounce of Witch Hazel cream, which is available in many pharmacies. Apply to the rectal area as needed.

- Myrtle Oil may help infections of the bladder and urinary tract. Add 4 drops of Myrtle Oil to warm bathwater, mixing it well, before you take a bath.

- A chest massage oil containing Myrtle Oil can help relieve discomfort associated with asthma, flu, colds, and coughs. Mix 3 drops each of Myrtle and Frankincense Oils with 1 ounce of Sweet Almond Oil and apply to the chest area as needed.

Take Care! Do not apply undiluted essential oil of Myrtle, or any essential oil, directly to your skin. It can cause an allergic reaction, skin irritation, and reddening, even in those who have normal skin. Pregnant women and epileptics should check with an aromatherapist before using Myrtle Oil.

Niaouli Oil

The essential oil of niaouli is extracted and distilled from the fresh leaves of evergreen trees. A member of the Myrtle family, niaouli, or *Melaleuca viridiflora*, is a close relative of the Cajeput tree. Originally from Australia, the niaouli is now cultivated in Malaysia and the Philippines. The tree's colorless to pale yellow oil has a fresh, camphor-like aroma that aids concentration. It can blend well with such essential oils as Eucalyptus, Ocean-Pine, Orange, Hyssop, Lemon, and Myrtle. The oil's wound-healing and antiseptic qualities, which were first discovered by the Australian Aborigines, are similar to Tea Tree Oil. Niaouli Oil is now used as a remedy for many infections of the reproductive and respiratory systems, such as vaginitis, yeast infections, colds, flu, and bronchitis. Niaouli is also an expectorant that thins mucus and helps to alleviate coughs. As an effective anti-inflammatory, the oil can relieve swollen membranes that accompany many types of ailments. It is also helpful as a treatment for athlete's foot, burns, and ear infections.

For Concentration and Mental Clarity

The slightly pungent scent of Niaouli Oil helps to clear the mind and enhance ordered, logical thinking. This blend in an aromatherapy lamp also helps you to maintain your cool in stressful situations.

4 drops Niaouli

2 drops Lime

1 drop Eucalyptus

Therapeutic Effect: The main components in Niaouli Oil are cineol, pinene, terpineol, and limonene, which have anti-inflammatory, antiseptic, and expectorant properties that reduce swelling, help to heal infections and relieve coughs. Niaouli

Oil also stimulates the immune system, which accelerates recovery from illness. Applied topically, niaouli helps tissue regenerate from burns and wounds.

For Antiviral Protection: The antiviral properties of the oil can protect the body by reducing the risk of infection by viruses, it can also treat flu and colds. Mix 5 drops each of Niaouli, Thyme, and Lemon Oils in an aromatherapy lamp for a disinfecting blend.

For Fresh Breath: For a mouthwash to freshen your breath and protect you from infections, including the herpes virus, blend 1 drop of Niaouli Oil with 4 ounces water. Shake it, and gargle.

For Coughs and Bronchitis: Niaouli's expectorant effect is useful in treating coughs and bronchitis. Add 2 drops each of Niaouli, Frankincense, and Eucalyptus Oils to a hot bath or an aromatherapy lamp. Or add them to 2 tablespoons of Sweet Almond Oil then massage your chest with the mixture.

For Insect Bites: Niaouli Oil relieves the itch of insect bites and helps reduce swelling. The bites heal faster, while the oil's skin softeners counteract scars. Mix 2 drops of Niaouli Oil in 2 tablespoons Witch Hazel, and apply to the affected areas.

For a Skin Moisturizer: For moisturizing body oil, mix 5 drops Niaouli Oil, 10 drops of Lavender Oil, and 2 tablespoons of Sweet Almond Oil. This mixture strengthens resistance to bacteria, viruses, and fungi, and keeps the skin from drying out.

! **Take Care!** The pungent and spicy aroma of the essential oil of Niaouli can irritate the delicate conjunctival mucous membranes of the eyes. When you are using the oil externally, especially while you are inhaling it, always keep your eyes closed to help protect them from the rising vapors.

Extra Tip: Niaouli Oil helps to relieve dizziness by stimulating circulation—refreshing the body and mind. Dab a few drops of the oil on a handkerchief, hold it to your nose, and deeply inhale the scent.

Applications

- Inhalations with Niaouli Oil and Lemon Oil help to reduce mucus and clear nasal congestion. Put 3 drops of Niaouli Oil and 2 drops of Lemon Oil in 2 quart of very hot water. Inhale vapors deeply for 10. Repeat as needed.

- A vaginal douche of Niaouli Oil helps to relieve vaginitis and yeast infections. Add 1 drop each of Niaouli Oil and Tea Tree Oils and 1 teaspoon of apple cider vinegar to a vaginal douche bottle that is filled with warm water. Mix it well, and use it to moisten the inside of the vagina. This works best when used at bedtime.

- For a topical salve for cuts and burns, add 2 drops Niaouli Oil, 2 drops of Tea Tree Oil, and 5 drops of Lavender Oil to 2 ounces each of Witch Hazel and purified water. Mix and apply. Or, add the oils to a base of unscented mineral-oil lotion and apply to cuts and burns.

Orange Oil

The essential oil of orange can be recognized by a fresh, sweet, citrusy aroma, just like the orange itself. The orange tree, *Citrus aurantium,* yields petigrain oil from its foliage, Neroli Oil from its flowers, and Orange Oil from its fruit. The oil improves the mood, calms anxiety, and lifts the spirit. It also stimulates circulation and aids digestion. As a cosmetic, Orange Oil can help maintain healthy, youthful skin, helping to boost collagen production, and reduce skin puffiness and blemishes. Orange Oil also works in harmony with other essential oils—cinnamon and flowery scents, such as Ylang-Ylang, to name a few. As a room freshener, these blends may induce a positive outlook and reduce everyday tension. Even furniture can benefit from Orange Oil. A few drops added to Linseed Oil will make a gentle wood protectant. Not even culinary use escapes this versatile oil. Orange extract—the familiar, delicious dessert flavoring—is derived from Orange Oil. Orange Oil is surprisingly inexpensive; because of its many uses, orange is a good choice when deciding which oils to buy.

For Fatigue and Exhaustion

Use a blend of Orange, Lime, and Lemongrass Oils in an aromatherapy lamp to dispel fatigue and exhaustion and instantly freshen a room. This blend will help create a cheerful and sunny mood:

    5 drops Orange

    3 drops Lime

    2 drops Lemongrass

Therapeutic Effect: Orange Oil has a refreshing and invigorating effect on the body and psyche. The primary components are limonene, linalool, geraniol, citronellol, terpineol, and vitamin C. Because of its regenerative and mildly firming properties, Orange Oil is frequently found as an ingredient in many cosmetics and is even thought to reduce cellulite.

As a Food Additive: An extract from Orange Oil diluted with alcohol is sold in stores for use as a food flavoring. Add 2 drops of Orange Oil to food—such as cream, for instance—for flavoring and to stimulate digestion. Add the oil just before beating and then use as you normally would. This makes even very rich cakes easily digestible.

For Circulation Disorders: Orange and Rosemary Oils, when mixed together, have an invigorating effect and may improve circulation. Try a hot and then cold shower, adding both essential oils to your regular unscented shower gel.

For a Gentle Massage: Add 8 drops of Orange Oil and 4 drops of Geranium Oil to 1 ounce of lotion or vegetable oil. The skin-softening and soothing properties of Orange Oil provide the skin with greater elasticity and help protect it against drying.

For Firm Skin: A mixture of Orange and Bergamot oils acts as a tonic for the skin, smoothing small wrinkles, and keeping the skin fresh and youthful looking. Add 5 drops of Orange Oil and 3 drops of Bergamot Oil to 2 ounces of water in a spritzer bottle; spray your body daily.

Extra Tip: Used in a massage or aromatherapy lamp, the fresh scent of Orange Oil is a good remedy for nausea during pregnancy, and it has no side effects.

Applications: External Use

- To help reduce cellulite, massage the area each day with a blend of 15 drops of Orange Oil, 4 drops of Geranium Oil, 4 drops of Cinnamon Oil, and 3 tablespoons of Sunflower Oil. A brush massage with soft natural bristles beforehand will increase circulation, intensifying the effect.

- Mouthwash containing Orange Oil supports the healing process in cases of inflamed gums and periodontal disease. Add 3 drops of Orange Oil and ½ tablespoon of apple cider vinegar to a glass of warm water and stir it well. Rinse your mouth thoroughly with this mixture after brushing your teeth. The mouthwash also fights sore throats and coughs.

Applications: Internal Use

- As a food flavoring, Orange Oil may help to increase the appetite and stimulate digestion: Add 1 drop of Orange Oil to puddings or cheesecakes or put it in a yogurt dressing for fruit salad. You can also place a drop of Orange Oil in 1 teaspoon of honey and take the mixture once daily before meals to improve digestion.

Take Care! Orange Oil may irritate the skin and cause a phototoxic effect. This can lead to sunburn and cause brown pigment spots to form on the skin that may last for years. Avoid using Orange Oil or skin-care products that contain Orange Oil whenever you're going to be exposed to the Sun. In addition, the pale yellow pigment in the oil leaves spots on textiles that are difficult, if not impossible, to remove.

Oregano Oil

Native to the entire Mediterranean area, oregano is a sweet, minty herb long valued for its myriad culinary and medicinal uses. In fact, the ancient Egyptians used oregano as a preservative for food and as an antidote to poison. The essential oil is extracted from the flowering plant, *Oregano vulgare*, a member of the mint family. The resulting pale-yellow oil has a potent camphoraceous, spicy aroma that strengthens the body and mind. Oregano Oil is considered one of the most antiseptic essential oils; it can treat parasites, digestive problems, and infections, as well as respiratory ailments, such as bronchitis, colds, and flu. When applied topically, Oregano Oil relieves eczema, psoriasis, and other chronic skin conditions and may help to reduce the formation of cellulite. Steam inhalations with the oil help loosen phlegm, promote expectoration, and quiet coughs. Massages with Oregano Oil soothe menstrual pain and muscle cramps as well. On an emotional level, Oregano Oil relieves fatigue, improves concentration, and helps ease depression.

For Renewed Energy and Increased Focus

The powerful, spicy aroma of Oregano Oil relieves weakness and improves circulation. The following mixture in your aromatherapy lamp provides fresh energy and stimulates both the body and the mind:

    3 drops Oregano
    2 drops Peruvian Balsam
    1 drop Basil

Therapeutic Effect: Oregano Oil contains thymol, carvacrol, cymene, terpinine, and menthene, which have expectorant, antiseptic, and antiviral effects. These properties help ease respiratory congestion, colds, bronchitis, and flu symptoms. The oil is also a mild laxative and thus relieves constipation. Oregano Oil boosts circulation as well, alleviating rheumatism, menstrual pain, and muscle cramps.

For Cellulite: A massage oil with 1 drop of Oregano Oil with 2 drops each of Rosemary and Orange Oils mixed in 2 tablespoons of Sweet Almond Oil reduces the formation of cellulite. Oregano Oil promotes blood flow while it drains toxins from the tissues. This reduces buildup of water, toxins, and fats beneath the skin, which helps loosen the appearance of cellulite.

For Asthma: Blend 1 drop of Oregano Oil and 2 drops each of Frankincense and Eucalyptus Oils, and add to a bowl of hot water. Drape a towel over your head and inhale the vapors. This eases coughing, loosens mucus, and relaxes the bronchial tubes to restore easy breathing.

For Menstrual Pain: Since Oregano Oil increases circulation, it eases menstrual pain. Add 1 drop of Clary Sage Oil to warm bathwater. Soak for 20 minutes to relax muscles and soothe cramps.

For Headaches: Oregano Oil's camphoraceous, pungent aroma helps relieve pressure headaches. Apply 2–3 drops of the oil to a cloth and inhale the scent deeply and calmly. However, be sure to avoid direct skin contact with the oil by holding the cloth away from your nose.

Extra Tip: For a massage oil for strained muscles, mix 1 drop of Oregano Oil and 2 drops each of Lavender and Roman-Chamomile Oils in 2 ounces of Jojoba Oil. Massage the blend into the affected muscles.

Applications

- Oregano Oil is an antiparasitic and can help get rid of head lice. Mix 5 drops of Oregano Oil in 2 tablespoons of Olive Oil. Massage the mixture into the scalp several times each day to alleviate itching, prevent infection, and eliminate the lice.

- Make a household disinfectant spray by blending 2 drops each of Oregano, Thyme, and Lavender Oils, 5 drops of Lemon Oil, 1 cup of warm water, and ½ cup of vodka. Add the mixture to a spray bottle. Spray the areas of the house where the germs tend to accumulate, such as the kitchen and the bathroom. Don't spray near furniture, however, as it can discolor fabric and wood.

- During a fasting regimen, warm "liver wraps" with Oregano Oil can assist the detoxification process. Mix 1 teaspoon of apple cider vinegar, 1 quart of warm water, and 1 drop of Oregano Oil. Dip a cloth in the mixture and place it below the rib cage on the right side of your body (the liver is located below this area). Next, put a hot-water bottle over the compress and cover it with a towel. Cover up with blankets and rest in bed for about an hour.

Take Care! Oregano Oil may irritate the skin and the mucous membranes, so dilute it before use. In addition, carvacrol, one of the oil's components, is slightly toxic, so the oil should be used in small doses. Since it can stimulate uterine bleeding, Oregano Oil shouldn't be used during pregnancy. Also, insist on pure Oregano Oil, as it is often confused with Marjoram Oil.

Palmarosa Oil

Although Palmarosa Oil is not among the most popular oils used in the United States, in Asia (where palmarosa grass grows wild and freely) the oil is highly regarded for its harmonizing effect on both the body and soul. It takes more than 154 pounds of dried, sweet grass to yield roughly 1 quart of yellow essential Palmarosa Oil, extracted through steam distillation. The oil's delicate scent is somewhat Rose-like, thanks to its high geraniol concentration. This aroma seems to have a calming effect, particularly in times of stress and anger. Applied topically, the oil is a good nutrient for your skin. It stimulates cell growth and regulates sebum production, supporting the regeneration of damaged tissue. Because palmarosa has antibacterial and antiseptic qualities, it is beneficial for oily skin and acne. Palmarosa Oil blends well with other oils and is a good moisturizer, especially for mature skin. The oil is also used often in Ayurvedic medicine; its antispasmodic properties help to promote muscle relaxation, as well as reduce muscle pain.

To Calm Nerves

To enhance the relaxing and antispasmodic properties of Palmarosa Oil, put this mixture in a simmer pot or diffuser. At the same time, the blend will perfume your room, awakening your mind with a stimulating, yet very delicate fragrance.

　6 drops Palmarosa
　2 drops Lemon Balm
　2 drops Sandalwood

Therapeutic Effect: Palmarosa Oil is good for both oily and dry, sensitive skin. Its main constituents are geraniol and limonene with citronellal, farnesol, and dipentene. Geraniol balances the oil and moisture levels in the skin. Limonene's gently invigorating properties help to ease muscle cramps and prevent the pain that can be caused by nervous tension.

For Neck Pain: Hot compresses made with Palmarosa Oil can ease pain that results from neck tension. Fill a small bowl with hot water, put 5 drops of Palmarosa oil on the water's surface. Touch the surface lightly with a cloth to absorb the oil, then fold the compress with the oil side in, to prevent any direct skin contact, and apply. If necessary, repeat 3–4 times.

Relaxing Bath: After a trying day, rejuvenate in a warm aromatherapy bath. Mix 5 drops of Palmarosa Oil, 3 drops of Bergamot Oil, and 3 tablespoons of Sweet Almond Oil; add to bathwater.

Natural Remedy For Pimples: The balancing effect of this essential oil helps regulate the activity of the sebaceous glands, easing skin disorders. Mix 5 drops of Palmarosa Oil into 1 ounce of your favorite face lotion. Make this lotion part of your daily routine, applying it to cleansed skin.

Emotional Consolation: Palmarosa Oil is an excellent soothing agent for anyone suffering from loss or the trauma of grieving. Put 5 drops of Palmarosa Oil with 3 drops of Lemon Balm Oil and 3 drops of Rose-Otto Oil in an aromatherapy lamp. For a quick pick-me-up, dab on a handkerchief and inhale.

Extra Tip: Palmarosa Oil has a light, citrus-floral aroma associated with love and healing. In a diffuser, its scent improves clarity of mind and can help you relax physically, as well as stimulate your mind.

Take Care! If you experience chronic tiredness or low blood pressure, this may not be the best choice for you. It may further lower blood pressure and could have a negative effect on the body. In some cases, even though this is a very mild oil, those who use it experience a decline in their performance and a lack of focus.

Applications: External Use

- Palmarosa is an effective oil for preventing scar formation. It helps strengthen the skin and stimulates the formation of new tissue, so developing scars are less dense. Mix 15 drops of Palmarosa Oil with approximately 3 tablespoons of Sweet Almond Oil and massage it into the affected area several times a day. This mixture can be especially beneficial for healing wounds and surgical scars.

- Massaging with Palmarosa Oil helps soothe muscle tension and ease pain. Mix 5 drops of Roman Chamomile Oil, 10 drops of Lavender essential oil, 20 drops of Palmarosa Oil, and ½ cup of Sweet Almond Oil. Blend the oils and massage the mixture into the affected areas of the body to help reduce muscle pain.

- For a gentle skin oil, mix 10 drops of Palmarosa Oil with 5 drops each of Sandalwood, Lavender, and Geranium Oils. Blend into ¼ cup of Sweet Almond Oil. This soothing blend helps to heal dry, sensitive skin and protects it from damage and inflammation. For best results, massage this oil blend into your skin just after a bath or shower—while your skin is still wet, to seal in moisture. Make a double batch of the oil if you plan to use it often.

Patchouli Oil

Patchouli Oil has as many uses as it has characteristics scents—musty and exotic, spicy and sweet, earthy and sensuous—all of which will improve with age. Native to Southeast Asia, the herb and its distilled essential oil are prized for their wide range of effects. Specifically, the herb, which is believed to kill fungi, has been effective against athlete's foot, while the essential oil's therapeutic properties have made it a favored skin-care aid in bath products, massage oils, and creams. The herb is also found in perfumes, where, some say, it is useful as an aphrodisiac. In aromatherapy, Patchouli Oil can be either stimulating or calming: the amount used controls the effects, which include lifting depression, calming anxiety, and relieving premenstrual complaints and menopausal symptoms. Patchouli, with its pungent aroma, was popular in the 1960s among the peace and love generation. When combined with other oils, such as Bergamot, Neroli or Rose Geranium, Patchouli becomes less overpowering. Used alone, it can be very a effective insect repellent.

For Exotic Dreams

The potent bouquet of scents in Patchouli Oil is believed to stimulate the reaming brain, opening the door to sweet and exotic visions. In combination with Ylang-Ylang Oil, it helps to drive away depression, lift your mood, and encourage your imagination to take flight. Blend the following oils and let the mixture evaporate in an aromatherapy lamp in the evening before going to bed.

> 5 drops Patchouli
> 4 drops Ylang-Ylang
> 4 drops Lavender

Therapeutic Effect: The main component is patchoulene, a particularly calming and relaxing substance. Patchoulene, similar to chamazulene found in chamomile, is anti-inflammatory and helps heal wounds, supporting the regeneration of injured tissue and keeping the skin toned. Patchouli is also antiviral and antifungal, so it's beneficial for ringworm, athlete's foot, and yeast infections. In an aromatherapy lamp, Patchouli Oil combats stress, lethargy, and mental and emotional fatigue.

For Well-Being: Patchouli Oil can be mentally energizing and yet not overstimulating physically. It is believed to release the neurotransmitters that control your mood and general well-being. Patchouli Oil blends well with Vanilla-Absolute Oil for enhancing your mood. The warmth of a bath scented with these oils is calming, restorative, and energizing at the same time.

For Good "Grounding": With its woodsy, earthy scent, it's no wonder Patchouli Oil has a reputation for keeping us centered, focused, and in touch with our feelings. To help keep your feet firmly planted on the proverbial ground, rub them daily with a simple mixture of Sunflower and Patchouli Oils. Blend 2 teaspoons of Sunflower Oil (or other carrier oil) with 5 drops of Patchouli Oil for a healing massage.

For Sore Skin: A body oil combining Jojoba or any other carrier oil with Patchouli Oil provides natural relief for stressed or chafed, cracked, sore skin. Gently massage the oil mixture into your skin twice a day.

! Take Care! Like other essential oils, Patchouli Oil should not be taken internally—the highly concentrated plant material could cause serious injury unless prescribed by a professional health-care provider. Combine the oils with a carrier oil for direct use on the skin. Whenever you purchase essential oils, check the labels for the addition of other substances—only pure oils give you the best therapeutic results.

Extra Tip: A sachet with a drop of potent, earthy Patchouli Oil prevents clothing from becoming moth-eaten and repels other insects as well.

Skin Care Applications

- The patchoulene contained in the oil helps care for damaged skin by reducing scarring and promoting the regeneration of the affected tissue. Skin-care oil containing Patchouli Oil may be especially helpful for eczema and allergic skin reactions. Mix 3 tablespoons of Sweet Almond Oil with 10 drops of Patchouli Oil, and gently apply the mixture to the affected areas 2 to 3 times daily.
- Toners made with Patchouli Oil help firm and tighten dry, tired, slack skin on the face. Add 3 drops of Patchouli Oil and 1 teaspoon apple cider vinegar to 2 cups of warm water; moisten a cotton pad or ball in the liquid, and generously apply to your face in the morning and in the evening after cleansing. Leave the mixture on to air-dry.
- For a spirit-reviving blend, combine 10 drops of Bergamot, 5 drops of Patchouli, and 2 drops of Rose-Absolute Oils in a 1-ounce bottle. Add the blend to a bath or combine a drop with a few drops of water in your hands and lace through your hair. Vary amounts of the oils if you prefer a stronger scent.

Peppermint Oil

Essential oil of Peppermint, which is distilled from the leaves of the peppermint plant, has become one of the most popular oils in aromatherapy. The plant has been popular for its pungent flavor and its curative powers since the seventeenth century, when it may have been brought from the Orient by way of North Africa. In all of its uses, Peppermint Oil is refreshing to the mind, body, and spirit. The distinctive scent of Peppermint Oil can improve a person's concentration and focus. The way this works is that the scent actually triggers the hippocampus, a part of the brain linked to memory. The oil relieves not only mental fatigue but also nausea and dizziness. As a healing oil, Peppermint is both antiseptic and anesthetic because of its high proportion of menthol. Thus, the essential oil, when inhaled, is extremely effective for fighting respiratory infections, from colds to bronchitis and sinusitis. When diluted and applied to the skin, the oil soothes and cools. The oil is particularly useful with older children.

Peppermint Oil

- Soothes respiratory infections
- Aids circulation
- Fights inflammation
- Relieves flatulence and indigestion

For Fatigue

If your mind is overtaxed and fatigued, you are likely to have trouble focusing and remembering. The good news is that you can reenergize your mind and memory by simply inhaling the fresh, pure scent of Peppermint Oil in an aromatherapy lamp. Combine Peppermint Oil for the greatest benefits.

  8 drops of Peppermint

  5 drops of Lemon

Therapeutic Effect: Peppermint Oil has cooling, fever-reducing, and antiseptic properties, largely due to high levels of menthol, which is an antibacterial and anesthetic. The oil helps cure colds, bronchitis, and sinus infections. It also aids healthy digestion by increasing digestive, liver, and gallbladder secretions and relaxes cramped intestinal muscles. Plus, the scent clears the mind and eases mental tension.

For Opening Nasal Passages: The high menthol content of Peppermint Oil reduces inflammation in the nasal passages during a cold, opening them up, and improving breathing.

For Focusing the Mind: Whenever you are weary and tense at the end of a taxing day, Peppermint Oil is a remedy that will revitalize you. It clears your thoughts and allows you to breathe deeply and freely again.

For Headaches: Mix a base oil, such as Sweet Almond Oil, with Peppermint Oil and rub a few drops on your forehead and the nape of your neck. This can rapidly alleviate the pain of a headache and migraine.

For a Cleansing Sauna: Regular visits to a sauna stimulate the body's own defenses. You can increase the detoxifying, fortifying effect of a sauna by adding a few drops of Peppermint Oil to the water poured on the sauna coals.

For Fresh Breath: Peppermint Oil is an excellent natural alternative to mouthwash. It has a disinfectant effect, inhibits infection, and prevents cavities and gum disease, while combating bad breath at the same time.

Extra Tip: For motion sickness and nausea, place a few drops of Peppermint Oil on a cloth. Hold the cloth in front of your mouth and nose, and breathe in deeply for a few seconds.

! **Take Care!** Do not treat children with Peppermint Oil, since the high menthol content can irritate sensitive mucosa. If you have chills, avoid Peppermint Oil, because of its intense cooling properties. Keep your eyes tightly shut when inhaling Peppermint Oil, as the vapors can irritate them. The oil may also irritate sensitive skin, Pregnant and nursing women should avoid using the oil altogether.

Applications: Packs and Compresses

- Cold packs with Peppermint Oil can reduce a fever. Mix 8 drops of Peppermint Oil and 1 tablespoon vinegar in 1 quart of cool water. Soak 2 packs in the mixture, wring them out, and place them on the calves of your legs. Replace as often as necessary until the fever abates.

- A compress with Peppermint Oil relieves the symptoms of a sinus infection. Mix 5 drops of Peppermint Oil in 2 cups of warm water. Lay a small cloth dampened with the mixture across your nose and over your cheekbones. Breathe deeply, keeping your eyes closed.

Applications: Beauty Benefits

- Peppermint Oil can help keep skin looking and feeling healthy. This oil reduces oiliness that can produce skin blemishes. It is also known to help minimize the redness of broken capillaries by constricting the vessel walls. Mix the essential oil with a base oil before applying.

- For a cool, refreshing bath, add 2–4 drops of Peppermint Oil to a tub of tepid water.

Petitgrain Oil

Petitgrain Oil, like Neroli Oil, is derived from the bitter-orange tree, or *Citrus aurantium*. Petitgrain Oil, however, comes from the leaves and stems, while Neroli Oil is from the blossoms. Historically, the oil was distilled from the tree's unripe fruit, hence its French name *petit grain*, or "little grain." While their fragrances are similar, petitgrain's aroma is stronger and more pungent than Neroli's scent. Petitgrain is also frequently substituted for its more expensive cousin. The oil is often used to scent cosmetics, soaps, aftershaves, and colognes and to flavor candies, alcoholic beverages, soft drinks, and desserts. The oil's antibacterial properties help alleviate numerous skin conditions, such as acne, dry skin, and blemishes. The oil also eases headaches, muscle tension and abdominal pain. On an emotional level, the refreshing, relaxing scent of petitgrain is very effective for treating depression, nervous exhaustion, insomnia, stress, and mood swings.

For a Refreshing Pick-Me-Up

Petitgrain Oil's relaxing and antidepressant effect is at its strongest when it is used in an aromatherapy lamp. If you're tired and worn out, allow the following blend to evaporate in your aromatherapy lamp:

4 drops Petitgrain
3 drops Bergamot
2 drops Grapefruit

Therapeutic Effect: Petitgrain Oil moisturizes the skin to help it maintain softness and elasticity. The oil's antibacterial property protects acne-prone skin from becoming infected and helps pimples heal faster. The refreshing scent can offer relief from depression. It contains linalyl acetate, linalool, geranyl acetate, farnesol, geraniol, terpineol, Nerolidol, limonene, and nerol.

For Depression: The mood-brightening effect of Petitgrain Oil helps drive off depression and dark thoughts. Blend 5 drops of Geranium, 3 drops of Petitgrain Oil, and 1 drop each of Jasmine and Rose-Otto Oils. Burn the mixture in your aromatherapy lamp to renew your sense of optimism.

For Migraines: Petitgrain Oil's relaxing effect can help relieve migraines or headaches caused by nerves. Place 2 drops of Petitgrain Oil on a handkerchief and inhale the scent deeply.

For Natural Skin Care: A skin-care oil with Petitgrain Oil keeps dry, sensitive skin soft. The oil nourishes tissue to protect against reddening and dry lines. Blend 5 drops of Petitgrain Oil, 3 drops of Lavender Oil, 2 drops each of Sandalwood and Frankincense Oils, and 1 drop of Neroli Oil in 2 ounces of Sweet Almond or Olive Oil. Wash your face and apply the mixture with the tips of your fingers.

For Restlessness: A warm bath with Petitgrain Oil can have a soothing effect if you have difficulty falling asleep due to nervousness. The following blend can help to promote relaxation and peace of mind, encouraging a deep, restorative sleep. Mix 2 drops each of Petitgrain and Lavender Oils with 1 drop each of Ylang-Ylang and Chamomile Oils, add this combination to warm bathwater, and soak 20 minutes before bedtime.

Extra Tip: Petitgrain Oil often replaces expensive Neroli Oil in hair tonics, perfumes, and both facial and body lotions. Add 3 drops of Petitgrain Oil to enhance a hair rinse or conditioner.

Applications

- Following physical exertion, add Petitgrain Oil and 3 drops of Rosemary Oil to a warm bath. Soak for at least 15–20 minutes. Wrap yourself warmly and rest in bed for one hour.

- A deodorant spray using Petitgrain Oil is refreshing and helps protect against unpleasant odor. Mix 5 drops of Petitgrain Oil and 2 drops of Clary Sage Oil in 3 tablespoons of orange-blossom water. Store the mixture in a spray bottle. Shake the blend thoroughly before each use and spray it onto your skin after bathing or showering. Keep the bottle in a dry, cool place.

- Add Petitgrain Oil to a facial mask to regulate the activity of the sebaceous glands and relieve oily skin and pimples. Combine 1 drop of Petitgrain Oil with 1 tablespoon of Witch Hazel extract and stir it into 1 tablespoon of facial clay or ground oats. Apply the mask to oily areas of your face and allow to dry. Keep it in place for 5 minutes and rinse off. For severe acne, apply the mask everyday.

! **Take Care!** When buying Petitgrain Oil, make sure it has been extracted from the bitter-orange tree by checking the Latin name. Impure Petitgrain Oil may be distilled from other types of citrus, such as Sweet Orange or Lemon.

Pine-Needle Oil

Also known as Scotch and Norwegian pine, *Pinus sylvertris* originated in northern Europe, the eastern United States, and the Baltic. This majestic, aromatic tree can grow to a height of 130 feet and bears brown cones, yellow-orange flowers, and blue-green candles. Pine is cultivated for tar, wood, cellulose, turpentine, pitch, and essential oil, which is extracted from the needles by steam distillation. The oil's many healing properties have been recognized ever since people discovered the fresh, invigorating scent released by pine needles crushed underfoot when stepped on in a forest. Pine-Needle Oil's crisp woodsy aroma can, in fact, clear the sinuses and help relieve bronchitis, colds, sore throats, and flu. It cools fevers, eases congestion, stimulates blood circulation, and soothes sore muscles and joints that accompany sciatica, arthritis, and rheumatism. Pine-Needle Oil also has antifungal and antiseptic properties that fight infection and help boost the immune system. It can restore both emotional and physical strength, and relieve general malaise and fatigue.

To Ease Breathing

Pine-Needle Oil helps open the respiratory passages and promotes expectoration. The oil also relieves swollen nasal mucosa. The following blend in an aromatherapy lamp will help you to breathe freely again.

3 drops Pine-Needle
2 drops Peppermint
2 drops Eucalyptus

Therapeutic Effect: The primary components in Pine-Needle Oil are sylvestrene, pinene, pumilone, dipentene, cadinene, and bornyl acetate. The oil has anti-inflammatory, antifungal, antiseptic, expectorant, diuretic, analgesic, decongestant, insecticidal, and antibacterial properties that are effective in treating respiratory and bladder infections, skin conditions, fever, and muscle spasms.

For Relieving Pain: A warm bath containing Pine-Needle Oil helps stimulate the circulation and alleviates pain associated with arthritis, gout, and rheumatisms. Add

3 drops each of Pine-Needle. Roman-Chamomile, and Lavender Oils to warm bathwater and soak.

For Boosting Immunity: To boost the immune system and help fight infections, add 3 drops each of Pine-Needle, Lemon, and Tea Tree Oils to a pot of hot water. Put a towel over your head and lean over the pot to let your lungs and skin absorb the rising steam.

For a Deep, Restorative Sleep: Pine-Needle Oil's fresh scent dispels nervous tension and insomnia. Put a few drops of Pine-Needle Oil on your pillow before going to bed. You'll wake up refreshed and invigorated the next morning.

For Foot Odor: A daily warm footbath with 3 drops of Pine-Needle Oil in 2 gallons of water regulates the production of sweat and prevents unpleasant foot odor. The oil also promotes blood circulation in the feet.

For Insect Bites: Pine-Needle Oil is a natural insect repellent that protects you from bug bites. During mosquito or black fly season, place a few drops of oil in a cloth and keep it near you, or take aromatherapy lamp outside.

Take Care! The penetrating aroma of Pine-Needle Oil can be irritating to the eyes, so keep them closed during inhalations to protect them from rising steam. Pine-Needle Oil can also irritate the skin. Handle with caution, and always mix well when creating an oil blend.

Extra Tip: Pine-Needle and Rosemary Oils improve concentration. Place 2 drops of each on a cloth, avoiding direct contact with the skin, and inhale.

Applications

- To promote better circulation: Massages with Pine-Needle and Rosemary Oils to relieve muscular pain after athletic exertion. Mix 4 drops of Pine-Needle and 3 drops of Rosemary Oils in 1 ounce of Olive Oil, and then massage the muscles with firm kneading motions.

- For the flu: Inhalations with Pine-Needle Oil can provide some relief when you are weakened by an infection. Add 3 drops of Pine-Needle Oil and 2 drops of Chamomile Oil to a pot with 1 quart of warm water. Cover your head with a towel as you inhale the rising steam slowly and deeply. Keep your eyes closed. Note: For a severe case of the flu, do this twice a day.

- To clean the home: Blend 5–10 drops of Pine-Needle Oil with 2 gallons of water. You can also add a cleaning soap if you wish. Use this mixture with a cloth or in a spray bottle to help disinfect your home and leave a fresh scent. Or, mix 5–7 drops of the oil in 2 cups of borax to use as a rug freshener. Wash your hands thoroughly after use.

- For holiday cheer: To add some holiday spirit to your home, mix 5 drops each of Pine-Needle and Cinnamon Oils in 1 quart of water, and let it simmer on the stove or in an aromatherapy lamp.

Rosemary Oil

The popular Rosemary bush is native to the coastal Mediterranean region but is cultivated throughout the world. The pungent herb has long been favored for its stimulating, medicinal effects, and ancient healers would often turn to Rosemary for its memory-enhancing qualities. Rosemary is also highly prized for use in aromatherapy and is in high demand. Long thought to be a rejuvenating tonic for both the body and the mind, Rosemary Oil aids mental clarity and stimulates the central nervous system. The spicy essential oil is also often used in bath and body products, such as soaps, shampoos, and bath salts. To produce the oil, the needlelike leaves must be harvested before the plant blossoms, and then dried. More than 200 pounds of leaves are used to produce about a quart of oil by steam distillation.

For Energy and Mental Clarity

The fragrance from Rosemary Oil helps renew energy levels and aids concentration. Use the following oil mixture in an aromatherapy lamp to clear your head and allow you to think clearly again.

3 drops Rosemary
1 drop Peppermint
1 drop Clary Sage

Therapeutic Effect: Rosemary Oil has a strong stimulating and anti-inflammatory effect. The substances contained in Rosemary Oil activate circulation and the nervous system.

For Grooming and General Well-Being: Because Rosemary Oil has a strong warming effect, a body oil containing the extract retains heat after a bath and energizes the circulatory system. The skin absorbs essential oils particularly well after baths or showers.

For Cold Feet: Pamper and warm cold feet with a footbath containing Rosemary Oil for quick and long-lasting results. Mix 9 drops of the oil with the warm water of the footbath. Be sure to mix well so that the oil disperses throughout.

For Cellulite: Adding Rosemary Oil to bathwater is helpful for removing water from tissue and improving circulation, which in turn diminishes the appearance of cellulite. Mix 10 drops of Rosemary Oil with 2–3 tablespoons of whipping cream or base oil as an emulsifier, and add to bathwater. While bathing, massage skin with a loofah to stimulate circulation.

For Hair Loss: Add 2 drops of Rosemary Oil to your shampoo. The oil will stimulate circulation to the scalp, giving it a bit of a "wake-up call" and, at the same time, improving the nutrient supply to the hair roots. The result will healthy and shiny hair.

! Take Care! Do not burn your aromatherapy lamp for more than four hours a day. Burning the lamp longer could overstimulate the nerves in the nose, resulting in a painful headache.

Caution! The camphor, thymol, and terpineol in Rosemary Oil are highly stimulating. Pregnant women should not use the herb as either an essential oil or a tea preparation, as either can cause premature labor. Those prone to asthma may be bothered by Rosemary Oil's strong scent, and the active ingredients can also cause seizures in epileptics. Rosemary Oil may cause skin irritation if nor diluted properly. Keep these precautions in mind when using Rosemary Oil around others.

Applications: External Use

- Clear toxins from the body with a warm Rosemary Oil compress. Mix 4 drops of Rosemary Oil with 2 cups of warm water and then moisten a hand towel with the mixture. To detoxify the body, apply the compress to the liver area; cover with wool cloth.

- To help control minor pain, add 9 drops of Rosemary Oil to 4 teaspoons of Sweet Almond Oil and gently rub the gallbladder area.

- Make a Hair Oil by adding 2 drops of Rosemary, 2 drops of Lavender, 2 drops of Clary Sage, and 2 drops of Jasmine-Absolute Oils to ½ ounce of a base oil. Add drop by drop to a wooden hairbrush before brushing. The treatment conditions hair and adds a pleasing scent.

- A natural alternative to coffee or other stimulants, Rosemary Oil can provide a lift during the day simply by adding it to a simmer pot or diffuser.

- For an energizing bath, add 3 drops of Rosemary Oil, 3 drops of Lemon Oil, and 2 drops of Eucalyptus Oil directly into a tub of warm water. Swirl the water until the oils are mixed.

Rosewood Oil

A member of the laurel family, the rosewood tree is native to South American rain forests, and like other species of that threatened region, it has an uncertain future.

Plantation-grown trees, however, are harvested for the commercial use of their wood and essential oil. The essential oil of the rosewood tree has a fresh, somewhat flowery, woodsy scent that aromatherapists consider to be calming and harmonizing for both the mood and the body. Rosewood Oil is often used to provide gentle relief for menstrual pains and for cramped or fatigued muscles. Skin-care preparations of all kinds—for minor irritations and wounds, daily health regimens, and dryness—will benefit from the oil, which is soothing and antibacterial. As for the emotional benefits of using Rosewood Oil, it is believed to assuage anxiety, reduce stress, and relieve depression. The balancing power of the oil may even help stabilize mood swings and diminish aggressiveness. Ongoing research will help us further understand the oil's therapeutic uses.

For Stress
When you find that you are agitated by the hectic pace of life, Rosewood Oil may help relax and soothe you. Let the following mixture evaporate in your diffuser:
   8 drops Rosewood
   5 drops Lavender

Therapeutic Effect: Among the primary components in Rosewood Oil are linalool and cineole. They are believed to give the oil its calming and balancing properties, which are beneficial for the improvement of emotional states. Because the components are antibacterial, the oil is valuable for relieving most skin irritations and blemishes. It is also considered very effective in toners and massage oils for maintaining the skin's oil balance and elasticity. In addition, Rosewood Oil seems to ease menstrual complaints.

For Headaches: Rosewood Oil will relieve headaches that are accompanied by nausea and linked to nervousness and tension in the muscles.

For Stretch Marks: A regular massage of the stomach, thighs, and hips with a cream or an oil containing Rosewood Oil will tighten the skin and may even assist in preventing stretch marks.

For Irritability: To help combat irritability—especially when it is related to premenstrual syndrome—add a mixture of sweet cream and 3 drops each of Rosewood Oil and Bergamot Oil to a hot bath. In addition, the bath will guard against infections and stimulate circulation. Avoid sun exposure for up to 12 hours after your bath, as Bergamot Oil is phototoxic (skin may blister or redden).

For Clear, Balanced Skin: After showering or bathing, massage your body with a mixture of Rosewood Oil and Sweet Almond Oil to soothe sensitive skin, help prevent wrinkles, and treat blemishes. It also effectively combats either oily or dry skin. To get optimal results, massage the oil in gently, circling upward from the feet (be sure your skin is still wet).

A Little Lore: Once known as *bois de rose*, Rosewood Oil was a popular choice of perfume, usually mixed with other scents. It was also believed to be an aphrodisiac that would cure impotence.

Take Care! Taking Rosewood Oil internally is not advised, as it is considered to be poisonous. There are few known dangers when the oil is used externally. Diluted with any base oil, such as Sweet Almond Oil, it will rarely irritate the skin.

Applications

- For nervous skin disorders: Put a few drops of Rosewood Oil on the outer corners of your pillow. When you lie down, you'll breathe in the relaxing oil, which may have a soothing effect, making it easier to fall asleep.

- For depression and blue moods: Combine 8 drops of fresh, flowery Rosewood Oil with up to 5 drops of fruity, zesty Grapefruit Oil in a diffuser. This will lift your mood and refocus your mind.

- For tired, tense muscles: Add 1 teaspoon apple cider vinegars and 5 drops of Rosewood Oil to 2 cups of cool water. Rinse sore, tight muscles with the mixture to help freshen tissues and re-tone muscles.

- For menstrual cramps: Gently massage the entire lower body; front and back, with a mixture of ½ cup Sweet Almond Oil and 25 drops Rosewood Oil. Place a covered hot-water bottle on the abdomen and rest. This will relax cramped muscles and may even ease the flow of menstrual blood. Repeat as needed.

- For acne and blemishes: Add 4 drops each of Rosewood and Lavender Oils to ½ cup distilled water. After cleaning your face, dab it with a cotton pad dipped in the solution to clear up acne and prevent blemishes. Shake the solution well with each use; the oil tends to separate out. Label and date the bottle.

Savory Oil

Savory has been a valuable medicinal and culinary herb for at least 2,000 years. The two varieties, summer savory and winter savory, have very similar therapeutic effects. The more common essential oil is made from the summer variety, or *Satureja hortensis,* but winter savory, or *Satureja montana*, is considered more potent. Extracted from the stems and leaves by steam distillation, savory has a fresh, herbal, slightly medicinal aroma that revitalizes a sluggish nervous system. In addition, the oil is an effective remedy for many digestive ailments, including bloating, cramps, flatulence, and diarrhea. For respiratory problems, such as bronchitis and asthma, inhalations with Savory loosen mucus and soothe irritated and inflamed bronchial tubes. Furthermore, the oil stimulates circulation, which helps flush toxins from the body and relieves muscle tension and pain. When the oil is applied topically, it has a beneficial effect on fungal infections, insect bites, acne, and inflamed oily skin. On an emotional level, the oil restores energy and relieves apathy and dejection.

For Exhaustion

The refreshing, stimulating fragrance of Savory Oil helps banish fatigue and malaise. Add the following blend to an aromatherapy lamp:

  3 drops Savory
  2 drops Lemon
  2 drops Oregano

Therapeutic Effect: Cymene, thymol, carvacrol, and phenol give the oil its stimulating properties and help to boost blood circulation, which eases muscle pain and tension. The oil's antiseptic quality helps treat intestinal ailments, respiratory conditions, and skin inflammations. Savory Oil also activates the adrenal glands. In addition, it is believed to be an aphrodisiac.

For Muscle Tension: To stimulate circulation and help alleviate muscle tension, add 2 drops each of Savory, Lavender, and Juniper Oils to 2 tablespoons of milk. Blend well and add to a warm bath.

For Oily Skin and Acne: Savory Oil is antiseptic and regulates the oil production of the sebaceous glands to help heal acne. Add 1 drop of Savory Oil and 2 drops of Lavender Oil to 2 tablespoons of aloe vera gel. Cleanse your face with it and rinse off.

For Itchy Insect Bites: Savory Oil alleviates swelling and relieves the itching of insect bites. Mix 1 drop each of Roman-Chamomile, Tea Tree, and Savory Oils with 2 ounces of Witch Hazel extract. Soak a cotton ball in the mix and dab on insect bites. This also protects the skin from infection due to scratching.

For Skin Fungus: To inhibit the growth of fungus and prevent re-infection, blend 1 drop of Savory and 2 drops each of Tea Tree and Lavender Oils in 2 ounces of unscented skin cream. Apply to the affected areas as often as needed until the symptoms have subsided. Wash your hands well after using to prevent spreading the fungal infection to other parts of your body.

Extra Tip: To ease coughs and labored breathing due to bronchitis, blend 2 drops each of Frankincense and Sandalwood Oils, plus 1 drop of Savory Oil, in a bowl of hot water. Deeply inhale the vapors.

Applications

- The antiseptic quality of Savory Oil helps treat inflammations of the mouth and gums. Combine 1 drop of Savory Oil with 1 teaspoon of vinegar and add to a glass of water. Mix well. Rinse your mouth three times a day. Repeat the procedure as needed until the symptoms have totally disappeared.

- For impaired hearing and mild tinnitus, or ringing in your ears, resulting from an ear infection, try the following remedy. Blend 1 drop of Savory Oil in 3 ounces of Sweet Almond Oil. Mix well and add to a dropper bottle. Put 3–4 drops in each ear canal once a day. Lie down on your side and let the oils soak into each ear. Even if you have symptoms in only one ear, you must treat both ears at the same time.

- For digestive complaints, such as bloating, flatulence, diarrhea, and abdominal cramps, blend 2 drops each of Savory, Roman-Chamomile, and Lavender Oils with 2 ounces of Sweet Almond Oil. Gently massage your abdomen with the mixture in a clockwise motion. Then rest in bed with a hot-water bottle for 20 minutes

- For a quick pick-me-up, put 1–2 drops of Savory Oil in a cloth or on your sleeve and inhale deeply.

! Take Care! Always dilute Savory Oil before using, as it may cause skin irritation in certain individuals. In addition, the oil should not be used by pregnant women, as it may cause premature contractions. If you develop any skin irritation while using the summer-Savory Oil variety, don't use the winter-savory variety since it's even more potent. Test a patch of skin first for sensitivity.

Tea Tree Oil

Native Australians were the first to discover that the tea tress is a remedy for many different ailments. The Aborigines used its leaves to make a medicinal tea that builds and strengthens the immune system. Today, because of its antiviral properties, Tea Tree Oil occupies a favored position in aromatherapy. It can counteract bacteria, fungi, and viruses, as well as eliminate parasites. It inhibits inflammation, eases pain, and protects the skin. The oil has also been shown to penetrate outer layers of the skin and attack infections, helping to heal wounds. The essential oil from the Tea Tree leaves—which has a scent similar to camphor—is extracted through steam distillation. It is sold in stores under two names: "Tea Tree Oil" and "*melaleuka oil.*" It is a popular ingredient in personal-care products, such as soaps and mouthwashes. Keep this versatile oil part of your home medicine chest.

Tea Tree Oil

- Acts as an antiseptic
- Is antiviral
- Is antibacterial
- Is antifungal
- Helps heal acne, sunburns, and even infections

Mosquito Repellent

To keep pesky mosquitoes out of your house in summer, try using Tea Tree Oil in a diffuser or a spray bottle of water (4 quarts of water and 10 drops of Tea Tree Oil). If the medicinal smell of the pure oil is strong for your taste, try the following scent mixtures instead:

3 drops Tea Tree
2 drops Lavender
2 drops Geranium

OR

4 drops Tea Tree
3 drops Bergamot

Therapeutic Effect: More than 50 rare, natural substances have been identified from the essence of Tea Tree leaves. Because Tea Tree kills viruses, bacteria, and fungi, it can heal internal and external infections, including athlete's foot and fungi that affect the nails. It is also believed that Tea Tree Oil alleviates acne and rashes and helps irritated skin and wounds to heal more quickly, Tea Tree Oil is fungicidal, antiseptic, and safe to use on most delicate parts of the body.

For Skin Care and Comfort: Run a Tea Tree Oil bath to relieve dry-cracked skin or muscle aches and pains.

For Sore Throat Pain: To ease a sore throat and inhibit inflammation, gargle a solution of 3–6 drops of Tea Tree Oil to one glass of water.

For Cold Sores: Once a person is infected with Herpes simplex virus, cold sores often appear on the face and, most frequently, on the lips when the immune system is weakened by infection, stress, or fatigue. To help relieve the discomfort, mix the essential oil with 10 times its volume of carrier oil (base oil, such as Jojoba or calendula), and dab on the affected area as soon as symptoms of a developing cold sore appear.

Extra Tips: For nasty spider bites, a combination of Tea Tree and Lavender Oils applied undiluted (neat) to the skin will help clear up and soothe the bites. To eliminate head lice, add a few drops of the oil on a fine-tooth comb and work well through hair. Tea Tree Oil is also helpful on plants: Gardeners will find that the oil eliminates aphids and ants and kills mildew. Add about 15 drops of Tea Tree Oil to 1 cup of water; spray plants.

! **Take Care!** While Tea Tree Oil is one of the few essential oils that is safe to use undiluted on the skin, never apply it undiluted near the eye. Also, undiluted oils are not recommended for use on pets, small children, the elderly, or babies. (Cats have an extreme reaction to Tea Tree Oil and it should not be used on them.)

Applications: External Use

- Tea Tree Oil can help clear up bronchitis. Put 5 drops of the oil on a damp, warm cloth; place the cloth on the chest and cover it with a dry hand towel. It is best to allow the compress to work overnight.

- For bleeding gums, put some Tea Tree Oil on a cotton swab and dab it on the affected areas. For irritated skin or shingles, mix Tea Tree Oil with Sweet Almond Oil in a 1:9 ratio. Warm the mixture and apply it to the affected skin three times a day.

- Highly antiseptic and antifungal, Tea Tree Oil is considered to be a reliable home remedy for athlete's foot. After showering, dry between the toes well— use a hair dryer for an extra-thorough job—and apply a couple of drops of undiluted Tea Tree Oil to the affected areas. It is important to only wear socks made of natural materials, such as cotton or wool.

Applications: Hygiene

- In an emergency situation, use pure Tea Tree Oil to disinfect your hands before treating an open wound. It's also good for cleaning hands following any contact with blood, pus, or vomit.

- With Tea Tree Oil, yeast infections are short-lived. To use, moisten a tampon with 10–15 drops of Tea Tree Oil and insert as directed. For best results, use this Tea Tree Oil treatment daily for 7 days.

Vetiver Oil

Native to the hot, tropical climates of India, vetiver grass is now cultivated in Indonesia, Haiti, Brazil, Angola, and China, as well as its country of origin. It is related to Lemongrass and citronella, with large tufts of long, narrow, aromatic leaves that can reach six feet in length. The plant's roots are extremely strong and extensive, making the plant useful for areas that are prone to soil erosion and flooding. The roots are also the source of the essential oil of vetiver, which has a deep, earthy scent reminiscent of a damp forest floor soon after a heavy rainfall. This fragrance often triggers contradictory reactions in different people—some feel that it is comforting, but others seem to think it is smelly. Regardless, Vetiver Oil has been shown to have a beneficial effect on health. It stimulates the production of red blood cells, which carry oxygen throughout the body, and improves circulation and immunity. The oil also eases muscular cramps. On an emotional level, Vetiver Oil calms nervousness, relieves tension, and helps induce deep, restful sleep.

For Insecurity and Anxiety

The warm, woodsy aroma of Vetiver Oil boosts courage and confidence. Try these oils in an aromatherapy lamp:

>   4 drops Vetiver
>   2 drops Lemon
>   1 drop Basil

Therapeutic Effects: Vetiver Oil has a number of therapeutic effects. It helps to fight infections and alleviates arthritic and rheumatic pain. It is also quite good for treating muscle spasms and strains. When used on the skin, the oil works to help regulate overactive sebaceous glands while replenishing moisture to drier areas. It can prevent stretch marks and speed healing of minor wounds. Vetiver Oil has a calming, soothing effect on the nerves; it may be very helpful for easing the emotional impact of menopause.

To Rehydrate Dry Skin: Added to creams and moisturizers, Vetiver Oil can help nourish dry and mature skin, leaving it ultra soft and smooth. Blend 2 drops each of Vetiver, Frankincense, and Rose-Otto Oils. Thoroughly mix them with about 1 ounce of a light, unscented cream or moisturizer; apply as needed to your body.

For a Stimulating Bath: Add a little Vetiver Oil to your bath to boost the production of your red blood cells, which help to strengthen immunity. Mix 2 drops each of Vetiver and Lavender Oils in a tub full of warm bathwater.

For a Deep, Woodsy Perfume: Vetiver Oil's unique fragrance is a staple in many perfumes. To make your own scent, mix 2 drops of Vetiver Oil in ½ cup of vodka for a perfume base. Then add 8 drops of either Orange, Sandalwood, Lemon Verbena, Geranium, or Ylang-Ylang Oil. Shake well before using.

To Calm Your Spirits: Insomnia and anxiety can be eased by an inhalation with Vetiver Oil. Add 2 drops each of Vetiver and Lavender Oils and 1 drop of Ylang-Ylang Oil to a bowl of steaming water. Inhale the vapors deeply.

Extra Tip: Since Vetiver Oil is very thick, it may be hard to measure in drops if it is at room temperature. Run hot water over the capped bottle for few minutes before use so it's easier to measure.

Applications

- A massage oil containing Vetiver Oil can help to alleviate cramps and indigestion. Mix 2 drops of Vetiver Oil and 2 tablespoons of Sweet Almond Oil and use this blend to massage your entire abdomen.

- Vetiver Oil's components help to condition the skin and prevent dryness. It is especially good for a healthy scalp. Blend 5 tablespoons of Jojoba Oil with 5 drops each of Vetiver and Rosemary Oils. Use the oil to thoroughly massage your scalp. Cover your hair with several sheets of regular plastic wrap, and then wrap a towel over the plastic. Leave it on for one hour, so the oil can work into your scalp. Then wash your hair with a mild shampoo until the oil is completely rinsed out. For best results, don't wet your hair before you apply the shampoo.

- A bath with Vetiver Oil alleviates menstrual cramps, as it helps to stimulate circulation and has an antispasmodic effect. Blend 2 drops of Vetiver Oil, 3 drops of Clary Sage Oil, and about 3 drops of heavy cream. Add the mixture to your bathwater.

- Vetiver Oil also repels insects. Mix 3 drops of Vetiver Oil, 2 drops of Patchouli Oil, and 5 drops of Lavender Oil. Sprinkle it over 4 ounces of dried flowers; use them as needed.

Take Care! Because Vetiver Oil has a stimulating effect on the circulation, it can induce contractions in pregnant women. Epileptics should also avoid this essential oil. Do not use Vetiver Oil, or any essential oil, internally. Also, store it well out of the reach of children. In addition, be careful not to let this oil touch your clothing, since it may stain.

Violet Oil

Viola odorata, originally from the Mediterranean region, has long been prized for its medicinal value. Hippocrates, the ancient Greek physician, recommended it for pain of any kind; indeed, violet does contain salicylic acid, which is the precursor of aspirin. Similarly, the plant's essential oil, which is extracted from the flowers at the height of their bloom, relieves muscle pain, cramps, and headaches. The oil's antiseptic properties can help treat colds, flu, and bladder inflammations. Violet Oil is especially beneficial in steam inhalations. The oil's expectorant qualities loosen mucus and stop dry, hacking coughs due to bronchitis and respiratory congestion. Used topically for skin conditions, the oil also soothes eczema, chapping, and dry flaky skin. On an emotional level, Violet Oil's fine, delicate scent eases nervous tension, depression, insomnia, and overwrought nerves. However, the oil is quite expensive and is often adulterated with other oils, so be sure to check the label for purity and use it sparingly.

An Aromatic Treasure

Violet Oil helps ease sexual dysfunction caused by stress, tension, and depression. Try burning this blend in your aromatherapy lamp to create a soothing, relaxing mood:

> 2 drops Violet
> 2 drops Jasmine
> 1 drop Neroli

Therapeutic Effect: Salicylic acid, violine, eugenol, and odoratine give Violet Oil its pain-relieving and antiseptic properties. Cooling compresses with the oil are effective in treating headaches and bruises. The oil's ability to promote expectoration and calm dry coughs relieves symptoms caused by colds and flu. Skin creams containing Violet Oil help heal eczema and chapping as well.

To Promote Sensuality: Violet Oil is thought to be an aphrodisiac. Blend 2 drops each of Violet, Clary Sage, and Jasmine Oils in a warm bath to stimulate your senses and promote a relaxing and erotic mood.

For Reddened Skin: Blend 2 drops of Violet Oil in 1 ounce of face cream. Apply to soothe dryness and prevent chapping. The oil's antiseptic quality may also heal acne outbreaks.

For Pain Relief: The salicylic acid in Violet Oil relieves pain and counteracts muscle cramps. Mix 4 drops of Violet Oil and 3 drops of Lavender Oil into 2 ounces of Sweet Almond Oil. Massage the blend onto affected areas as often as needed.

For Bloating: To alleviate painful intestinal bloating and gas, massage your abdomen in clockwise circles with 2 drops of Violet Oil blended with 1 ounce of Sweet Almond Oil. Then put a hot-water bottle on your stomach and rest in bed. This technique has a mild laxative effect to promote elimination.

For Bladder Inflammations: Violet Oil's antiseptic property relieves inflammations of the ureters and bladder. Blend 1 drop each of Violet Oil and Lavender Oil in a sitz bath an soak for 20 minutes to flush bacteria from the urinary tract.

Extra Tip: Since Violet Oil is so expensive, it is frequently stretched with other oils. To make sure that you buy only pure essential oil, read the label carefully.

Applications

- To help calm coughs and loosen mucus, add 1 drop of Violet Oil to 2 quarts of hot water. Pour into a bowl, drape a towel over your head and bend over the bowl. Inhale the vapors for 2–3 minutes.

- Violet Oil can help heal broken capillaries and stimulates the flow of blood to help alleviate congestion in the fine blood vessels of the skin. Mix 2 drops of Violet and 1 drop of Rose-Otto Oils in 4 ounces of distilled water. Add the blend to a spray bottle. Shake well; apply to your face each morning and evening.

- If you have a raw, painful nipples from nursing, blend 2 drops of Violet Oil and 1 drop of Roman-Chamomile in 1 ounce of Sweet Almond Oil or Avocado Oil. Gently rub onto breasts several times daily. Wash off before nursing.

- A cooling compress of Violet Oil helps relieve headaches. Blend 1 drop of Violet Oil with 1 quart of cold water. Moisten a compress or a soft washcloth with the solution and place it on your forehead. Then lie down and relax for at least 30 minutes. Breathe calmly and deeply. Repeat as needed.

- To ease depression, anxiety and insomnia, place a few drops of Violet Oil on a cloth and inhale, avoiding direct skin contact.

Take Care! Violet Oil may cause severe nausea and vomiting, so it shouldn't be used internally. When applying the oil to your skin, do not exceed the recommended dosages and always dilute it first. Apply with light dabs to sensitive skin.

White-Camphor Oil

There are more than 250 species of camphor trees, but only one, *Cinnamomum camphora*, or White-Camphor, produces useful essential oil. Other types, including brown and yellow camphor, however, contain higher levels of safrole, which is toxic; small amounts of White-Camphor, however, are safe. Extracted from the wood and leaves of trees more than 50 years old, camphor has been used as a tonic in East Asia for two millennia and was once an ingredient in smelling salts. Its powerfully medicinal scent is known, in fact, to stimulate breathing, promote circulation, and strengthen the heartbeat. It can, therefore, be used as an emergency treatment for heart failure or shock, before medicinal help arrives. White-Camphor Oil's invigorating properties make it useful remedy for colds, flu, and respiratory infections, though it may be too strong for those with asthma. In addition, its antispasmodic and analgesic effects help to relieve muscle and joint pain. It can also lift a depressed mood, alleviate fatigue, rejuvenate the senses, and enhance memory.

For Viral Infections

White-Camphor Oil has strong anti-inflammatory, antiseptic, and antispasmodic qualities that make it a great remedy for bronchitis and flu. Add this blend to your aromatherapy lamp to disinfect the air:

3 drops White-Camphor

2 drops Eucalyptus

2 drops Lemon

2 drops Thyme

Therapeutic Effect: White-Camphor Oil contains camphor, azulene, and pinene, which have anti-inflammatory and antiseptic effects. A small amount of safrole is also present. The oil stimulates the circulatory, respiratory, and nervous system, which can have a beneficial effect on mood, heart rate, breathing, and blood flow.

For Fatigue: The invigorating scent of White-Camphor Oil provides quick relief from exhaustion due to a hectic pace of life. As needed, place a few drops on a handkerchief and inhale deeply, being careful not to touch the oil to the skin.

For Cold Feet: A warm footbath of White-Camphor and Peppermint Oils can stimulate circulation. Add 1 drop of each oil to 1 gallon of warm water. Mix well and soak feet for 10 minutes. Dry feet well and put on warm socks.

For Muscle Strain: Blend 2 drops each of White-Camphor and Lavender Oils and 1 drop of Rosemary Oil in 2 tablespoons of Sweet Almond Oil. Rub the mixture on tender muscles or tendons before working out to help relieve muscle tension and prevent injuries and strains.

For Memory Recall: Memory and the sense of smell are linked in the brain. Add 2 drops each of White-Camphor and Rosemary Oils to an aromatherapy lamp while studying for a test. Add the blend to a small bottle and take it to your exam. Inhale the aroma to help recall the information that was studied.

For Depression: White-Camphor Oil brightens the spirits and invigorates the nervous system. A blend of 2 drops each of White-Camphor, Peppermint, and Lemon Oils in an aromatherapy lamp helps combat depressed moods.

Extra Tip: To help revive a person who has fainted or is in shock, put 2–3 drops of White-Camphor Oil on a handkerchief and hold to the nose, away from skin.

Applications

- For bronchitis and respiratory infections, add 1 drop of White-Camphor Oil to a bowl of warm water. Drape a towel over the head and inhale the vapors, keeping eyes closed.

- The warming effect of White-Camphor Oil enhances blood circulation and gently soothes the joint pain of rheumatism and arthritis. Blend 4 drops of White-Camphor Oil and 3 drops each of Rosemary and Lavender Oils with 2 ounces of sweet cream. Pour this mixture into a warm bath and soak for about 20 minutes. Then rest and keep well covered to promote circulation.

- Make a chest balm for adults to help alleviate coughing. Blend 2 drops of White-Camphor Oil and 3 drops each of Eucalyptus and Thyme Oils in 2 ounces of lotion. This balm strengthens the lungs, has a very powerful anti-inflammatory effect on the respiratory tract and helps to expectorate mucus.

- You can buy camphor ointment at pharmacies and health-food stores. Apply ointment to calf cramps, bruises, and muscle strains. Or mix the ointment with 3 tablespoons of Sweet Almond Oil and massage it into the skin to relieve aches.

! Take Care! White-Camphor Oil can be toxic when inhaled in large quantities. The oil may also cause allergic reactions and irritation; direct skin contact is not recommended. Do not use White-Camphor Oil during pregnancy or on children younger than 6 years. Since camphor can induce convulsions, it should not be used by epileptics or the elderly. Wash hands thoroughly after each use.

Yarrow Oil

Yarrow, once a sacred plant in ancient China, was valued as the perfect unification of yin and yang energies, since the hard, strong stem is filled with a soft substance. In fact, the 64 wooden sticks in the I-Ching ritual, which is used in China to make key decisions, were made from the yarrow stem. Yarrow's Latin name, *Achillea millefoium*, honors Achilles, a Greek hero of the Trojan wars. It's said he cured his injured Achilles tendon with this powerful plant. Native to both Europe and Asia, this perennial grows to a height of three feet and bears fragrant, feathery leaves with yellow, pink, or white flowers. The oil, which is extracted by steam distillation, is an age-old remedy for fevers, skin irritations, wounds, varicose veins, arthritic pain, digestive problems, nervous tension, and respiratory infections. Vapors from Yarrow Oil are also believed to help balance opposing energies, assist in setting goals and increase a sense of security, making it useful during life transitions. Used during meditation, the oil strengthens mental clarity and supports intuitive energy.

For Skin Conditions

Yarrow Oil helps relieve skin inflammation, blemishes, acne, itching, and sunburn. Like all of the essential oils, Yarrow Oil is soluble in both alcohol and oil and imparts its scent in water. It makes an ideal addition to cosmetics, skin lotions or creams due to its antiseptic, astringent, and anti-inflammatory properties. The camphoraceous oil also makes a great toner for skin when added to either lotion or spring water.

5 drops Yarrow

5 drops Lavender

4 ounces spring water

Therapeutic Effect: The flavonoids present in Yarrow Oil dilate the peripheral arteries and induce sweating, while alkaloids help to lower blood pressure. The astringent property of the tannins in Yarrow Oil assist in healing wounds. Cyanidin, azulene, and salicylic acid possess anti-inflammatory effects. Yarrow Oil also contains volatile oils borneol, camphor, isoartemesia ketone, cineole, and terpineol as well as amino acids, lactones, saponins, coumarins, and sterols. In addition, Yarrow Oil possess valuable laxative, analgesic antispasmodic, carminative, expectorant, stimulant, and antiseptic effects.

For Acne: Add 3 drops each of Yarrow and Bergamot Oils to a pot of boiling water. Simmer for two minutes; place the pot on a safe surface and lean over it, with a towel draped over your head. Let the vapors clean the pores for as long as possible. Or, prepare a warm compress with 2 drops each of Yarrow, Bergamot, and Chamomile Oils, and apply to affected areas.

For Stretch Marks: To help reduce stretch marks and scars, rub several drops of Yarrow Oil on the affected areas every day.

For Digestive Complaints: For constipation or sluggish digestion, blend a few drops of Yarrow Oil in 1 ounce of Sweet Almond Oil, and gently massage it into the abdomen. Repeat as needed.

To Support Meditation: Yarrow Oil's balancing effect on the mind assists meditation and can deepen awareness. To help support a more insightful meditation, put 3–4 drops in a diffuser or on a light bulb ring.

Take Care! Yarrow Oil can cause skin irritation in people with sensitive skin. It can also cause allergic reactions in some individuals. For those with sensitive skin, it's best to do a patch test to identify sensitivity before using Yarrow Oil.

Applications

- For first aid: Yarrow Oil is a good addition to a first aid kit. It aids in blood clotting and heals minor skin wounds. The oil also helps soothe itching from insect bites. Put 3 drops of Yarrow Oil on a warm compress and apply to cuts as soon as possible after an injury. For bruises, put 5-7 drops of oil on the affected area several times a day. Follow with a cold compress with 10 drops of Yarrow Oil for 10 minutes.

- For fevers, head colds, and sinus discomfort: Yarrow Oil induces sweating to help break fevers. The vapors also rid the body of excess mucus from respiratory infections. Add 3 drops each of Yarrow, Eucalyptus, and Tea Tree Oils to a pot of boiling water (*don't use aluminum pot*). Place the pot on a safe surface and lean over it, with a towel draped over your head, and deeply in hale the vapors.

- A circulatory stimulant, the oil's analgesic properties provide pain relief. It eases swelling and expands blood vessels. As a massage for rheumatism and for arthritis: Add 3 drops each of Yarrow, Chamomile, Lavender, and Eucalyptus Oils to 8 ounces of Sweet Almond Oil, and massage it into the shoulders, chest, hips, legs, feet, neck, hands and arms, paying attention to any stiff or inflamed areas.

Ylang-Ylang Oil

The Ylang-Ylang tree, native to the Philippines, can reach heights of over 60 feet. The gently drooping branches bear yellowish white, highly fragrant flowers, which are harvested before sunrise to retain their precious essential oil. About 135 pounds of the blossoms are needed to make 1 quart of essential oil, which is extracted through steam distillation. These blossoms from Ylang-Ylang, or "flower of flowers," are considered a very special wedding gift in Indonesia. Freshly picked blossoms, with the flowery, sweet fragrance, are strewn on the newlyweds' bed for their wedding night. The soft scent is believed to enhance erotic moods and intensify emotions. Ylang-Ylang Oil has a relaxing effect, making it useful as an antidepressant. It also eases spasmodic pains, stress levels, and high blood pressure. In addition, Ylang-Ylang Oil is valuable for body care products, as it softens skin and balances moisture.

An Exotic Scent for the Home

The gentle, sweet scent of Ylang-Ylang Oil can help calm nerves and raise spirits. Adding this fragrant blend to an aromatherapy lamp is sure to put you in a relaxed frame of mind.

    3 drops Ylang-Ylang

    2 drops Orange

    2 drops Patchouli

Therapeutic Effects: The main components of Ylang-Ylang Oil include linalool, safrole, geraniol, methylbenzoates, salicylate, and pinene, which give the oil beneficial stimulant properties. The oil helps to encourage the production of mood-lifting endorphins and is helpful in reducing pain, raising spirits, and relieving tension. Ylang-Ylang Oil acts as a skin antiseptic and moisturizer.

To Invigorate the Body: The intense yet relaxing fragrance of Ylang-Ylang Oil is especially suited for use in the bath. The invigorating, sensuous aroma stimulates both the body and mind. Add 3–5 drops to bathwater just before you enter the tub.

For Skin Care: Ylang-Ylang Oil helps balance and moisturize both dry and oily skin. Mix 1 drop each of Ylang-Ylang, Frankincense, and Lavender Oils in 1 tablespoon of cream or Sweet Almond Oil. Massage a small amount into the face. Do not use on inflamed or irritated skin.

For Menstrual Cramps: Painful menstrual cramps can be eased by a warm bath. Add 2 drops each of Ylang-Ylang and Clary Sage Oils to your bathwater just before you enter the tub. The oils help promote menstrual flow and soothe the lower abdomen.

A Breath of the Orient: Many perfumes with a strong Oriental note contain Ylang-Ylang Oil. Combine 2 drops each of Ylang-Ylang, Jasmine, Patchouli, and Rose Oils with at least 2 tablespoons of Sweet Almond Oil for a unique and erotic feminine scent.

For Gentle Relaxation: Ylang-Ylang Oil is wonderful for easing stress after along day at work. Add 1 drop each of Ylang-Ylang and Lavender Oils and 2 drops each of Vanilla and Clary Sage Oils to an aromatherapy lamp for a soothing scent.

Extra Tip: Ylang-Ylang Oil is often considered heavy by itself; blend it with other essences such as Lavender, Jasmine, and Rose Oils.

Applications

- Ylang-Ylang Oil is wonderful for sunburned skin, as it soothes inflammation, eases pain, and supports the formation of new skin tissue. Add 3 drops each of Ylang-Ylang and Lavender Oils, 1 drop of Frankincense Oil, and 1 teaspoon of apple cider vinegar to 1 quart of cold water. Soak a towel in the solution and apply to affected areas. Replace the compress often to gain the maximum benefit.

- To relax the facial muscles, try using a massage oil consisting of 2 drops Ylang-Ylang Oil, 1½ tablespoons of Sweet Almond Oil, and 1 drop each of Sweet Orange and Roman-Chamomile oils. After thoroughly cleansing your skin, apply 1 teaspoon of the blend to your face, neck, and chest, and rub with your fingers in a gentle circular motion. This facial mixture smoothes and conditions your skin and also relaxes with its uplifting, sweet fragrance. However, caution is advised when using this oil during exposure to the Sun.

- Ylang-Ylang Oil can help lower high blood pressure and elevate your spirits. Apply 1 drop to the pillow before you go to sleep, or on your sleeve or handkerchief during the day, for a refreshing and soothing fragrance with a beneficial effect on your mood and your health.

! **Take Care!** Be careful when buying Ylang-Ylang Oil. Select only "complete" Ylang-Ylang Oil for therapeutic purposes at home. This designation refers to the un-separated flower essence, which is diluted for at least 24 hours. *Note:* Using Ylang-Ylang Oil in high concentrations or over extended periods of time can result in severe headaches, mild nausea, and even some vomiting.

Magical Intent

Have you ever cast a spell that you thought was absolutely perfect, but then it turned out all wrong? Maybe someone gave you a spell that they said had worked for them, but when you tried it, it had exactly the opposite effect of what you were trying to accomplish! What happened?

Well, did you make sure that when you cast the spell, you gave all the exact instructions on exactly what you wanted it to do—and not to do? Not only do you have to tell the spell what you want it to do, you also have to remember to tell it what you don't want it to do! Let's not ever forget that part! This is the *Magical Intent*.

Words and the intent that you have when you create an oil also have their own power!

Let's go back to your childhood for a moment. You are in love with a toy you saw in a shop. You dream about it, wish for it, desire it, and this toy is in your every thought. That is the energy we are talking about. The way that you focus on the toy, the emotions you project when telling someone you want it, that is intent.

The way that you thought about that toy is the energy you wish to use for your magic to work correctly. *Magical Intent* is passion—manifest. Remember the thought about having that toy in your hands, how it made you feel? When you specifically think about the outcome of your work, the oil you are crafting will manifest your desires.

What would happen if you crafted what you thought was the perfect love oil to bring you your perfect love, but you weren't specific enough in what you asked for—and asked not to have? It's possible that suddenly you'd be flirting dangerously with a married man, or worse, your best friend's other half!

Intent binds the practitioner to the task and enables elemental energies to effectively interact with them.

Make sure that you don't forget to put specific limits on what you want when you're creating your oil. Of course, you can always make another oil if the first one goes bad, but wouldn't it be better to get it right the first time?

The following is a list of herbs and their intent to assist you.

Magical Intent	*Herbs*
Astral Projection	Dittany, Mugwort, Poplar
Beauty	Avocado, Catnip, Ginseng, Maidenhair, Yerba Santa
Chastity	Cactus, Camphor, Coconut, Cucumber, Fleabane, Hawthorn, Lavender, Pineapple, Sweet Pea, Vervain, Witch Hazel
Courage	Borage, Black Cohosh, Columbine, Masterwort, Mullein, Poke, Ragweed, Sweet Pea, Tea, Thyme, Tonka, Wahoo
Divination	Broom, Camphor, Cherry, Dandelion, Fig, Goldenrod, Ground Ivy, Hibiscus, Meadowsweet, Orange, Orris, Pomegranate
Employment	Devil's Shoestring, Lucky Hand, Pecan
Exorcism	Angelica, Arbutus, Asafetida, Avens, Basil, Beans, Birch, Boneset, Buckthorn, Clove, Clover, Cumin, Devil's Bit, Dragon's Blood, Elder, Fern, Fleabane, Frankincense, Fumitory, Garlic, Heliotrope, Horehound, Horseradish, Juniper, Leek, Lilac, Mallow, Mint, Mistletoe, Mullein, Myrrh, Nettle, Onion, Peach, Peony, Pepper, Pine, Rosemary, Rue, Sagebrush, Sandalwood, Sloe, Snapdragon, Tamarisk, Thistle, Witch Grass, Yarrow
Fertility	Agaric, Banana, Bistort, Carrot, Cuckoo Flower, Cucumber, Cyclamen, Daffodil, Dock, Fig, Geranium, Grape, Hawthorn, Hazel, Horsetail, Mandrake, Mistletoe, Mustard, Myrtle, Nuts, Oak, Olive, Date Palm, Patchouli, Peach, Pine, Pomegranate, Poppy, Rice, Sunflower, Wheat
Fidelity	Chickweed, Chili Pepper, Clover, Cumin, Elder, Licorice, Magnolia, Nutmeg, Rhubarb, Rye, Skullcap, Spikenard, Vetch, Yerba Mate
Friendship	Lemon, Love Seed, Passion Flower, Sweet Pea
Gossip, to end	Clove, Slippery Elm
Happiness	Catnip, Celandine, Cyclamen, Hawthorn, High John the Conqueror, Hyacinth, Lavender, Lily of the Valley, Marjoram, Meadowsweet, Morning Glory, Purslane, Quince, Saffron, St. John's Wort, Witch Grass

Healing	Adder's Tongue, Allspice, Amaranth, Angelica, Apple, Balm, Balm of Gilead, Barley, Bay, Bittersweet, Blackberry, Burdock, Calamus, Carnation, Cedar, Cinnamon, Citron, Cowslip, Cucumber, Dock, Elder, Eucalyptus, Fennel, Figwort, Flax, Gardenia, Garlic, Ginseng, Goat's Rue, Goldenseal, Groundsel, Heliotrope, Hemp, Henna, Hops, Horehound, Horse Chestnut, Ivy, Job's Tears, Life Everlasting, Lime, Mesquite, Mint, Mugwort, Myrrh, Nettle, Oak, Olive, Onion, Peppermint, Pepper Tree, Persimmon, Pine, Plantain, Potato, Rose, Rosemary, Rowan, Rue, Saffron, Sandalwood, Wood Sorrel, Spearmint, Thistle, Thyme, Ti, Tobacco, Vervain, Violet, Willow, Wintergreen, Yerba Santa
Health	Anemone, Ash, Camphor, Caraway, Coriander, Fern, Galangal, Geranium, Groundsel, Juniper, Knotweed, Larkspur, Life Everlasting, Mandrake, Marjoram, Mistletoe, Mullein, Nutmeg, Oak, Pimpernel, Rue, St. John's Wort, Sassafras, Wood Sorrel, Spikenard, Tansy, Thyme, Walnut
Hexes, counteracting	Bamboo, Chili Pepper, Datura, Galangal, Huckleberry, Hydrangea, Poke, Thistle, Holy Thistle, Toadflax, Vetiver, Wahoo, Wintergreen
Legal Matters	Buckthorn, Cascara, Celandine, Hickory, Marigold, Skunk Cabbage

Love	Adam and Eve, Wood Aloes, Apple, Apricot, Aster, Avens, Avocado, Bachelor's Buttons, Balm, Balm of Gilead, Barley, Basil, Beans, Bedstraw, Beet, Betony, Bleeding Heart, Blood-root, Brazil Nut, Caper, Cardamom, Catnip, Chamomile, Cherry, Chestnut, Chickweed, Chili Pepper, Cinnamon, Clove, Clover, Black Cohosh, Coltsfoot, Columbine, Copal, Coriander, Crocus, Cubeb, Cuckoo Flower, Daffodil, Daisy, Damiana, Devil's Bit, Dill, Dogbane, Dragon's Blood, Dutch-man's Breeches, Elecampane, Elm, Endive, Eryngo, Fig, Gardenia, Gentian, Geranium, Ginger, Ginseng, Grains of Paradise, Hemp, Hibiscus, High John the Conqueror, House-leek, Hyacinth, Indian Paint Brush, Jasmine, Joe Pye Weed, Juniper, Kava Kava, Lady's Mantle, Lavender, Leek, Lemon, Lemon Verbena, Licorice, Lime, Linden, Liverwort, Lobe-lia, Lotus, Lovage, Love Seed, Maidenhair Fern, Male Fern, Mallow, Mandrake, Maple, Marjoram, Mastic, Meadow Rue, Meadowsweet, Mimosa, Mistletoe, Moonwort, Myrtle, Nuts, Oleander, Orange, Orchid, Pansy, Papaya, Pea, Peppermint, Periwinkle, Pimento, Plum, Plumeria, Poppy, Prickly Ash, Primrose, Purslane, Quince, Raspberry, Rose, Rosemary, Rue, Rye, Saffron, Sarsaparilla, Skullcap, Sienna, Black Snakeroot, Southernwood, Spearmint, Spiderwort, Strawberry, Sugar Cane, Tamarind, Thyme, Tomato, Tonka, Trillium, Tulip, Va-lerian, Vanilla, Venus Flytrap, Vervain, Vetiver, Violet, Willow, Witch Grass, Wormwood, Yarrow, Yerba Mate, Yohimbe
Luck	Allspice, Aloe, Bamboo, Banyan, Bluebell, Cabbage, Cala-mus, China Berry, Cinchona, Cotton, Daffodil, Devil's Bit, Fern, Grains of Paradise, Hazel, Heather, Holly, Houseleek, Huckleberry, Irish Moss, Job's Tears, Linden, Lucky Hand, Male Fern, Moss, Nutmeg, Oak, Orange, Persimmon, Pine-apple, Pomegranate, Poppy, Purslane, Rose, Snakeroot, Star Anise, Straw, Strawberry, Vetiver, Violet
Mental Ability	Caraway, Celery, Eyebright, Grape, Horehound, Lily of the Valley, Mace, Mustard, Periwinkle, Rosemary, Rue, Savory, Spearmint, Walnut

Peace	Eryngo, Gardenia, Lavender, Loosestrife, Meadowsweet, Morning Glory, Myrtle, Olive, Passion Fruit, Pennyroyal, Skullcap, Vervain, Violet
Power	Carnation, Club Moss, Devil's Shoestring, Ebony, Gentian, Ginger, Rowan
Prophetic Dreams	Bracken Fern, Cinquefoil, Heliotrope, Jasmine, Marigold, Mimosa, Mugwort, Onion, Rose
Prosperity	Alfalfa, Alkanet, Allspice, Almond, Ash, Banana, Basil, Benzoin, Bergamot, Blackberry, Bladder Wrack, Blue Flag, Bryony, Buckwheat, Calamus, Camellia, Cascara, Cashew, Cedar, Chamomile, Cinnamon, Cinquefoil, Clove, Clover, Comfrey, Cowslip, Dill, Dock, Elder, Fenugreek, Fern, Flax, Fumitory, Galangal, Ginger, Goldenrod, Goldenseal, Gorse, Grains of Paradise, Grape, Heliotrope, High John the Conqueror, Honesty, Honeysuckle, Horse Chestnut, Irish Moss, Jasmine, Lucky Hand, Mandrake, Maple, Marjoram, May Apple, Mint, Moonwort, Moss, Myrtle, Nutmeg, Nuts, Oak, Oats, Onion, Orange, Oregon Grape, Patchouli, Pea, Pecan, Periwinkle, Pine, Pineapple, Pomegranate, Poplar, Rattlesnake Root, Rice, Sassafras, Sesame, Black Snakeroot, Snakeroot, Snapdragon, Sweet Woodruff, Tea, Tomato, Tonka, Trillium, Tulip, Vervain, Vetiver, Wheat

Protection	Acacia, African Violet, Agrimony, Ague Root, Aloe, Althea, Alyssum, Amaranth, Anemone, Angelica, Anise, Arbutus, Asafetida, Ash, Balm of Gilead, Bamboo, Barley, Basil, Bay, Bean, Betony, Birch, Bittersweet, Blackberry, Bloodroot, Blueberry, Boneset, Bryony, Broom, Buckthorn, Burdock, Cactus, Calamus, Caraway, Carnation, Cascara, Castor, Cedar, Celandine, Chrysanthemum, Cinchona, Cinnamon, Cinquefoil, Clove, Clover, Club Moss, Coconut, Black Cohosh, Cotton, Cumin, Curry, Cyclamen, Cypress, Datura, Devil's Bit, Devil's Shoestring, Dill, Dogwood, Dragon's Blood, Ebony, Elder, Elecampane, Eucalyptus, Euphoria, Fennel, Fern, Feverwort, Figwort, Flax, Fleabane, Foxglove, Frankincense, Galangal, Garlic, Geranium, Ginseng, Gorse, Grain, Grass, Hazel, Heather, Holly, Honeysuckle, Horehound, Houseleek, Hyacinth, Hyssop, Irish Moss, Ivy, Juniper, Kava Kava, Lady's Slipper, Larch, Larkspur, Lavender, Leek, Lettuce, Lilac, Lily, Lime, Linden, Liquid Amber, Loosestrife, Lotus, Lucky Hand, Mallow, Mandrake, Marigold, Masterwort, Meadow Rue, Mimosa, Mint, Mistletoe, Mugwort, Mulberry, Mullein, Mustard, Myrrh, Nettle, Oak, Olive, Onion, Orris, Papaya, Papyrus, Parsley, Pennyroyal, Peony, Pepper, Pepper Tree, Periwinkle, Pilot Weed, Pimpernel, Pine, Plantain, Plum, Primrose, Purslane, Quince, Radish, Ragwort, Raspberry, Rattlesnake Root, Rhubarb, Rice, Rose, Rosemary, Rowan, Sage, St. John's Wort, Sandalwood, Southernwood, Spanish Moss, Sweet Woodruff, Tamarisk, Thistle, Ti, Toadflax, Tomato, Tulip, Turnip, Valerian, Venus Flytrap, Vervain, Violet, Wax Plant, Willow, Wintergreen, Witch Hazel, Wolf's Bane, Wormwood, Yerba Santa, Yucca
Psychic Powers	Acacia, Althea, Bay, Bistort, Bladder Wrack, Borage, Celery, Cinnamon, Citron, Elecampane, Eyebright, Flax, Galangal, Grass, Honeysuckle, Lemon Grass, Mace, Marigold, Mastic, Mugwort, Peppermint, Rose, Rowan, Saffron, Star Anise, Thyme, Uva Ursi, Wormwood, Yarrow, Yerba Santa

Purification	Alkanet, Anise, Asafetida, Avens, Bay, Benzoin, Betony, Bloodroot, Broom, Cedar, Chamomile, Coconut, Copal, Euphorbia, Fennel, Gum Arabic, Horseradish, Hyssop, Iris, Lavender, Lemon, Lemon Verbena, Mimosa, Parsley, Peppermint, Pepper Tree, Rosemary, Sagebrush, Shallot, Holy Thistle, Thyme, Tobacco, Turmeric, Valerian, Vervain, Yucca
Sex	Avocado, Caper, Caraway, Carrot, Cattail, Celery, Cinnamon, Daisy, Damiana, Deer's Tongue, Dill, Endive, Eryngo, Galangal, Garlic, Ginseng, Grains of Paradise, Hibiscus, Lemon Grass, Licorice, Maguey, Mint, Nettle, Olive, Onion, Parsley, Patchouli, Radish, Rosemary, Saffron, Sesame, Black Snakeroot, Southernwood, Vanilla, Violet, Witch Grass, Yerba Mate, Yohimbe
Sleep	Agrimony, Chamomile, Cinquefoil, Datura, Elder, Hops, Lavender, Lettuce, Linden, Passion Fruit, Peppermint, Purslane, Rosemary, Thyme, Valerian, Vervain
Spirituality	African Violet, Wood Aloes, Cinnamon, Frankincense, Gardenia, Gum Arabic, Myrrh, Sandalwood
Strength	Bay, Carnation, Masterwort, Mugwort, Mulberry, Pennyroyal, Plantain, Saffron, St. John's Wort, Sweet Pea, Tea, Thistle
Success	Ash, Balm, Cinnamon, Clover, Frankincense, Garlic, Ginger, High John the Conqueror, Mistletoe, Rowan, Vervain, Wahoo, Winters Bark
Wisdom	Clary-Sage, Eyebright, Hazel, Iris, Peach, Sage, Sunflower

Herbal Correspondence Charts

Elemental Correspondences

Element	Herbs
Water	Apple Blossom, Lemon Balm, Calamus, Chamomile, Camphor, Catnip, Cardamom, Cherry, Coconut, Comfrey, Elder, Eucalyptus, Iris, Gardenia, Heather, Hyacinth, Jasmine, Lemon, Licorice, Lilac, Lily, Lotus, Myrrh Resin, Orris Root, Passion Flower, Sandalwood, Peach, Plumeria, Rose, Spearmint, Stephanotis, Sweet Pea, Tansy, Thyme, Tonka Beans, Vanilla Beans, Violet, Ylang-Ylang
Fire	Allspice, Angelica, Asafetida, Basil, Bay, Carnation, Cedar, Cinnamon, Clove, Copal Resin, Coriander, Deer's Tongue, Dill, Dragon's Blood Resin, Fennel, Juniper, Lime, Marigold, Nutmeg, Orange, Peppermint, Rosemary, Rose Geranium, Sassafras Bark, Tangerine, Tobacco, Woodruff
Earth	Bistort, Cypress, Fern, Honeysuckle, Horehound, Magnolia, Mugwort, Narcissus, Oakmoss, Patchouli, Primrose, Rhubarb, Vervain, Vetiver
Air	Acacia, Gum Arabic, Almond, Anise, Gum Benzoin, Bergamot, Citron Peel, Lavender, Lemon Grass, Lemon Verbena, Mace, Marjoram, Mastic Resin, Parsley, Peppermint, Sage, Star Anise

Planetary Correspondences

Planet	Herbs
Sun	Acacia, Angelica, Gum Arabic, Ash, Bay, Gum Benzoin, Carnation, Cashew, Cedar, Celandine, Centaury, Chamomile, Chicory, Cinnamon Bark, Citron Peel, Copal Resin, Eyebright, Frankincense, Ginseng, Goldenseal, Hazel, Heliotrope , Juniper, Lime, Liquid Amber, Oak, Lovage, Marigold, Mastic Resin, Mistletoe, Olive, Orange, Peony, Palm, Pineapple, Rice, Rosemary, Rowan, Rue, Saffron, St. John's Wort, Sandalwood, Sesame, Sunflower, Tangerine, Tea, Walnut, Witch Hazel
Moon	Adders Tongue, Aloe, Lemon Balm, Bladder Wrack, Cabbage, Calamus, Camellia, Camphor Resin, Chickweed, Club Moss, Coconut, Cotton, Cucumber, Eucalyptus, Gardenia, Gourd, Grapes, Honesty, Irish Moss, Jasmine, Lemon, Lettuce, Lily, Loosestrife, Lotus, Mallow, Mesquite, Moonwort, Myrrh, Papaya, Poppy, Potato, Sandalwood, Purslane, Turnip, Willow, Wintergreen
Mercury	Almond, Aspen, Beans, Orange Bergamot, Bittersweet, Bracken Fern, Brazil Nuts, Caraway, Celery, Clover, Dill, Elecampane, Fennel, Ferns, Fenugreek, Filberts, Flax, Goats Rue, Horehound, Lavender, Lemon Grass, Lemon Verbena, Lily of the Valley, Mace, Male Fern, Mandrake, Marjoram, May Apple, Mint, Mulberry, Papyrus, Parsley, Pecans, Peppermint, Pimpernel, Pistachio, Pomegranate, Summer Savory, Sienna, Southernwood

Venus	Alder, Alfalfa, Aloes Wood, Apple, Apricot, Aster, Avocado, Bachelor's Buttons, Balm of Gilead, Banana, Barley, Bedstraw, Birch, Blackberry, Bleeding Heart, Blue Flag Iris, Buckwheat, Burdock, Capers, Cardamom, Catnip, Cherry, Coltsfoot, Columbine, Corn, Cowslip, Crocus, Cyclamen, Daffodil, Daisy, Dittany of Crete, Elder, Feverfew, Foxglove, Geranium, Goldenrod, Groundsel, Heather, Hibiscus, Huckleberry, Hyacinth, Indian Paint Brush, Iris, Lady's Mantle, Larkspur, Licorice, Lilac, Magnolia, Maidenhair Fern, Mugwort, Myrtle, Oats, Orris, Passion Flower, Pea, Peach, Pear, Periwinkle, Persimmon, Plantain, Plum, Plumeria, Primrose, Ragwort, Raspberry, Rhubarb, Rose, Rye, Sagebrush, Wood Sorrel, Spearmint, Spikenard, Strawberry, Sugar Cane, Sweet Pea, Tansy, Thyme, Tomato, Tonka Beans, Trillium, Tulip, Valerian, Vanilla, Vervain, Vetiver, Violet, Wheat, Willow
Mars	Allspice, Anemone, Asafetida, Basil, Black Snakeroot, Blood Root, Bryony, Broom, Cactus, Carrot, Chili Pepper, Coriander, Cubeb, Cumin, Curry Leaf, Damiana, Deer's Tongue, Dragon's Blood Resin, Galangal Root, Garlic, Gentian, Ginger Root, Gorse, Grains of Paradise, Hawthorn, High John the Conquerer, Holly, Hops, Horseradish, Hound's Tongue, Leek, Masterwort, Maguey, Mustard, Nettle, Onion, Pennyroyal, Pepper, Peppermint, Pepper Tree, Pimento, Pine, Poke Root, Radish, Reed, Shallots, Snapdragon, Thistle, Toadflax, Tobacco, Woodruff, Wormwood, Yucca
Jupiter	Agrimony, Anise, Avens, Banyan, Wood Betony, Borage, Cloves, Chestnuts, Cinquefoil, Dandelion, Dock, Endive, Fig, Honeysuckle, Horse Chestnut, Hens and Chickens, Hyssop, Linden, Liverwort, Meadowsweet, Maple, Nutmeg, Sage, Sarsaparilla, Sassafras, Star Anise, Witch Grass
Saturn	Aconite, Amaranth, Asphodel, Beech, Beet, Belladonna, Bistort, Boneset, Buckthorn, Comfrey, Cypress, Datura, Elm, Euphorbia, Fumitory, Hellebore, Hemlock, Hemp, Henbane, Horsetail, Ivy, Morning Glory, Pansy, Patchouli, Poplar, Quince, Skullcap, Skunk Cabbage, Slippery Elm, Solomon's Seal, Tamarind, Tamarisk, Yew

Astrological Correspondences

Sign	Herbs

Aries	Allspice, Carnation, Cedar, Cinnamon, Clove, Copal Resin, Cumin, Deer's Tongue, Dragon's Blood Resin, Fennel, Frankincense, Galangal Root, Juniper, Musk, Peppermint, Pine
Taurus	Apple Blossom, Cardamom, Daisy, Honeysuckle, Lilac, Magnolia, Oakmoss, Patchouli, Plumeria, Rose, Thyme, Tonka Beans, Vanilla Beans, Violet
Gemini	Almond, Anise, Bergamot, Citron Peel, Clover, Dill, Lavender, Horehound, Lemon Grass, Lily, Mace, Mastic Resin, Parsley, Peppermint
Cancer	Calamus, Eucalyptus, Gardenia, Jasmine, Lemon, Lemon Balm, Lilac, Lotus, Myrrh Resin, Rose, Sandalwood, Violet
Leo	Acacia, Gum Benzoin, Cinnamon, Copal Resin, Frankincense, Heliotrope, Juniper, Musk Oil, Nutmeg, Orange, Rosemary, Sandalwood
Virgo	Almond, Bergamot, Cypress, Dill, Fennel, Honeysuckle, Lavender, Lily, Mace, Moss, Patchouli, Peppermint
Libra	Apple Blossom, Catnip, Lilac, Magnolia, Marjoram, Mugwort, Plumeria, Rose, Spearmint, Sweet Pea, Thyme, Vanilla Bean, Violet
Scorpio	Allspice, Basil, Clove, Cumin, Deer's Tongue, Galangal Root, Gardenia, Ginger Root, Myrrh Resin, Pine, Vanilla Bean, Violet
Sagittarius	Anise, Carnation, Cedar, Clove, Copal Resin, Deer's Tongue, Dragon's Blood Resin, Frankincense, Ginger Root, Honeysuckle, Juniper, Nutmeg, Orange, Rose, Sage, Sassafras Bark, Star Anise
Capricorn	Cypress, Honeysuckle, Magnolia, Mimosa, Oakmoss, Patchouli, Vervain, Vetiver
Aquarius	Acacia, Almond, Gum Benzoin, Citron Peel, Cypress, Lavender, Gum Mastic, Mace, Mimosa, Patchouli, Peppermint, Pine
Pisces	Anise, Calamus, Catnip, Clove, Eucalyptus, Gardenia, Honeysuckle, Jasmine, Lemon, Mimosa, Nutmeg, Orris Root, Sage, Sandalwood, Sarsaparilla, Star Anise, Sweet Pea

Language of Flowers

Flower	*Meaning*
Acacia	Friendship
Amaryllis	Beautiful but Timid
Anemone	Go Away

Aster	Memories, Elegance, and Love
Anemone	Expectations
Alstroemeria	Devotion
Baby's Breath	Innocence
Bachelor Button	Hope
Begonia	A Fanciful Nature
Bells of Ireland	Good Luck
Calla Lily	Magnificent Beauty
Camellia	Perfection and Loveliness, Gratitude
Carnation	Devoted Love
Chrysanthemum	General=Abundance and Wealth (Red=I Love You; White=Truth)
Daffodil	Regard
Dahlia	Dignity and Elegance
Daisy	Gentleness, Innocence, Loyalty, and Romance
Delphinium	Flights of Fancy, Ardent Attachment
Forget Me Not	Faithful Love, Undying Hope, Memory, Do Not Forget
Freesia	Innocence
Gardenia	Purity and Sweet Love
Gladiolus	Generosity
Heather	Admiration and Beauty
Hibiscus	Delicate Beauty
Hyacinth	Playful Joy
Iris	Faith, Wisdom, Valor, and Promise
Ivy	Wedded Love, Fidelity, Friendship, and Affection
Jasmine	Amiability
Jonquil	Affection Returned
Larkspur	An Open Heart
Lemon Leaves	Everlasting Love
Lilac	First Emotion of Love
Lily	Innocence/Purity of the Heart
Lily of the Valley	Humility, Sweetness, Return of Happiness
Morning Glory	Affection
Myrtle	Duty and Affection

Orange Blossom	Innocence, Eternal Love, Marriage, and Fruitfulness
Orchid	Love, Beauty, and Magnificence
Pansy	Thoughtful Reflection
Peony	Happy Marriage and Prosperity
Primrose	Young Love
Ranunculus	Radiant, Charming
Rose, Pink	Perfect Happiness
Rose, White	Charm and Innocence
Rose, Red	Love and Desire; Single Red Rose=I Love You
Rose, White/Red Striped	Unity
Rose, Orange	Passion
Rose, Yellow	Joy and Gladness
Rosebud	Beauty and Youth
Rosemary	Remembrance
Star of Bethlehem	Purity
Stephanotis	Marital Happiness
Stock	Lasting Beauty
Sweet Pea	Blissful Pleasure
Tuberose	Dangerous Pleasure
Tulip	Love and Passion
Violet	Faithfulness

Bibliography

Ashley, Leonard R.N. *The Complete Book of Spells, Curses and Magical Recipes*. New York: Barricade Books Inc., 1997.

Baer, Randall, and Vicki Baer. *Windows of Light*. San Francisco: Harper and Row, 1984.

Beyerl, Paul. *Master Book of Herbalism*. Custer, WA: Phoenix Publishing, 1984.

———. *A Compendium of Herbal Magic*. Custer, WA: Phoenix Publishing, 1998.

———. *The Holy Books of the Devas*. Kirkland, WA: The Hermit's Grove, 1994.

Bias, Clifford. *Ritual Book of Magic*. York Beach, ME: Samuel Weiser, 1982.

Cunningham, Scott. *The Complete Book of Incense, Oils, and Brews*. St. Paul: Llewellyn Publications, 1989.

———. *Encyclopedia of Magical Herbs*. St. Paul: Llewellyn Publications, 1994.

———. *Magical Aromatherapy*: St. Paul: Llewellyn Publications, 1993.

Dodt, Colleen K. *The Essential Oils Book*. Pownal, VT: Storey Communications, 1996.

Drury, Nevill. *The Elements of Shamanism*. Rockport, MA: Element Books, 1989.

Eason, Cassandra. *The Handbook of Ancient Wisdom*. New York: Sterling Publishing, 1997.

Goodwin, Joscelyn. *Mystery Religions in The Ancient World*. San Francisco: Harper and Row, 1981.

Green, Marion. *A Witch Alone*. Wellingborough, England: The Aquarian Press, 1991.

———. *The Elements of Natural Magic England*. Rockport, MA: Element Books, 1992.

Heath, Maya. *Handbook of Incense, Oils, and Candles*. Merlyn Press, 1996.

Heisler, Roger. *Path To Power: It's All In Your Mind*. York Beach, ME: Samuel Weiser, 1990.

Holland, Eileen. *Grimoire of Magical Correspondences: A Ritual Handbook*. New Page Books, 2006.

Huson, Paul. *Mastering Herbalism, A Practical Guide*. First Madison Books, 1974.

———. *Mastering Witchcraft*. New York: Perigree/G. P. Putnam and Sons, 1970.

Katzeff, Paul. *Full Moons*. Secaucus, NJ: Citadel Press, 1981.

Keville, Kathi. *Pocket Guide to Aromatherapy*. The Crossing Press, 1996.

Lady Rhea with Eve LeFey. *The Enchanted Formulary*. Citadel Press, 2006.

Lewis, J. R., and E. D. Oliver. *Angels A to Z*. Detroit: Visible Ink Press, 1996.

Liddell, S., and MacGregor Mathers. *The Key of Solomon The King*. York Beach, ME: Samuel Weiser, 1974.

Meyer, Marvin W. *The Ancient Mysteries: A Source Book*. San Francisco: Harper and Row, 1987.

Riva, Anna. *Golden Secrets of Mystic Oils*. International Imports, 1990.

———. *Magic with Incense* and *Powders*. International Imports, 1985.

Sabrina, Lady. *Cauldron of Transformation*. St. Paul: Llewellyn Publications, 1996.

———. *Reclaiming the Power: The How and Why of Practical Ritual Magic*. St. Paul: Llewellyn Publications, 1992.

Sawyer, Pat Kirven. *Ancient Wisdom—The Master Grimoire*. Seventh House Publishing, 2005.

Skelton, Robin. *Spell Craft*. York Beach, ME: Samuel Weiser, 1978.

———. *Talismanic Magic*. York Beach, ME: Samuel Weiser, 1985.

———. *The Practice of Witchcraft Today*. Secaucus, NJ: Citadel Press, 1990.

Smith, Steven. *Wylundt's Book of Incense*. York Beach, ME: Samuel Weiser, 1989.

Starhawk. *The Spiral Dance*. San Francisco: Harper and Row, 1979.

Tarostar. *The Witch's Formulary and Spellbook*. Original Publications, 1980.

Valiente, Doreen. *Witchcraft for Tomorrow*. New York: St. Martin's Press, 1978.

Watson, Franzesca. *Aromatherapy Blends and Remedies*. Thorsons/Harper Collins, 1995.

Index

To Write to the Author

If you wish to contact the author or would like more information about this book, please write to the author in care of Llewellyn Worldwide Ltd. and we will forward your request. Both the author and publisher appreciate hearing from you and learning of your enjoyment of this book and how it has helped you. Llewellyn Worldwide Ltd. cannot guarantee that every letter written to the author can be answered, but all will be forwarded. Please write to:

Celeste Rayne Heldstab

℅ Llewellyn Worldwide

2143 Wooddale Drive

Woodbury, MN 55125-2989

Please enclose a self-addressed stamped envelope for reply,

or $1.00 to cover costs. If outside the U.S.A., enclose

an international postal reply coupon.

Many of Llewellyn's authors have websites with additional information and resources. For more information, please visit our website at http://www.llewellyn.com.

GET MORE AT LLEWELLYN.COM

Visit us online to browse hundreds of our books and decks, plus sign up to receive our e-newsletters and exclusive online offers.

- Free tarot readings • Spell-a-Day • Moon phases
- Recipes, spells, and tips • Blogs • Encyclopedia
- Author interviews, articles, and upcoming events

GET SOCIAL WITH LLEWELLYN

Find us on 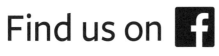 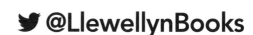 @LlewellynBooks

www.Facebook.com/LlewellynBooks

GET BOOKS AT LLEWELLYN

LLEWELLYN ORDERING INFORMATION

 Order online: Visit our website at www.llewellyn.com to select your books and place an order on our secure server.

 Order by phone:
- Call toll free within the US at 1-877-NEW-WRLD (1-877-639-9753)
- We accept VISA, MasterCard, American Express, and Discover.

 Order by mail:
Send the full price of your order (MN residents add 6.875% sales tax) in US funds plus postage and handling to: Llewellyn Worldwide, 2143 Wooddale Drive, Woodbury, MN 55125-2989

POSTAGE AND HANDLING

STANDARD (US): (Please allow 12 business days)
$30.00 and under, add $6.00.
$30.01 and over, FREE SHIPPING.

CANADA:
We cannot ship to Canada. Please shop your local bookstore or Amazon Canada.

INTERNATIONAL:
Customers pay the actual shipping cost to the final destination, which includes tracking information.

Visit us online for more shipping options. Prices subject to change.

FREE CATALOG!

To order, call 1-877-NEW-WRLD ext. 8236 or visit our website

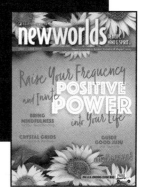